# Praeger Handbook of
# Asian American Health

# Praeger Handbook of Asian American Health

## Taking Notice and Taking Action

### Volume 2: Parts 5–8

Edited by William B. Bateman, MD,
Noilyn Abesamis-Mendoza, MPH, and
Henrietta Ho-Asjoe, MPS

**PRAEGER**

*An Imprint of ABC-CLIO, LLC*

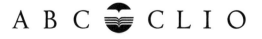

A B C 🝰 C L I O

Santa Barbara, California • Denver, Colorado • Oxford, England

**Library of Congress Cataloging-in-Publication Data**

Praeger handbook of Asian American health : taking notice and taking action /
William Baragar Bateman, Noilyn F. Abesamis, Henrietta Ho-Asjoe, editors.
    p. cm.
  Includes bibliographical references and index.
  ISBN 978-0-313-34701-6 (hard copy : alk. paper) — ISBN 978-0-313-34702-3 (ebook)
  ISBN 978-0-313-34703-0 (v. 1 : alk. paper) — ISBN 978-0-313-34704-7 (ebook)
  ISBN 978-0-313-34705-4 (v. 2 : alk. paper) — ISBN 978-0-313-34706-1 (ebook)
  1.  Asian Americans—Health and hygiene—Handbooks, manuals, etc.
2.  Asian Americans—Medical care—Handbooks, manuals, etc.  I. Bateman,
William B. (William Baragar) II. Abesamis, Noilyn F. III. Ho-Asjoe, Henrietta.
IV. Title: Handbook of Asian American health.
  RA448.5.A83P73 2009
  362.1089′95073—dc22          2009010075

13 12 11 10 09  1 2 3 4 5

This book is also available on the World Wide Web as an eBook.
Visit www.abc-clio.com for details.

ABC-CLIO, LLC
130 Cremona Drive, P.O. Box 1911
Santa Barbara, California 93116-1911

This book is printed on acid-free paper ∞
Manufactured in the United States of America

# Contents

# Abbreviations List

| | |
|---|---|
| A | Asians |
| a.k.a. | Also known as |
| A4D | Therapeutic code used for ACE Inhibitors |
| A4F | Therapeutic code used for Angiotensin Receptor Blockers |
| A9A | Therapeutic code used for Calcium Channel Blockers |
| AA | Asian Americans |
| AAFS | Asian American Family Services |
| AAHC | Asian American Health Coalition |
| AANCART | Asian American Network for Cancer Awareness, Research, and Training |
| AAPCHO | The Association of Asian Pacific Community Health Organizations |
| AAPI | Asian American and Pacific Islander |
| AASPI | Asian American Suicide Prevention Initiative |
| ACEI | ACE Inhibitor |
| ACGs | Adjusted Clinical Groups |
| ACIP | Centers for Disease Control Advisory Committee on Immunization Practices |
| ADD Health | National Longitudinal Study of Adolescent Health |
| ADH | Alcohol Dehydrogenase |
| ADHD | Attention Deficit Hyperactivity Disorder |
| AED | Automated External Defibrillator |
| AFDC | Aid to Families with Dependent Children |
| AHA | American Health Association |
| AHRQ | Agency for Healthcare Research and Quality |
| AIAN | American Indian and Alaskan Native |
| AIDS | Acquired Immunodeficiency Syndrome or Acquired Immune Deficiency Syndrome |

| | |
|---|---|
| ALDH | Aldehyde Dehydrogenase |
| ANOVA | Analysis of variance |
| Anti-HBs | Also referred to as HBsAg; Antibody to the Hepatitis B Surface Antigen |
| APA | Asian Pacific American |
| API | Asian Pacific Islander |
| APIAHF | Asian and Pacific Islander American Health Forum |
| APICHA | Asian and Pacific Islander Coalition on HIV/AIDS |
| APIPGTF | Asian Pacific Islander Taskforce on Problem Gambling |
| APIWHANN | Asian and Pacific Islander Women's HIV/AIDS National Network |
| APPEAL | Asian Pacific Partners for Empowerment, Advocacy and Leadership |
| ARB | Angiotensin Receptor Blocker |
| AsANA | Asian American Health Needs Assessment |
| ASH | Assistant Secretary of Health |
| AsPIRE | Asian American Partnership in Research and Empowerment |
| BB | Beta Blocker |
| BCG | Bacillus Calmette-Guerin (a vaccine to prevent Tuberculosis) |
| BDI | Beck Depression Inventory |
| BMI | Body Mass Index (weight in kilograms divided by the height in meters squared) |
| BPSD | Behavioral & Psychiatric Symptoms in Dementia |
| CACF | Coalition for Asian American Children and Families |
| CAGE | A pneumonic used to screen for alcoholism (Cutting down, Angry, Getting Annoyed, Eye opener) |
| CAM | Complementary and Alternative Medicine (also used as Cultural and Alternative Medicine in this text) |
| CAPES | Chinese American Psychiatric Epidemiologic Study |
| CAPI | Child Abuse Potential Inventory |
| CBDI | Chinese Beck Depression Inventory |
| CBO | Community Based Organization |
| CBPR | Community-based Participatory Research |
| CCB | Calcium Channel Blocker |
| CCCNY | Council of Churches of the City of New York |
| CCPGP | Chinese Community Problem Gambling Project |
| CCR | California Cancer Registry |
| CDC | Centers for Disease Control |
| CDR | Clinical Dementia Rating |
| CES-D | Center for Epidemiologic Studies Depression Scale |
| CHAIN | New York City Community Health Advisory and Information Network |
| CHD | Coronary Heart Disease |

| | |
|---|---|
| CHF | Congestive Heart Failure |
| CHIS | California Health Interview Survey |
| CHW | Community Health Worker |
| CIA | Central Intelligence Agency |
| CIND | Cognitive Impairment Not Dementia |
| CLEAN | Capacity building, Leadership development, Education, Advocacy and Network development (an approach to community organizing) |
| CPR | Cardiopulmonary Resuscitation |
| CRMH | Center for Research on Minority Health |
| CVD | Cardiovascular Disorders (includes heart attacks and strokes) |
| CXR | Chest X-Ray |
| CYP2A6 | Cytochrome P4502A6 |
| DASA | Dignity in All Schools Act |
| DHHS | Department of Health and Human Services |
| DOH | Department of Health |
| DOHMH | Department of Health and Mental Hygiene |
| DOT | Directly Observed Therapy |
| DSD | Scale for Depression |
| DSHEA | Dietary Supplement Health and Education Act (passed in 1994) |
| DSM | Diagnostic and Statistical Manual of Mental Disorder |
| DSM-III | Diagnostic and Statistical Manual of Mental Disorders, Third Version |
| DSM-IV | Diagnostic and Statistical Manual, Fourth Edition |
| DSM-IV-TR | Diagnostic and Statistical Manual, Fourth Edition, text revision |
| ECA | Epidemiological Catchment Area |
| ER | Emergency Room |
| FAHSI | Filipino American Human Services, Inc. |
| FBO | Faith-based Organization |
| FFQ | Food Frequency Questionnaire (a method for assessing diets) |
| FFS | Fee for Service |
| GAD | Generalized Anxiety Disorder |
| GAD-7 | Generalized Anxiety Disorder, seven questions screening for an anxiety disorder |
| GAVI | Global Alliance for Vaccines and Immunization |
| GI | Gastrointestinal |
| GRACE | Genetics Response & Cognitive Enhances |
| H1B Visa | A visa allowing entry into the United States for scholarly work |
| HAAHC | Houston Asian American Health Collaborative |

| | |
|---|---|
| HbA1c | Hemoglobin A1c (a laboratory test used in the management of diabetes mellitus that measures the average blood glucose) |
| HBIG | Hepatitis B Immune Globulin |
| HBM | Health Belief Model |
| HBV | Hepatitis B Virus |
| HCC | Hepatocellular Carcinoma |
| HCV | Hepatitis C Virus |
| HDL | High Density Lipoprotein ("good" cholesterol) |
| Hep B | Hepatitis B |
| HIPAA | Health Insurance Portability and Accountability Act |
| HIV | Human Immunodeficiency Virus |
| HIV/AIDS | Human Immunodeficiency Virus/Acquired Immuno-deficiency Syndrome |
| HMO | Health Maintenance Organization |
| HPV | Human Papilloma Virus |
| HRSA | Health Resources and Services Administration |
| IDT | Interdisciplinary Team |
| IGRA | Interferon Gamma Release Assay |
| IMGs | International Medical Graduates |
| INH | Isoniazid |
| IOM | Institute of Medicine |
| IPV | Intimate Partner Violence |
| IRS | Internal Revenue Service |
| J7C | Therapeutic code used for Beta-Adreneric Blocking Agents |
| JACL | Japanese American Citizen's League |
| JNC VII | Joint National Committee on the Prevention, Detection, Evaluation, and Treatment |
| KC | Kalusugan Coalition |
| LAAMP | Leadership and Advocacy Institute to Advance Minnesota's Parity for Priority Populations |
| LDL | Low Density Lipoprotein ("bad" cholesterol) |
| LEP | Limited English Proficiency |
| LGBT | Lesbian, Gay, Bisexual and Transgender |
| LPR | Legal Permanent Resident ("Green Card" holders) |
| LSM | Life-style Modification |
| LTBI | Latent Tuberculosis Infection |
| M.tb | Myobacteria Tuberculosis |
| MAA | Mutual Assistance Association |
| MBH | Mental & Behavioral Health |
| MDACC | MD Anderson Cancer Center |
| MDR-TB | Multi-drug Resistant Tuberculosis |
| MEPS | Medical Expenditure Survey |
| MLBW | Moderately Low Birth Weight |

| MMSE | Mini-mental Status Examination (an assessment of knowledge and memory) |
| MMWR | Morbidity and Mortality Weekly Report |
| MSA | Master Settlement Agreement (1998 decision between 46 states and the tobacco industry to pay damages for smoking-related disease) |
| MSQ | Mental Status questionnaire |
| NAMI | National Alliance on Mental Illness |
| NAPAFASA | National Asian Pacific American Families Against Substance Abuse |
| NCCAM | National Center for Complementary and Alternative Medicine |
| NCHS | National Center for Health Statistics |
| NCQA | National Committee for Quality Assurance |
| NCVS | National Crime and Victimization Survey |
| NESARC | National Epidemiologic Survey on Alcohol and Related Conditions |
| NGO | Non-governmental Organization |
| NH | Native Hawaiian |
| NHANES | National Health and Nutrition Examination Survey |
| NHDR | National Healthcare Disparities Report |
| NHIS | National Health Interview Survey |
| NHL | Non-Hodgkin's Lymphoma |
| NHLBI | National Heart, Lung, and Blood Institute |
| NHPI | Native Hawaiian and Other Pacific Islander |
| NHSDA | National Household Survey on Drug Abuse |
| NICOS | North East Medical Services, Independent Practitioners Association, Chinese Community Health Care Association, Chinese Hospital, On Lok Lifeway & Self Help for Elderly |
| NIH | National Institutes of Health |
| NLAAS | National Latino and Asian American Study |
| NLAES | National Longitudinal Alcohol Epidemiologic Survey |
| NLMS | National Longitudinal Mortality Study |
| NPH | Normal Pressure Hydrocephalus |
| NVAWS | National Violence against Women Survey |
| NVNM | Non-vitamin, Non-mineral supplements (includes herbals, tonics etc.) |
| NYAWC | New York Asian Women's Center |
| NYC | New York City |
| NYS-AI | New York State Department of Health, AIDS Institute |
| NYU | New York University |
| OCF | Outline for Cultural Formulation |
| OIS | Office of Immigration Statistics |
| OMB | Office of Management and Budget |

| OPG | Office of Problem Gambling |
|---|---|
| PACE | Program of All-Inclusive Care for the Elderly |
| PCP | Primary Care Provider (your "regular" or "personal doctor," usually a specialist in General Internal Medicine, Pediatrics or Family Practice) |
| PCP | Pneumocystis Carinii Pneumonia |
| PED NSS | Pediatric Nutrition Surveillance System |
| PHQ | Patient Health Questionnaire |
| PHQ-9 | Patient Health Questionnaire containing 9 questions screening for depression |
| PI | Pacific Islander |
| PPO | Preferred Provider Organization |
| PRUCOL | Permanently Residing Under Color of Law |
| PTA | Parent Teacher Association |
| PTSD | Post-traumatic Stress Disorder |
| PWA | People with AIDS |
| R1F | Therapeutic code used for Thiazide Diuretics |
| RAMS | Richmond Area Multi-Service |
| RD | Registered Dietician |
| RN | Registered Nurse |
| SAALT | South Asian Americans Leading Together |
| SAFE | Shelter Alternatives: Fostering Empowerment |
| SARS | Severe Acute Respiratory Syndrome |
| SD | Standard Deviation |
| SEARAC | Southeast Asia Resource Action Center |
| SEER | Surveillance Epidemiology and End Results |
| SES | Socioeconomic Status |
| SIJS | Special Immigrant Juvenile Status |
| SPSS | Statistical Package for the Social Sciences |
| STD | Sexually Transmitted Diseases |
| STI | Sexually Transmitted Infection |
| TANF | Temporary Assistance to Needy Families |
| TB | Tuberculosis |
| TEMIS | Team and Technology Enhanced Medical Interpreting System |
| TST | Tuberculin Skin Test |
| U.S. | United States |
| UCLA | University of California, Los Angeles |
| US | United States |
| USA | United States of America |
| USDA | Untied States Department of Agriculture |
| VAT | Visceral Abdominal Fat |
| VLBW | Very Low Birth Weight |
| WHO | World Health Organization |
| XDR-TB | Extensively Drug-Resistant Tuberculosis |

# PART V

---

# Child Health

# Chapter 27

# The Health of Asian American Children in the United States

*Joyce R. Javier and Taryn R. Liu*

The population of Asian Pacific Islander (API) children in the United States is expected to more than double by 2025, rising from just 4 percent of the child population in 1996 to about 7 percent (Stoddard et al. 2000) (see Figure 27.1). Despite the growth of this population, we have only a limited understanding of the health and health care issues that characterize these children. Even less is known regarding child health status for API subgroups. Among Asian American children, Filipino and Chinese make up the largest subgroups (see Figure 27.2).

This chapter will first describe a conceptual framework for understanding factors affecting the health status of Asian American children. It will then review what is known about the health of Asian American children in multiple clinical areas. Finally, we will make recommendations for research and policy with the goal of improving the health of Asian American children.

The term *Asian American* denotes any U.S. resident whose origins are in any of the original people of the Far East, Southeast Asia, or the Indian subcontinent, including the Philippine Islands. Also, we do not use the terms *API* and *Asian American* interchangeably. *API* refers to Asian Americans and Pacific Islanders together as one group. When we refer to these two groups separately, the term *Asian American* does not include Pacific Islanders. A Pacific Islander is a person whose origins are in any of the original peoples of Hawaii, Guam, Samoa, or other Pacific Islands. Pacific Islanders are a separate category from Asian Americans, although they are sometimes included with Asian Americans or relegated to another category.

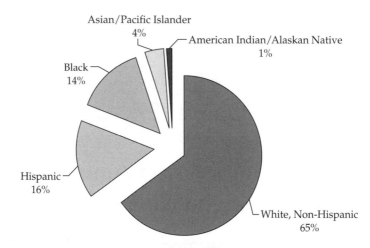

**Figure 27.1** Percentage of U.S. Children (Aged 0–18) by Racial or Ethnic Group, 2000. All categories include those of mixed race or mixed ethnicity (7). Calculated by Joyce R. Javier from U.S. Census Bureau, Census 2000 Summary File 2 (SF 2) 100-Percent Data files.

The majority of Asian American children in the United States are growing up in immigrant families, which are defined as having at least one parent born outside the United States (Hernandez and Macartney 2007a) (see Table 27.1). According to Hernandez and colleagues, along with other children in immigrant families, they are leading the racial-ethnic transformation

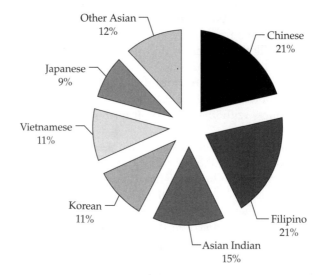

**Figure 27.2** U.S. Asian American Children (Aged 0–18) by Subgroup, 2000. All categories include those of mixed race or mixed ethnicity (7). Calculated by Joyce R. Javier from U.S. Census Bureau, Census 2000 Summary File 2 (SF 2) 100-Percent Data files.

**Table 27.1** Percent and Number of Children Ages 0–17, by Immigrant Country or Race/Ethnic Origin, United States, Census 2000

| Immigrant Country, Race/Ethnic Origin | Percent | Number | Immigrant Country, Race Ethnic Origin | Percent | Number |
|---|---|---|---|---|---|
| Total | 100.0 | 68,331,476 | Children in Immigrant Families (cont'd) | | |
| Children in Native-Born Families | 80.5 | 54,999,156 | China | 0.4 | 246,401 |
| White | 58.9 | 40,235,860 | Hong Kong | 0.1 | 92,254 |
| Black | 13.2 | 8,991,858 | Taiwan | 0.2 | 108,641 |
| Puerto Rican, Mainland Origin | 0.7 | 500,166 | Philippines | 0.8 | 540,304 |
| Puerto Rican, Island Origin | 0.8 | 526,228 | Hmong | 0.1 | 71,598 |
| Mexican | 3.4 | 2,315,406 | Cambodia | 0.1 | 80,812 |
| Other Hispanic/Latino | 1.5 | 1,048,439 | Laos | 0.1 | 87,264 |
| Asian American | 0.6 | 377,028 | Thailand | 0.1 | 60,487 |
| Hawaiian/Pacific Islander | 0.1 | 92,941 | Vietnam[a] | 0.6 | 386,645 |
| Native American | 1.3 | 911,230 | Indochina[a] | 1.0 | 686,806 |
| Children in Immigrant Families | 19.5 | 13,332,320 | India | 0.5 | 328,386 |
| Mexico | 7.6 | 5,165,982 | Pakistan/Bangladesh | 0.2 | 136,621 |
| Central America | 1.4 | 939,082 | Afghanistan | 0.0 | 17,879 |
| Cuba | 0.4 | 248,584 | Iran | 0.2 | 99,756 |
| Dominican Republic | 0.5 | 350,101 | Iraq | 0.1 | 39,298 |
| Haiti | 0.3 | 201,981 | Israel/Palestine | 0.1 | 72,306 |
| Jamaica | 0.3 | 230,808 | Other West Asia | 0.3 | 190,760 |
| Caribbean, English Speaking | 0.3 | 226,786 | Former USSR | 0.4 | 238,403 |
| South America | 1.0 | 647,643 | Other Europe, Canada[a] | 1.9 | 1,287,693 |
| Japan | 0.2 | 104,677 | Africa, Blacks | 0.4 | 237,078 |
| Korea | 0.5 | 321,866 | Africa, Whites[a] | 0.2 | 128,221 |
| | | | Other | 0.7 | 444,003 |

[a] "Vietnam" includes Indochina not specified; "Indochina, total" includes the following: Hmong, Cambodia, Laos, Thailand, Vietnam; "Other Europe, Canada" includes Australia and New Zealand; "Africa, Whites" includes Asian American Africans.

Calculated from Census 2000 5pct microdata (IPUMS) by Donald J. Hernandez, Nancy A. Denton, and Suzanne E. Macartney, Center for Social and Demographic Analysis, University at Albany, State University of New York with funding from the William and Flora Hewlett Foundation.

of America. The emergence of racial and ethnic minorities as the majority U.S. population is occurring rapidly and will first become a reality among children. In just twenty-three years, the U.S. Census Bureau projects that the proportion of children who identify as non-Hispanic white will fall steadily and drop below 50 percent after 2030. Along with other children of color, Asian American children will grow up to become working-age adults and will provide the majority of economic support to American society in coming years (Hernandez and Macartney 2007b).

## FACTORS SHAPING OUR UNDERSTANDING OF THE HEALTH OF ASIAN AMERICAN CHILDREN

### Data Availability

There are currently five national surveys and one regional survey that are used to assess the health of API children. However, national and state datasets that include API children often report aggregated results that mask key variations in health status among API subgroups (Brahan and Bauchner 2005). For example, the National Health and Nutrition Examination Survey and National Survey for Children with Special Health Care Needs place Asian American children into one category. Fortunately, others, including the National Health Interview Survey, the National Center for Health Statistics Vital Statistics, the National Longitudinal Survey of Adolescent Health, and the California Health Interview Survey (CHIS), are dividing APIs into subgroups, allowing for disaggregated analysis of the population. CHIS, a random-digit dial telephone survey designed to produce reliable estimates of California's diverse racial and ethnic groups, is unique in that it was conducted in six languages: English, Spanish, Chinese, Korean, Vietnamese, and Khmer (Ponce et al. 2004). The UCLA Center for Health Policy Research conducts the survey every other year and uses community-based participatory research principles to develop each cycle of the survey (Brown 2005).

In this chapter, we performed a literature search using the following terms in several different combinations: *Asian, Asian American, children, adolescents, United States, health, asthma, birth outcomes, cancer, cardiovascular disease, communicable diseases, health care access, hypertension, mental health, nutrition, obesity, overweight, physical activity, oral health, sexually transmitted disease, substance use,* and *violence.* Search results were limited to those published between 1985 and April 2008. This search resulted in identification of 276 peer-reviewed articles on API children, which are listed and organized by topic in Table 27.2.

### Conceptual Framework for Understanding Health Status of Asian American Children

Given that the majority of Asian American children in the United States are growing up in immigrant families, they are often studied in the context

**Table 27.2** Peer-Reviewed Articles in the Original Database Regarding Asian American Child Health

| Topic | # |
|---|---|
| Acculturation/Culture | 15 |
| Asthma | 16 |
| Cancer | 8 |
| Cardiovascular Disease/Hypertension | 2 |
| Communicable Diseases/Vaccinations | 8 |
| Diseases of Other Organs | 7 |
| Health-care Access | 7 |
| Mental Health | 43 |
| Nutrition/Obesity/Physical Activity | 79 |
| Oral Health | 3 |
| Pregnancy/Birth | 50 |
| STD/HIV | 6 |
| Substance Use | 25 |
| Violence and Abuse | 7 |
| **TOTAL** | **276** |

of other immigrant children. Coll and Szalacha's integrative model of child development (2004), provides a conceptual framework for understanding how the health of all children is influenced not only by family systems but by other institutions in which the child and family interact (see Figure 27.3). The model identifies eight major constructs hypothesized

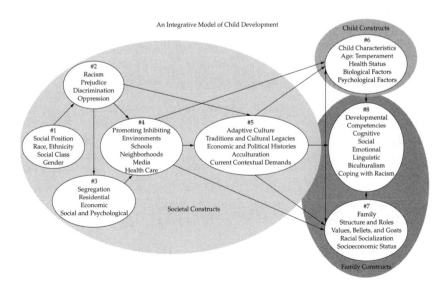

**Figure 27.3** An Integrative Model of Child Development.

to influence developmental processes for children of color and children of immigrant families. It assumes that cognitive, emotional, and behavioral development are profoundly affected by the child's social position within society. Using this model to identify unique sources of risk and protective factors for children in immigrant families can provide a new base on which to build social policies and implement effective prevention and intervention programs.

## Strengths of Asian Immigrant Families

Asian American children benefit from several strengths in their families. First, similar to children living in other immigrant families, Asian American children are more likely than non-Hispanic white children to live in two-parent families (U.S. Census Bureau 2004; Hernandez and Macartney 2007c). They also tend to live with other relatives or nonrelatives who can provide the child additional social support and resources (Hernandez and Macartney 2007c). For example, grandparents often provide childcare, nurturing, and economic resources in Asian American families (Kataoka-Yahiro and Yoder 2004). Finally, Asian American adults have high labor force participation rates overall (U.S. Census Bureau 2004).

Another strength of Asian immigrant families is a strong sense of ethnic and cultural identity. Research among immigrant groups indicate a link between ethnic identity and well-being (Phinney 2007). For instance, a study examining a large sample of adolescents from a variety of backgrounds (e.g., Vietnamese, Chinese, Indian, and Pakistani), showed positive correlations between ethnic identity and self-esteem, coping, mastery, and optimism, and negative correlations with depression and loneliness. Interventions promoting ethnic identity have been used to address teen pregnancy prevention in the Filipino population (Javier et al. 2006a).

## Challenges Faced by Asian American Children

Risk factors for poor health among immigrant children in general include poverty, generational status, and English proficiency. These factors also apply to Asian American children (Mendoza and Burgos 2007).

Poverty is a significant issue for many Asian American children in the United States. According to the 2000 U.S. census, Asian American children have a higher poverty rate than non-Hispanic white children (14.3 versus 9.3), but a lower poverty rate than Pacific Islanders (22.7), Latinos (27.8), and African Americans (33.1) (Lai et al. 2003). Among Asian Americans, Southeast Asians particularly, Vietnamese, Hmong, Cambodian, and Lao children are more likely to live in poverty than other API groups (Hernandez and Macartney 2007c).

Children growing up in immigrant families tend to have better health outcomes than children of U.S.-born parents. This phenomenon has been

**Table 27.3** Poverty Status by Age and Race, 1999, U.S. Census 2000

| Total Population | General Population | Non-Hispanic White Alone | Hispanic Alone | Black Alone | Asian Alone | Native Hawaiian/ Pacific Islander |
|---|---|---|---|---|---|---|
| Child poverty rate (<18 years of age) (%) | 16.6 | 9.3 | 27.8 | 33.1 | 14.3 | 22.7 |

Lai, E., Arguelles, D., and eds. *The New Face of Asian Pacific America: Numbers, Diversity, and Change in the 21st Century.* 2003, San Francisco: Asian Week.

termed the "immigrant paradox"; that is, despite higher levels of poverty and limited access to health care, children in immigrant families are less likely than children in nonimmigrant families to have poor health outcomes. This is primarily seen in the area of birth outcomes, in infant mortality and low birth weight, and in adolescent risk behaviors (Guendelman et al. 1999; Harris 1999). However, the immigrant paradox cannot be applied to all health conditions. For example, children with asthma in immigrant families are more likely to report poor health than children of U.S.-born parents. This finding was associated with higher rates of poverty and limited English proficiency in immigrant families (Javier and Mendoza 2007a).

Children with parents who do not speak English or have limited English proficiency tend to have less access to care (Yu et al. 2004a) and are more likely to report dissatisfaction with the care that they receive (Weech-Maldonado et al. 2001). Moreover, limited English proficiency populations are more likely to receive poor quality care (Flores et al. 2003).

Although Asian American children share many of the risk and protective factors affecting the health of children in other immigrant families, it is important to recognize that important differences exist depending on various factors, including country of origin, socioeconomic status, culture and acculturation, residential status, and economic opportunity (Mendoza and Burgos 2007).

Given the rapid growth of the Asian American child population, it is important to accurately assess its health to ensure that interventions and services adequately meet the goal of improving their quality of life. The following section describes what is known about Asian American child health disparities from birth to adolescence. Overall, health disparities in Asian American child health are manifest in two major areas: health and health care. The chapter first examines health care by looking at access to quality health care. Then it will describe the health of Asian American youth in the following categories: birth outcomes, chronic illness, mental health, obesity, and adolescent risk factors.

## ASIAN AMERICAN CHILD HEALTH AND HEALTH CARE

### Quality of Health Care

According to the Agency for Health Care Research and Quality, quality health care is care that is "effective, safe, timely, patient-centered, equitable, and efficient" (Agency for Healthcare Research 2007). Health-care quality is measured in several ways, including clinical performance measures of how well providers deliver specific services, assessments by patients of how well providers meet health-care needs from the patient's perspective (i.e., patient centeredness), and outcome measures. We were able to assess the quality of medical care provided to Asian American children by examining studies addressing access to care, utilization of care, and the level of patient-centeredness provided. Research is needed in the other aforementioned areas of health-care quality for Asian American children.

### Access to Quality Health Services

According to the California Health Interview Survey 2001 and 2003 (Laverreda and Ponce 2005), 9 percent of API children are uninsured all or part of the year. However, insurance coverage for children varies by Asian American subgroup. The percentage of children uninsured all or part of the year ranged from as low as 6.9 percent in Chinese to as high as 27.7 percent in Koreans. Korean and Vietnamese children had the lowest rates of continuous coverage from job-based insurance, at 40.5 percent and 42.6 percent, respectively, compared to 71.9 percent of Filipino children and 62.7 percent of API children overall. Despite their low rate of employment-based insurance coverage, Vietnamese children are protected by Medi-Cal and Healthy Families. Korean children, however, have half the rate of public coverage enrollment and, consequently, twice the rate of uninsurance (see Table 27.4). Data from the National Health Interview Survey 1997–2000 found that Chinese, Asian Indian, and other API children were more likely to be without insurance at the time of interview than non-Hispanic white youth (Yu et al. 2004b). All Asian American children were more likely to lack a usual source of care and more likely to be without contact with a health-care professional within the past twelve months (see Table 27.5) (Yu et al. 2004b).

### Use of Health Care Services

Disparities in utilization of care have been documented in Asian American children for acute appendicitis, asthma, and congenital heart defects. Compared with non-Hispanic white children with acute appendicitis in studies in California and New York, Asian American have a higher probability of rupture or perforated appendicitis. Along with Latino and African American children, APIs experience higher rates of hospital

**Table 27.4** Asian Ethnic Group by Health Insurance Coverage During the Last Twelve Months, Ages 0–18, California 2001/2003 (California Health Interview Survey)

| Ethnic Group | Uninsured All or Part Year (%) | Employment-Based Insurance All Year (%) | Medi-Cal or Healthy Families All Year (%) | Population in 2003 |
|---|---|---|---|---|
| Filipino | 7.8 | 71.9 | 13.1 | 327,000 |
| Korean | 27.7 | 40.5 | 16.7 | 99,000 |
| Chinese | 6.9 | 65.4 | 19.3 | 246,000 |
| Vietnamese | 9.4 | 42.6 | 42.1 | 142,000 |
| South Asian | *** | 72.0 | 13.6 | 124,000 |
| Japanese | *** | 77.1 | 5.8 | 82,000 |
| Other Single or Multiple Asian Group | 5.1 | 58.3 | 31.5 | 176,000 |
| Total Asian American and Pacific Islander Population | 9.0 | 62.7 | 20.4 | 1,196,000 |

admissions for appendicitis with a perforated appendix than non-Hispanic white children (Jablonski and Guagliardo 2005; Guagliardo et al. 2003). Increased rates of rupture and hospitalization for rupture in Asian American children may be due to various factors, such as delayed emergency care or language barriers.

**Table 27.5** Health Status and Health Services Utilization Characteristics of Asian American and Pacific Islander Children: United States 1997–2000 (National Health Interview Survey)

| | Non-Hispanic White | Chinese | Filipino | Asian Indian | Other API |
|---|---|---|---|---|---|
| Without health insurance at time of interview (%) | 8.4 | 11.3 | 7.0 | 14.9 | 13.9 |
| Without a usual place for health care (%) | 1.7 | 3.8 | 3.6 | 1.9 | 6.3 |
| Without contact with a doctor or health professional in the past 12 months | 19.3 | 24.2 | 28.1 | 28.1 | 26.1 |

Asthma is an important disease because it is one of the most common chronic conditions of childhood. API children are more likely (OR: 1.59; CI: 1.24–2.59) than non-Hispanic white children to experience an adverse asthma outcome such as intubation, cardiopulmonary arrest, and death (Calmes et al. 1998). Also, the proportion of high-severity asthma cases among children hospitalized with asthma substantially increased for Asian American or Pacific Islanders, adolescents, girls, self-pay children, and lowest income families and during spring months (Meurer et al. 2000). Finally, Californian annual asthma hospitalization rates from 1983 through 1996 increased for Hispanics and Asian Americans whereas it decreased for non-Hispanic whites and remained constant for African Americans (Von Behren et al. 1999).

Mortality from heart defects remains a major cause of death in infancy and childhood (Boneva et al. 2001). A delay in diagnosis of a congenital heart defect can lead to delayed surgical repair, which in turn may lead to increased mortality. In a study using data from the 1995 and 1996 Office of Statewide Health Planning and Development, compared with non-Hispanic white, African American, and other ethnicities, Asian American children tended to be older at surgery repair for heart defects, including ventriculoseptal defects, tetralogy of fallot, and atrioventricular canal. The authors propose that this difference between Asian American children and other ethnicities could be attributed to poor access to care or to the cultural background of the Asian American population (Change et al. 2000). The above studies highlight the need for more research to better understand differences among ethnic groups regarding utilization of care for children with acute appendicitis, asthma, and congenital heart disease.

## Patient Centeredness

*Patient centeredness*, a term used to describe an approach to improving the relationship between a provider and a patient, is an essential component of quality care. In a study conducted in Southern California, Asian American parents reported the poorest interpersonal relationships between their child and their child's physician and were the most affected by managed care policies. Asian American children experienced significant deficits in the relationship domain across each managed care policy, regardless of the source of insurance data. These findings are consistent with previous research documenting tenuous patient-provider relationships for Asian American adults (Taira et al. 1997). This is concerning because Asian American children are at greater risk than non-Hispanic whites of having poor health, being under-immunized, and contracting preventable illnesses such as hepatitis B (Centers for Disease Control 1998, 2000; Weigers and Cohen 1998). Asian Americans are also more likely than non-Hispanic whites to experience difficulty communicating with their physician, to feel that they are treated with disrespect when receiving health care, to experience barriers to access to care such as lack of insurance or not having a regular doctor, and to feel they would receive better care if they were of a different race or ethnicity. In addition, parental assessment of pediatric Medicaid managed care reveals that Asian American non-English-speakers score staff helpfulness, timeliness of care, provider communication, plan service, and getting needed care lower than non-Hispanic whites (Weech-Maldonado et al. 2001).

Inappropriate use of antibiotics is a major public health concern, and discussion of this topic can strain the patient-doctor relationship. A study of community pediatric practices in Los Angeles, California, revealed that Asian Americans tend to go to physicians who make few bacterial diagnoses for non–Asian Americans, but tend to make substantially more bacterial diagnoses for Asian Americans. The source of this difference is unknown, but the authors propose that it may be due to Asian American parents more forcefully communicating a belief that their child's illness requires antibiotics. They also raise the concern that this may represent physician bias in the management of patients belonging to different racial/ethnic groups (Mangione-Smith et al. 2004).

## HEALTH STATUS

The health status of Asian American children is a mixed picture. According to national data from the Agency for Healthcare Research and Quality, compared to non-Hispanic white youth, Asian American children are more likely to report that they are in poor health (Weigers and Cohen 1998). Also, Asian American children are at greater risk for underimmunization and contracting preventable illnesses such as hepatitis B (Yu et al.). Yet, APIs are less likely to report a school absence, learning disability, use of prescription medications, and chronic conditions (Fuler 2001).

### Birth Outcomes

Infant mortality, defined as death in the first year of life, now accounts for almost 60 percent of all deaths from birth through age eighteen (Wise 2004). Neonatal mortality, defined as deaths occurring in the first twenty-eight days of life accounts for nearly 40 percent. Also, death associated with premature birth, low birth weight, congenital anomalies, and genetic disorders is becoming increasingly important (Wise 2004). Thus, any assessment of child health must examine birth outcomes.

Infant and neonatal mortality rates for detailed API subgroups are only available in eleven states (California, Hawaii, Illinois, Minnesota, Missouri, New Jersey, New York, Texas, Virginia, Washington, and West Virginia). Data from the year 2002 revealed that in these eleven states, the infant mortality rates (4.6 versus 5.4 deaths per 1000 live births) and neonatal mortality rate (3.1 versus 3.6) for APIs is less than non-Hispanic whites. However, disaggregated data reveal that infant mortality rates vary by

Asian American subgroup. Filipinos and Hawaiians had higher infant and neonatal mortality rates than non-Hispanic whites, whereas Chinese, Japanese, Vietnamese, Asian American Indian, Korean, and other APIs had lower rates (Mathews et al. 2004).

Using California data from 1991 to 2001, unadjusted neonatal mortality rates for Chinese, Japanese, and Koreans were significantly less than non-Hispanic whites. When risk factors (i.e., pregnancy complications, congenital anomalies, etc.) are taken into consideration, adjusted neonatal mortality rates for Thai infants are statistically significantly worse than outcomes for infants born to Cambodian, Chinese, Filipino, Indian, Japanese, Korean, Laotian, and Vietnamese mothers (Baker et al. 2007).

Low birth weight is an important predictor of infant morbidity and mortality (Committee to Study the Prevention of Low Birth Weight 1985). In a study of California births during 1992, very low birth weight (VLBW) (500–1499 g) was more likely among infants of Filipino women and less likely among infants of Chinese women, relative to infants of non-Hispanic white women. Moderately low birth weight (MLBW) (1500–2499 g) was more likely among Cambodian, Filipino, Indian, Japanese, Laotian, and Thai infants and was less likely among Korean infants, relative to non-Hispanic whites. In multivariate analyses, Filipino women remained at increased risk of both very low and moderately low birth weight, whereas Cambodian, Asian Indian, and Laotian infants had elevated odds of moderately low birth weight. In addition, Filipino women have an unrecognized high rate of gestational diabetes (59.8 per 1000 compared with 30.4 per 1000 for black women) (Martin et al. 2003). In summary, perinatal outcomes among Asian Americans vary by national origin, and accepted risk factors only partially explain this variation (Fuentes-Afflick and Hessol 1997).

## Teen Births

Weitz et al. examined teen pregnancy among API subgroups and reported that in aggregate, fewer than 6 percent of births to APIs in California are teen births. When data on APIs are disaggregated, Filipinos have the highest percentage of births to teens among California's six largest API groups (Chinese, Filipino, Vietnamese, Korean, Indian, and Japanese). Compared with non-Hispanic white teens, Filipino teens are more likely to request a pregnancy test and no other services from a provider, suggesting that they are sexually active but not looking for birth control. Taking all API subgroups into account, Laotian (18.9%), Hawaiian (14.1%), and Other Asian American (13.4%) have a higher percentage of births to teens than non-Hispanic whites (12%) (Weitz et al. 2001).

According to a study of births in New York City between 1987 and 1993, infants of Asian American adolescents had increased risk for both MLBW and VLBW. Also, a significantly elevated risk for VLBW was found for infants of Asian American teens born in the United States (Madan et al. 2002). The above studies demonstrate the need for culturally appropriate teen pregnancy prevention programs for diverse population of Asian American youth.

## Chronic Illness

The prevalence of chronic childhood illness has increased during the past several decades (Newacheck and Halfon 1998). While injuries remain the major cause of childhood illness and death, among noninjury causes, chronic illness now accounts for the majority of children's hospital days and deaths. The reasons for the apparent increase in childhood chronic illness are unclear. Wise suggests that this increase may be related to changes in survey procedures, improvements in diagnosis, and a greatly expanded public awareness of behavioral and developmental disorders. Also, certain important chronic child health conditions have been on the rise (Wise 2004). These include asthma, mental health disorders, developmental and behavioral disorders such as autism and attention deficit and hyperactivity disorder (ADHD), and childhood obesity. With the exception of asthma, we were unable to identify any studies examining the prevalence of chronic conditions and developmental and behavioral disorders in Asian American children. Thus, we will focus on what is known about Asian American children in the areas of asthma, obesity, and mental health conditions.

## Asthma

Asthma is one of the most common chronic childhood conditions. Among California children, the prevalence of active asthma varies by ethnic groups, with the highest prevalence among African Americans (17%) and American Indians/Alaska Natives (17%), followed by whites (10%), Latinos (7%), and Asian Americans (7%) (Meng et al. 2007). However, lifetime asthma diagnosis among eleven API subgroups ranged from 10.9 percent among Koreans to 23.8 percent among Filipinos (Davis et al. 2006). There are no national prevalence data available on API subgroups for asthma.

As mentioned earlier, Asian Americans are more likely to have an adverse outcome when they are hospitalized for asthma. A study comparing asthma knowledge for Asian Americans, predominantly recent Chinese immigrants and non-Asian populations, found that lower socioeconomic status and being Asian American were independent predictors of less asthma knowledge. This study pointed out the importance of developing asthma education programs tailored to recent Asian American immigrants and testing them for efficacy (Lee et al. 2007).

## Obesity

Childhood and adolescent obesity is a major health problem for American youth because of its associated morbidities and tendency to persist into adulthood. In Table 27.6, data for Asian American youth are

**Table 27.6** Overweight and Obesity

| Author (Year) | Data Source/ Age or Grade of Population | Measurement | Ethnicity | Male | Female | Combined |
|---|---|---|---|---|---|---|
| Gordon-Larsen (1999) | Add Health (Wave II-1996)/ 12–20 years | % BMI≥ 85th percentile/ % BMI≥ 95th percentile | Asian | 22.78 | 10.37 | — |
| | | | non-Hispanic white | 26.53 | 22.24 | — |
| | | | Asian | 23/7 | 11/4 | — |
| | | | non-Hispanic white | 28/12 | 22/10 | — |
| Popkin (1998) | Add Health (Wave II-1996)/ 12–22 years | % Obese-BMI≥ 85th | Asian | 25.7 | 15 | 20.6 |
| | | | non-Hispanic white | 25.8 | 22.6 | 24.2 |
| | | | Filipino | 22.6 | 12.8 | 18.5 |
| | | | Chinese | 18.9 | 10.9 | 15.3 |
| | | | Other: Korean, Japanese, Southeast Asian, Indian American | 35.9 | 20.6 | 28.2 |
| | | | 1st generation | 15.6 | 8.3 | 11.6 |
| | | | 2nd generation | 30.8 | 22.0 | 27.2 |
| | | | 3rd generation | 34.6 | 20.3 | 28.0 |

| Study | Data source | Measure | | | | |
|---|---|---|---|---|---|---|
| **Gordon-Larsen (2004)** | Add Health (Wave III-2001)/ 19–26 years | % BMI≥ 30/ % BMI≥ 40 | **Asian** | 19.1/1.3 | 7.7/0.8 | 14.1/1.1 |
| | | | Became obese | 13.2 | 6.5 | — |
| | | | Remained obese | 5.9 | 1.2 | — |
| | | | Became non-obese | 0.1 | 1.2 | — |
| | | | Remained obese | 80.8 | 91.1 | — |
| | | | **non-Hispanic white** | 20.8/3.3 | 21.0/4.3 | 22.1/4.3 |
| | | | Became obese | 11.6 | 12.5 | — |
| | | | Remained obese | 9.2 | 8.5 | — |
| | | | Became non-obese | 2.2 | 1.1 | — |
| | | | Remained non-obese | 77.0 | 78.0 | — |
| **Harris (2006)** | Add Health (Waves I-III)/ Ages 12–26 | Proportion of Obesity: BMI≥ 30 (Wave I-II to Wave III) | **Asian** | 0.10–0.21 | 0.04–0.09 | — |
| | | | **non-Hispanic white** | 0.14–0.19 | 0.10–0.21 | — |
| **Haas (2003)** | Medical Expenditure Panel Survey (MEPS) Household Component/ 6–17 years | Overweight: Odds Ratio (95% Confidence Interval) | **Asian** | | | |
| | | | 6–11 years | — | — | 0.83 (0.34, 2.01) |
| | | | 12–17 years | — | — | 4.35 (1.89–10.00) |
| | | | **non-Hispanic white** | — | — | Reference |

**Table 27.6** *(Continued)*

| Author (Year) | Data Source/ Age or Grade of Population | Measurement | Ethnicity | Male | Female | Combined |
|---|---|---|---|---|---|---|
| PedNSS (2009) | 2007 Pediatric Nutrition Surveillance-California/ 2–19 years | % BMI 85th–95th percentile/ % BMI≥ 95th percentile | **Asian** | | | |
| | | | 2–5 years | | | 13.0/12.7 |
| | | | 5– <20 years | | | 13.8/13.5 |
| | | | **Filipino** | | | |
| | | | 2–5 years | | | 13.3/12.3 |
| | | | 5– <20 years | | | 14.6/18.9 |
| | | | **Pacific Islander** | | | |
| | | | 2–5 years | | | 21.4/25.4 |
| | | | 5– <20 years | | | 21.5/38.3 |
| | | | **non-Hispanic white** | | | |
| | | | 2–5 years | | | 15.2/13.7 |
| | | | 5– <20 years | | | 17.0/20.0 |
| Beets (2004) | 2002 California FITNESSGRAM/ 10–15 years | Odds Ratio of Overweight *P<0.01 | **Asian** | 1.08 (1.05-1.11)* | 0.78 (0.76-0.81)* | — |
| | | | **Filipino** | 1.66 (1.60-1.73)* | 1.23 (1.17-1.28)* | — |
| | | | **non-Hispanic white** | reference | reference | |

| Johnson (2006) | 1999 Los Angeles Area middle schools/ seventh grade | Adjusted OR of overweight (% BMI 85th–95th percentile) or obese (% BMI ≥ 95th percentile)—% overweight or obese | Asian | — | — |
|---|---|---|---|---|---|
| | | | non-Hispanic white | | Reference |
| | | | Chinese | | Reference |
| | | | Filipino | | 1.60 (.82–3.13) |
| | | | Korean | | 2.10 (1.05, 4.20) |
| | | | Vietnamese | | .91 (.40, 2.04) |
| | | | Other Asian | | 1.80 (1.10, 2.96) |

0.68
(.49, .96)

presented using national, state, or local county/city data from several different regions of the United States. National data is limited regarding overweight and obesity rates for Asian American youth. In addition, definitions of overweight are not universal and consistent with the terms *at risk for overweight*, *overweight*, and *obesity* being used interchangeably to denote BMI ranges between the eighty-fifth and ninety-fifth percentile or above the ninety-fifth percentile. Studies aggregating Asian Americans with Pacific Islanders are difficult to interpret, because PIs are known to have the highest rates of obesity in the world (Barbes et al. 2004). Nevertheless, data suggests that Asian Americans are at increasing risk of overweight and obesity.

## National Data

National studies have shown mixed findings regarding the prevalence of overweight for Asian American children. The National Longitudinal Study of Adolescent Health (Add Health) is the primary data source used to report national prevalence rates of overweight and obese for Asian Americans adolescents. According to Add Health, Asian American female adolescents have lower rates of overweight (BMI ≥ eighty-fifth percentile) than both their Asian American male counterparts and female counterparts from other ethnic groups (Popkin and Udry 1998; Gordon-Larsen et al. 1999, 2003, 2004). In addition, Asian Americans of later generations have significantly higher obesity rates than first-generation Asian Americans (Popkin and Udry 1998). Both Asian American males and females have significant increases in rates of obesity over time during adolescence and from adolescence into young adulthood (Gordon-Larsen et al. 2004; Harris et al. 2006).

In contrast to Add Health, a separate nationally representative survey, the 1996 Medical Expenditure Panel Survey (MEPS), found API adolescents (twelve to seventeen years) were more than four times as likely to be overweight (BMI ≥ ninety-fifth percentile) compared to non-Hispanic white counterparts.

The Pediatric Nutrition Surveillance System (PedNSS) monitors the nutritional status of low-income children participating in federally funded maternal and child heath programs (Polhamus et al. 2007). National data from 2006 showed API (3% of surveyed children) children aged two to five years had prevalence rates of overweight (BMI ≥ ninety-fifth percentile) and at risk of overweight (BMI between eighty-fifth and ninety-fifth percentile) similar to non-Hispanic whites and African Americans (see Figure 27.4). However, APIs are the only ethnic group among this age group that did not see an increase in obesity over time (Polhamus et al. 2007a).

Beginning in 2005, the state of California separated Filipino Americans and Pacific Islanders from Asian Americans in its Pediatric Nutrition Surveillance (Paulhamus et al. 2007b). California data from 2006 show

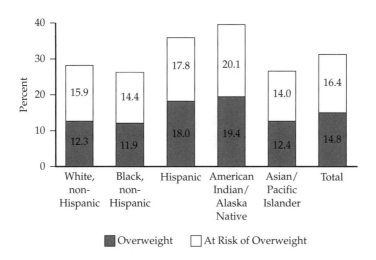

**Figure 27.4** Prevalence of Obesity* and Overweight† among Children Aged 2 to <5 Years, by Race and Ethnicity.

* Obesity: ≥ 95th percentile BMI-for age.
† Overweight: ≥ 85th to <95th percentile BMI-for-age, CDC growth charts, 2000.
*Source:* 2007 National PedNSS Data Table BD. Available at http://www.cdc.gov/pednss/pednss_tables/tables_numeric.htm.

that Asian Americans and Filipino Americans have slightly lower prevalence rates of overweight (BMI ≥ ninety-fifth percentile) and at risk of overweight (BMI between eighty-fifth and ninety-fifth percentile) compared to non-Hispanic whites, with Filipino American youth overweight prevalence rates in between (Paulhamus et al. 2007b).

## Local Data: Regional, State, and County

Local studies have also shown mixed findings regarding the prevalence of overweight for Asian American children and reveal that these rates vary according to age, generational status, and gender. In a California study that separated Asian Americans from Filipino Americans, being an Asian American male and a Filipino American (male or female) adolescent was associated with an increased risk for being overweight (BMI ≥ ninety-fifth percentile) compared to non-Hispanic whites. In contrast, being an Asian American female was shown to be a protective factor (Betts and Pitetti 2004). In Southern California, seventh grade Asian Americans as a whole had a lower risk of being overweight (BMI between eighty-fifth and ninety-fifth percentile) compared to non-Hispanic whites. However, when examining Asian American subgroups, Korean Americans and Other Asian Americans were more likely to be overweight than Chinese American youth (Johnson et al. 2006). Several smaller studies conducted in other states, including Florida, New York, and Texas, found at risk for overweight (BMI between eighty-fifth and ninety-fifth percentile) and actual overweight (BMI ≥ ninety-fifth percentile) rates were slightly lower or very similar for Asian Americans compared to non-Hispanic whites (Stettler et al. 2005; Johnson et al. 2007; Thorpe et al. 2004; Sorof et al. 2004). In contrast, one study found the odds of having a BMI greater than the ninety-fifth percentile are 1.78 times higher (95% CI 1.02, 3.08) for Asian American children compared to non-Hispanic whites (Rappaport and Robbins 2005).

The variability in the national and local data suggests more research is needed that includes a representative number of Asian Americans and its subgroups for comparison. In addition, given that overweight and obesity rates rise with longer residence in the United States (Bates et al. 2008; Smith et al. 2005), it is imperative to implement culturally tailored prevention methods before overweight and obesity rates rise further among Asian American children.

## Body Mass Index and Risk for Complications Related to Obesity

The use of BMI to define overweight and obesity across populations has been questioned in numerous studies because the relationship between BMI and risk for diabetes, hypertension, and metabolic syndrome in Asian American adults differs from that in non-Hispanic whites (Javier et al. 2007). At the same age, sex, and BMI, Asian Americans carry comparatively more body fat and/or visceral fat than non-Hispanic whites (Barbes et al. 2004; Smith et al. 2005; Daida et al. 2006). Asian American adults also have a 60 percent higher rate of type 2 diabetes mellitus when compared to non-Hispanic whites at the same BMI (APIOPA 2005). This is important because increased visceral fat is associated with increased rates of metabolic syndrome, insulin resistance, hypertension, and diabetes (Smith et al. 2005). South Asian Americans commonly suffer from metabolic syndrome, even with body mass indices lower than 25 $kg/m^2$ (Smith et al. 2005), and Asian Americans have a higher proportion of risk factors for cardiovascular disease and type 2 diabetes mellitus below the BMI cutoff of 25 $kg/m^2$ (Barbes et al. 2004).

This suggests that when using current BMI cutoffs as a trigger point for risk factors of obesity comorbidities (i.e., diabetes, cardiovascular disease), Asian Americans of lower BMIs may be overlooked, and Asian Americans at higher BMIs may be more at risk than previously thought. In fact, the World Health Organization has suggested changing BMI cutoff points for Asian American adults so that more attention can be given to obesity prevention in Asian American populations (see Table 27.7 and compare to current WHO BMI cutoffs in Figure 27.5.) (Barbes et al. 2004). More research examining specific BMI characteristics among Asian American youth is needed.

**Table 27.7** World Health Organization (WHO) Suggested Additional Body Mass Index Trigger Points for Public Health Action for Asian Populations

| | |
|---|---|
| < 18·5 kg/m² | Underweight |
| 23–27·5 kg/m² | Increased risk |
| ≥ 27·5 kg/m² | High risk |

*Source: WHO Expert Consultation.* Appropriate body-mass index for Asian populations and its implications for policy and intervention. *Lancet.* 2004 Jan 10; 363 (9403): 157–63.

## Physical Activity

Physical activity and inactivity research and data are limited for Asian American youth, and younger children are particularly understudied. Table 27.8 summarizes the major studies assessing physical fitness of Asian American children.

## National Data

In a study examining national data from 1995 and 1996, Asian American males had a significantly greater increase in inactivity as measured by TV/video viewing and game playing. They also had a decrease in moderate to vigorous physical activity compared to non-Hispanic whites (Gordon-Larsen et al. 2002). Asian American adolescent females also increased their TV/video viewing more than non-Hispanic whites of the same sex (Gordon-Larsen et al. 2002). Asian American adolescents were also less physically active compared to non-Hispanic whites (Gorden-Larsen et al. 1999). Asian American females are the least physically active,

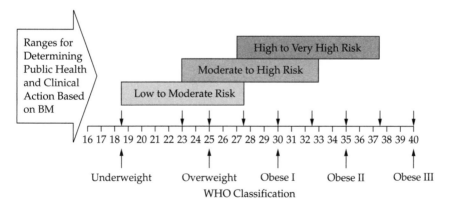
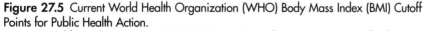

**Figure 27.5** Current World Health Organization (WHO) Body Mass Index (BMI) Cutoff Points for Public Health Action.

Reprinted from The Lancet, 363, WHO Expert Consultation, Appropriate body-mass index for Asian populations and its implications for policy and intervention strategies, 157–63, 2004, with permission from Elsevier.

**Table 27.8** Physical Activity

| Author (Year) | Data Source/ Age or Grade of Population | Measurement | Ethnicity | Male | Female | Combined |
|---|---|---|---|---|---|---|
| Gordon-Larsen (2002) | Add Health (Wave I-II 1995–1996/ 12–22 years) | *(significantly different from NHW p < .01) +(within ethnicity gender difference P < .01) | | | | |
| | | Increase in TV/video _7 h/wk (% (SEM)) | Asian | 26.6* (1.73) | 26.2* (2.31) | — |
| | | | non-Hispanic white | 21.5+ | 18.2 (0.84) | — |
| | | Increase in games _1 h/wk (% (SEM)) | Asian | 35.8*+ (1.53) | 26.5 (2.22) | — |
| | | | non-Hispanic white | 30.4+ (0.73) | 21.5 (1.00) | — |
| | | Change in moderate to vigorous physical activity (bouts/wk) (%(SEM)) | Asian | −0.25* (0.11) | −0.57 (0.15) | — |
| | | | non-Hispanic white | −0.24 (0.05) | −0.11 (0.05) | — |
| Gordon-Larsen (1999) | Add Health (Wave II-1996/ 12–20 years) | Mean (SEM) hours of television per week* *Weighted to be nationally representative with the error terms corrected for design effects. | Asian | 15.0 (1.02) | 12.8 (1.09) | 14.0 (.87) |
| | | | non-Hispanic white | 14.4 (.40) | 11.9 (.43) | 13.1 (.37) |

| | Col 1 | Col 2 | Col 3 |
|---|---|---|---|
| Mean (SEM) composite inactivity hours per week based on TV and video viewing and computer and video game playing* | | | |
| **Asian** | 23.7 (1.45) | 18.6 (1.67) | 21.3 (1.20) |
| **non-Hispanic white** | 22.1 (.58) | 16.5 (.52) | 19.3 (.50) |
| The adjusted proportion of adolescents participating in given tertiles of composite inactivity* (low/medium/high) | | | |
| **Asian** | | | |
| Low | 23.1 | 41.2 | |
| Medium | 31.6 | 26.6 | |
| High | 45.3 | 32.2 | |
| **non-Hispanic white** | | | |
| Low | 31.4 | 47.6 | |
| Medium | 34.1 | 30.6 | |
| High | 34.5 | 21.7 | |
| The adjusted proportion of adolescents participating in given tertiles of moderate to vigorous physical activity* (low/medium/high) | | | |
| **Asian** | | | |
| Low | 25.3 | 44.5 | |
| Medium | 36.8 | 43.0 | |
| High | 37.9 | 12.5 | |
| **non-Hispanic white** | | | |
| Low | 27.2 | 39.5 | |
| Medium | 35.0 | 34.9 | |
| High | 42.1 | 25.6 | |
| **Asian** | | | |
| | −0.26 (−0.35, −0.18)* | −0.45 (−0.52, −0.39)* | |

*Change over time (estimated time 1 level [wave I or II] minus estimated time 2 level [wave III]) was significantly different from 0 ($P$_.01).

**Harris (2006)**

**Add Health (Waves I-III)/ 12–26 years**

**Table 27.8** (Continued)

| Author (Year) | Data Source/ Age or Grade of Population | Measurement | Ethnicity | Male | Female | Combined |
|---|---|---|---|---|---|---|
| | | Prevalence of no exercise | **Asian** | | | |
| | | | Wave I-II | 0.04 (0.02, 0.06) | 0.08 (0.05, 0.10) | |
| | | | Wave III | 0.31 (0.20, 0.41) | 0.53 (0.44, 0.62) | |
| | | | **non-Hispanic white** | | | |
| | | | Wave I-II | 0.05 (0.04, 0.06) | 0.06 (0.05, 0.07) | |
| | | | Wave III | 0.35 (0.33, 0.37) | 0.46 (0.43, 0.48) | |
| Wolf (1999) | 1991 Lynn, Mass/ Grades 5–12 (female only) | % Strenuous activity (h/wk) | **Asian** | | | |
| | | | " 1 | — | 37.5 | — |
| | | | 1–3 | — | 62.5 | — |
| | | | >3 | — | 0.0 | — |
| | | | **non-Hispanic white** | | | |
| | | | " ≤1 | — | 27.6 | — |
| | | | 1–3 | — | 57.2 | — |
| | | | >3 | — | 15.2 | — |
| | | % Minimum strenuous activity (15 min, >3 times/wk) | **Asian** | — | 16.7 | — |
| | | | **non-Hispanic white** | — | 40.7 | — |

**Beets (2004)**

**2002 California FITNESSGRAM/ 10–15 years**

Adjusted 1-mile run/walk time (seconds) mean difference between each ethnic group in comparison with white non-Hispanics
* Significantly different than white non-Hispanics at $P \le 0.01$.

**Asian**

| Age | | |
| --- | --- | --- |
| 10 years | 31.2* (27.0–35.5) | 10.2* (6.1–14.4) |
| 11 years | 26.2* (21.9–30.4) | 11.2* (6.8–15.5) |
| 12 years | 13.4* (9.9–17.0) | 8.3* (4.9–11.6) |
| 13 years | 7.8* (4.1–11.4) | 6.6* (2.9–10.4) |
| 14 years | 6.1* (2.2–10.1) | 1.9 (–2.0–5.7) |
| 15 years | 8.4* (4.3–12.4) | 4.6 (0.2–8.9) |

**Filipino**

| Age | | |
| --- | --- | --- |
| 10 years | 38.4* (31.6–45.1) | 14.4* (7.7–21.1) |
| 11 year | 21.3* (14.8–27.8) | 13.6* (7.0–20.2) |
| 12 years | 5.1 (–0.6–10.8) | 15.4* (10.0–20.9) |
| 13 years | 3.2 (–2.6–9.0) | 21.7* (15.7–27.6) |
| 14 years | _0.4 (–6.4–5.5) | 13.9* (7.9–19.9) |
| 15 years | 3.1 (–3.0–9.1) | 15.9* (9.3–22.5) |

**Table 27.8** (Continued)

| Author (Year) | Data Source/ Age or Grade of Population | Measurement | Ethnicity | Male | Female | Combined |
|---|---|---|---|---|---|---|
| | | | **non-Hispanic whites** | | | |
| | | | 10 years | 633.8 – 148.96 | 693.1 – 139.53 | |
| | | | 11 years | 620.8 – 149.49 | 678.6 – 141.58 | |
| | | | 12 years | 586.0 – 138.67 | 638.9 – 129.75 | |
| | | | 13 years | 567.4 – 137.26 | 633.0 – 130.48 | |
| | | | 14 years | 543.2 – 133.17 | 631.1 – 133.93 | |
| | | | 15 years | 527.2 – 130.03 | 629.7 – 136.21 | |

and Asian American males participate in the highest amount of inactive past times (Gordon-Larsen et al. 1999), while still being more physically active than Asian American females (Gordon-Larsen et al. 2002). As Asian adolescents move into young adulthood, their levels of inactivity significantly increase (Harris et al. 2006), suggesting an increased risk for related health risks such as obesity and its related chronic diseases.

## State and Local Data

Published state and local data regarding physical activity are limited. These studies reveal trends similar to national data, including Asian American females being less physically active than peers (Wolf et al. 1999) and acculturation being associated with lower levels of physical activity (Unger et al. 2004). In an assessment of fitness, Beets and Pitetti found that Asian American males and Filipino American females were significantly slower than non-Hispanic white counterparts at all age groups (ten to fifteen years) in a test of mile walk-run times (2004). Filipino American males, on the other hand, were only significantly slower than non-Hispanic white males for age groups ten and eleven years. While Asian American females were slower than non-Hispanic white females at age groups ten to thirteen years, they caught up in age groups fourteen and fifteen.

Again, these results show variability, suggesting that more efforts need to be taken to include Asian Americans in national and local studies in numbers, allowing the ability to look at the various Asian American subpopulations.

## Nutrition

As a partial explanation for the better health found in new immigrants, children growing up in immigrant families have been found to adopt poorer eating habits compared with their immigrant parents (Fuentes-Afflick 2006). However, in California, Asian Americans have a tendency to maintain or improve preventative health behaviors across generations, including consumption of more fruits, vegetables, and dairy (Allen et al. 2007; Wiecha et al. 2001). Asian American children also have diets lower in energy density (fewer calories per ounce of food) (Mendoza et al. 2006) and typically consume more fruits and/or vegetables compared to non-Hispanic white counterparts (Allen et al. 2007; Larson et al. 2006; Reynolds et al. 1999). In addition, Asian American youth report consuming fewer soft drinks than non-Hispanic white and Hispanic adolescents (Allen et al. 2007; Novotny et al. 2003; Giammettei et al. 2003). However, it is important to note that although Asian Americans tend to fair better than non-Hispanic whites in fruit and vegetable consumption, this does not mean that they are meeting the recommended dietary allowances for these food groups (see Table 27.9). For example, in California, it is

**Table 27.9** Dietary Guidelines

| Food Groups and Subgroups | USDA Food Guide Amount |
|---|---|
| **Fruit Group** | **2 cups (4 servings)** |
| **Vegetable Group** | **2.5 cups (5 servings)** |
| • Dark green vegetables | 3 cups/week |
| • Orange vegetables | 2 cups/week |
| • Legumes (dry beans) | 3 cups/week |
| • Starchy vegetables | 3 cups/week |
| • Other vegetables | 6.5 cups/week |
| **Grain Group** | **6 ounce-equivalents** |
| • Whole grains | 3 ounce-equivalents |
| • Other grains | 3 ounce-equivalents |
| **Meat and Beans Group** | **5.5 ounce-equivalents** |
| **Oils** | **24 grams (6 tsp)** |
| **Discretionary Calorie Allowance**[a] | **267 calories** |
| Example of distribution: | |
| Solid fat | 18 grams |
| Added sugars | 8 tsp |

Children and adolescents. Consume whole grain products often; at least half the grains should be whole grains. Children two to eight years should consume two cups per day of fat-free or low-fat milk or equivalent milk products. Children nine years of age and older should consume three cups per day of fat-free or low-fat milk or equivalent milk products.

Children and adolescents. Keep total fat intake between 30 to 35 percent of calories for children two to three years of age and between 25 to 35 percent of calories for children and adolescents four to eighteen years of age, with most fats coming from sources of polyunsaturated and monounsaturated fatty acids, such as fish, nuts, and vegetable oils.

[a]All servings are per day unless otherwise noted. USDA vegetable subgroup amounts and amounts of DASH nuts, seeds, and dry beans are per week.
*Source:* Dietary Guidelines for Americans 2005. U.S. Department of Health and Human Services, U.S. Department of Agriculture. Available at: www.healthierus.gov/dietaryguidelines.

estimated that over half (51.4%) of Asian American adolescents consume fast food every single day (Hastert et al. 2005), a known risk factor for low fruit and vegetable consumption. Larson et al. found that Asian American youth are significantly more likely to be involved in food preparation and grocery shopping compared to other ethnic groups. This was associated with better vitamin and mineral intake, but higher rates of overweight (2006).

Similar to other immigrant groups in the United States, it is important to note that Westernization of diet puts Asian American children at risk for poor nutrition. For some who immigrate to the United States who were previously underweight or malnourished, catch-up growth does occur (Javier et al. 2007), and nutrition disparities decrease with length of residence in the United States (Allen et al. 2007). However, snacking patterns that are not typical in their native land put Asian Americans at risk for excess calorie consumption, hence overweight and related risk factors (Adair and Popkin 2005). This suggests that preventative measures should reinforce the healthy aspects of traditional Asian diets and encourage consumption of Western foods in moderation.

Eating disorders have been reported among Asian American youth. In a review of eating patterns among ethnically diverse youth, Asian Americans girls had the highest incidence of binge eating, whereas Hispanic girls reported the greatest use of diuretics, and African American girls were more likely to report vomiting to lose or maintain weight (Bronner 1996). Furthermore, Robinson et al. reported that Asian American girls may be at higher risk for eating disorders than previously recognized (1996).

In summary, although Asian Americans tend to fair better in overall obesity rates and fruit and vegetable consumption, there is great variability among different subgroups. In addition, there is an unfavorable negative trend overall for Asian Americans with longer residence in the United States regarding overweight and diet patterns. Also of concern is the fairly consistent trend in lower physical activity rates among Asian Americans. Attention from health-care professionals and public policy makers needs to focus on culturally competent preventative measures to help curb the rising rates of overweight and obesity and help reverse the trends of physical inactivity.

## MENTAL HEALTH

### Prevalence of Mental Health Conditions

Overall, an individual's mental health is influenced by several factors, including cultural beliefs and religion, acculturation patterns, socioeconomic status, education, traumatic experiences, family dynamics, help-seeking behaviors, historical context of immigration patterns (Lu et al. 2002), indigenous traits, coping styles (Sanchez and Gaw 2007) and discrimination. Furthermore, understanding the development of mental illness in children requires an understanding of child development. Coll's integrative model of child development (Coll and Szalacha 2004) (see Figure 27.3) provides a model for understanding how mental illness is influenced, not only by family systems but by other institutions in which the child and family interact.

### Prevalence and Service Use

The mental health needs of Asian American children are not well identified. Furthermore, a stereotype persists for Asian Americans that presents youth as a "model minority," doing well in school and having few social problems (Su 1999). This model minority stereotype reinforces an assumed idea that Asian Americans do not suffer from the same mental and social issues that other minorities have. Depressive symptoms are no less among Asian American youth than other ethnic groups; however, expression may differ. For example, in the northeastern United States, Asian American students aged sixteen to twenty years reported higher levels of depressive symptomology, withdrawn behavior, and social problems compared to non-Hispanic white peers, even though they performed better academically and had fewer delinquent behaviors. These Asian Americans also perceived themselves more poorly and were more dissatisfied with their social support (Lorenzo et al. 2000). This highlights the unique mental health needs of older Asian American adolescents and the false assumptions of the model minority myth in terms of overlooking at-risk groups.

Yeh et al. reported that Asian Americans have higher unmet mental healthcare needs compared to non-Hispanic whites. However, limited prevalence data shows mixed results regarding depression and mental health issues among Asian American youth. Some researchers indicate mental health problems among this population are similar to non-Hispanic white peers (Chen 1995). In contrast, another study of API youth (five to eighteen years) in the state of Washington who were Medicaid-covered were less likely to have depression diagnosis than non-Hispanic white youth (Richardson et al. 2003).

Asian American children and adolescents underutilize mental health-care services (Sanchez and Gaw 2007; Garland et al. 2005; Bui and Takeuchi 1992), and when they do use the services it is more often for crisis intervention (Sanchez and Gaw 2007; Snowden et al. 2008). Chow et al. found that Asian American adults and children living in New York were half as likely to have used mental health services but three times more likely to be diagnosed with schizophrenia than non-Hispanic whites, and more likely to use public mental health services, including emergency mental health services (2003). Among elementary school-aged children, Asian Americans, along with Hispanic youth, had a significantly lower relative risk of being hospitalized for psychiatric diagnosis compared to white children (Chabra et al. 1999). However, among hospitalized adolescents, APIs have been found to have more psychiatric diagnosis related groups compared to non-Hispanic white, black, and Hispanic adolescents, but less than American Indian and Alaskan natives (Leal 2005).

## Parental Perception

Parents of API youth report significantly fewer barriers to mental health-care usage, even when data suggests that API youth have higher unmet mental health care needs (Yeh et al. 2003). Reasons for higher unmet mental health care needs include social stigma regarding mental illness and lack of knowledge regarding available mental services by immigrant parents who did not have such services in their native country. Stigma can lead to unwillingness to voice complaints or seek help due to traditional Asian cultural values (Yeh et al. 2003). Ultimately, it is important to assess the rates of psychiatric disorders among Asian American youth to truly decipher if underutilization is due to actual lower prevalence or more barriers to access and utilization.

## Medication Use

Findings regarding medication use for mental health conditions reveal mixed conclusions. Among children with attention-deficit hyperactivity disorder (ADHD), Asian Americans were less likely to receive ADHD-related medication, and those who did received fewer days' supply (Ray et al. 2006). Another study found that, among Medicaid youth, APIs were as likely as non-Hispanic whites and African-Americans to fill an antidepressant prescription or have a mental health visit within six months of a new episode of depression.

## Diagnostic Scales and Ethnocentrism

There has been some debate over whether or not psychiatric diagnostic scales are reliable and valid for the Asian American population. Some researchers have noted that the measures of depressive symptoms may be ethnocentric toward Western symptomology and thus do not properly capture depression among different ethnic groups. When using the Center for Epidemiologic Studies Depression Scale (CES-D), a self-administered instrument designed to measure the level of depressive symptomology in community populations, factors that correlate with depression vary by ethnic group. Depression in African American and non-Hispanic whites relates to four factors: depressed affect, somatic retardation, positive affect, and interpersonal. However, Filipino American adolescents present two factors, with the first factor combining depressed affect, somatic retardation, and interpersonal (containing fifteen of twenty CES-D items), and the second factor being the positive affect (Edman et al. 1999). Similarly, Koreans have been found to conclude the same two-factor solution, whereas Chinese and Japanese have a three factor-solution, combining only somatic retardation and the depressed affect (Edman et al. 1999). The CES-D has also shown that Filipino adolescents did not differ from non-Hispanic white adolescents in patterns of depression symptomology (Edman et al. 1999). These results suggest that Koreans, Chinese, and Japanese American youth may express symptoms of depression differently, but that the CES-D is a reliable tool in measuring these symptoms.

The *Diagnostic and Statistical Manual of Mental Disorders* (DSM) Scale for Depression (DSD) is a scale created to measure childhood depression. The DSD has been shown to be appropriate for Korean, Chinese, and Japanese American adolescents (Choi 2002). In addition, the DSD found striking similarities between Chinese and non-Hispanic white adolescents regarding the magnitude of association between measures of mental distress (Chen. et al. 1998).

The Western diagnostic framework has been recognized as the golden standard, and Western symptoms are considered to be central patterns of mental illness (Choi 2002). Therefore, tools like the CES-D and the DSD should continue to be used to study ethnic and cultural variations in depression among children and adolescents but should also be validated when being used to measure depression among Asian Americans and its subgroups.

## Cultural Differences

In general, Asian American cultures differ from Western ideology by emphasizing communalism and collectivism as opposed to individualism. This focus on the family as "center," as opposed to the individual, may affect whether or not a family accesses mental health services because of fear of shame or stigma that may be placed on the family as a whole. Individually, Asian American subgroups are different from one another, and the cultural and historical context of each individual needs to be considered when assessing mental health. Cultural variables influencing mental health and the variation among major Asian subgroups are shown in Table 27.10. These differences play into the psychological development of Asian American children and adolescents.

## Asian American Indian

Among Asian American Indians, family and religion are forms of support for individuals. Eighty percent of Asian American Indians are Hindu, which perceives suffering as a result of past deeds. Even for non-Hindu Asian American Indians, fatalism and animism are common beliefs. This belief system can impede or postpone seeking help for mental distress (Conrad and Pacquiao 2005). In addition, a traditional patriarchal family organization and family involvement can also act as a barrier for the advocacy of the individual (Conrad and Pacquiao 2005). For children of this culture, preferential treatment for male children can add to mental distress. Asian Indians and other South Asians, including people from Bangladesh, Pakistan, and Sri Lanka, use the inculcation of shame and guilt in child rearing, and delinquency problems, drugs, and mental health are all seen as sources of great shame for the family (Ahmed and Lemkau 2000).

## Chinese

Chinese, having roots in Confucian values, value the role of relationships, social order, and constraint on communication. Direct confrontation is avoided in order not to cause shame or loss of face (Ozer and McDonald

**Table 27.10** Ethnic Differences in Mental Health

| Author (year) | Asian Subgroup | Cultural Variables that Affect Mental Health |
|---|---|---|
| — | Asian Indian | – fatalism and animism are common beliefs<br>– traditional patriarchal family structure<br>– preferential treatment of male children<br>– the use of shame in child rearing<br>– delinquency problems, drugs, and mental health issues bring shame to the family |
| — | Chinese | – constraint of communication to maintain social order<br>– avoidance of shame or losing face<br>– common needs of family and social relationships are more important than individual needs |
| — | Filipino | – *pakikisama*—conceding to the wishes of the collective<br>– *hiya*—devastating shame<br>– *amor propio*—sensitivity to criticism<br>– fatalisitic attitudes/strong religious beliefs (Catholicism)<br>– children with mental health issues may be seen as dangerous and unpredictable |
| — | Japanese | – seeking mental help may mean alienation and feelings of loneliness<br>– influenced by Shinto, Buddhist, and Confucian philosophies<br>– introspection is preferred |
| — | Korean | – influenced by Confucian, Buddhist, and Taoist philosophies<br>– "non-doing" may influence individual to wait it out and let nature take its course |
| — | Southeast Asian (Cambodian, Hmong, Laotian, Vietnamese) | – family is the primary social unit<br>– inferiority of women<br>– Buddhist ideas of fatalism and karma<br>– refugee status |

2006). Children and adolescents with mental distress will push individual needs aside for the better of the family (Hwang and Myers 2007).

## Filipino

Filipinos are family oriented and believe in *pakikisama* (conceding to the wishes of the collective), *hiya* (roughly translated as shame, shyness,

hesitation, or reluctance), and *amor propio* (sensitivity to criticism). Filipinos also have a fatalistic attitude and a strong sense of religion. Deep
religious faith often turns them toward alternative forms of healing, and,
although children with mental health issues are sometimes viewed as
bringers of good luck, they are also thought to be dangerous and unpre-
dictable (Sanchez and Gaw 2007). These cultural concepts can impede
treatment-seeking behaviors.

## Japanese

Japanese value an unofficial social network and may avoid seeking
professional help because it may signify that they are alone and alienated
in their own community. Japanese society is deeply influenced by Shinto,
Buddhist, and Confucian philosophies. They respect introspection and
mediation to gain insight about mental problems and tend to not
exchange ideas or problem solve using Western logic (Kozuki and
Kennedy 2004).

## Korean

Korean culture has adopted some Western values but is also influenced
by Confucian values in addition to Buddhism and Taoism. Confucian
values have instilled the notion of personal responsibility for behavior
and the need to control behavior for the sake of the group. The Taoist idea
of "non-doing" also influences the individual to wait and let nature and
time take its course (Park and Bernstein 2008).

## Southeast Asian

Southeast Asian American families, such as those with Cambodian,
Hmong, Laotian, and Vietnamese heritage, share some similar qualities
as the Asian American groups mentioned above, such as family being
the primary social unit, inferiority of women, and Buddhist ideas of
fatalism and karma. However, an important factor unique to Southeast
Asian American families is refugee status (Hsu et al. 2004). Whereas the
majority of other Asian Americans immigrate to the United States by
choice, some Southeast Asian American refugees were forced out of
their countries of origin, and children were sometimes separated from the
larger family unit. The Hmong and Laotian, in particular, have historically less Western influence in their homeland and are rooted in tribal,
agrarian, and preliterate societies (Hsu et al. 2004). In the United States,
Southeast Asian American communities remain among the poorest
(Ho 2008). Negative life events experienced in their homeland during
times of war and negative life events living in refugee camps and in
mainstream America have severe consequences for psychological health
(Ho 2008).

Although it is important to take the above cultural descriptions into consideration, it is imperative to assess to what extent an individual or family adheres to their traditional cultural values in order to avoid stereotyping.

## Somatization

Somatization is a common result of mental distress or depression found among several different Asian American populations (Chen et al. 1998; Conrad and Pacquiao 2005; Willgerodt and Thompson 2006). When comparing Chinese middle school students to non-Hispanic white middle school students, somatic-retarded activity, such as insomnia and lack of concentration, better discriminated depression severity of the Chinese group, whereas energy loss and guilt were better discriminates of depression among the white students (Chen et al. 1998). In Houston, Texas, Korean adolescents were found to have higher DSM Scale for Depression (DSD) scores and scores regarding loneliness and somatic symptoms. In addition, foreign-born Korean adolescents had significantly more somatic symptoms than those born in the United States (Choi et al. 2002). Willgerodt and Thompson found that third-generation Chinese adolescents showed less somatic symptoms than Filipinos and non-Hispanic whites but more than first- or second-generation Chinese adolescents (2006). Being Filipino, however, was significantly associated with higher depression and delinquency scores. These mixed results suggest that although somatization is common among Asian Americans, variability among subgroups and individuals exist.

## Acculturation

Acculturation is the process of adopting values, languages, and norms of the dominant group in a society (Mossakowski 2003). Levels of acculturation can be positively correlated with mental health status in which the individual successfully adapts and becomes a member of mainstream society (Shen and Takeuchi 2001). It can also have a negative effect in which acculturation may cause a greater sense of struggle and psychological stress when an individual strives to maintain a balance between two cultures. A third possibility is one of active struggle, in which those that are in between, or halfway through the acculturation process, may be at greatest risk for mental distress (Shen and Takeuchi 2001).

For children and adolescents, the myriad of issues that must be dealt with after reaching the United States can be overwhelming. Dealing with issues of discrimination, language, cultural adjustments, and culture shock regarding the idea of self can be difficult. Asian Americans have the added pressure of the model minority stereotype. In addition, because children often adapt to a new culture at a faster rate than their parents, intergenerational strain may frustrate the process (Ahmed and Lemkau 2000). As the children strive to blend into their new surroundings, their parents may strive to retain and preserve native cultural values. Acculturative processes can also be affected by ethnic identity (Mossakowski 2003) and bicultural orientation (Ho 2008). For example, among Cambodian and Vietnamese youth, those with higher bicultural orientation had lower self-reported externalizing aggression (Ho 2008).

## Adolescent Health Risk Behaviors

Whether adolescents from immigrant and ethnic minority families will make a successful transition to adulthood depends on their educational achievement, their acquisition of employable skills and abilities, and their physical and mental health. In general, immigrant youth appear to be healthier and are less likely to engage in high-risk behaviors compared with non-Hispanic white youth. For Asian Americans in aggregate, this appears to hold true, but it is important to note that, when the data are disaggregated, certain API subgroups are more likely to engage in high-risk behaviors and thus do not conform to the model minority myth.

## Tobacco, Alcohol, and Substance Abuse

Substance abuse is a major public health concern in the United States. Substance abuse costs the United States more than $484 billion dollars per year (NIDA 2008). This is more than the costs of diabetes and cancer combined. Adolescents are highly vulnerable to substance use and abuse. Given that many minority youth are also at increased risk, it is important to understand the patterns of use among all ethnicities, including Asian American adolescents. Table 27.11 summarizes the major available data concerning substance use in Asian American children.

## Smoking Prevalence

When compared to other ethnic groups, APIs in aggregate have lower smoking rates, except for African Americans, who show similar or slightly lower smoking rates (Chen and Unger 1999; Chen et al. 1999; Grunbaum et al. 2000). Studies examining smoking prevalence rates among Asian American subgroups reveal mixed findings, except for two common trends among Chinese and Filipino youth. Chinese Americans almost consistently have the lowest smoking rates compared to other Asian American subgroups, while Filipino adolescents tend to have the highest rates (Chen and Unger 1999; Chen et al. 1999; Wong et al. 2004; Price et al. 2002). Age of smoking onset was found to be earlier among "Other" Asian Americans (12.4 years), and later among Japanese (14 years), with Chinese (13 years), Filipino (13.1 years), and Koreans (13.1 years)

**Table 27.11** Substance Abuse

| Author (Year) | Data Source/ Age or Grade of Population | Measurement | Ethnicity | Male | Female | Combined |
|---|---|---|---|---|---|---|
| Chen (1999) | 1990–1991, 1992, and 1993 California Tobacco Survey, 1994, 1995, and 1996 California Youth Tobacco Surveys/12–17 years | Lifetime smoking prevalence (%) *(p < .01 Asian< NWH) **(p < .05 Chinese lowest among Asian American subgroups) ***(p < .05 Filipino highest among Asian American subgroups) ****(p < .05 within ethnicity gender difference) | **Asian** **non-Hispanic white** **Chinese** **Filipino** **Japanese** **Korean** **Other Asian** | — 29.8 13.4 19.0 14.3**** 18.8 13.1**** | — 28.5 8.3**** 18.9 18.6 15.9**** 19.3 | 16.1* 29.2 11.0** 18.9*** 17.3 16.3 13.7 |

**Table 27.11** (*Continued*)

| Author (Year) | Data Source/ Age or Grade of Population | Measurement | Ethnicity | Male | Female | Combined |
|---|---|---|---|---|---|---|
| Wong (2004) | 1998 California Healthy Kids Survey (CHKS)/ Grades 7, 9, 11 1998 Hawaii Student Alcohol and Other Drug Use Survey (HSAD)/Grades 6, 8, 10, 12 | Lifetime usage rates (%) CHKS (Grade 9)/ HSAD (Grade 10) | | | | **CHKS** **HSAD** |
| | | | **Chinese** | | | |
| | | | Alcohol | | | 37.4    54.9 |
| | | | Cigarettes | | | 21.2    33.8 |
| | | | Marijuana | | | 6.4    15.4 |
| | | | Cocaine | | | 3.0    3.1 |
| | | | Meth-amphetamine | | | 3.1    2.2 |
| | | | **Filipino** | | | |
| | | | Alcohol | | | 56.9    73.5 |
| | | | Cigarettes | | | 44.8    64.8 |
| | | | Marijuana | | | 18.5    35.4 |
| | | | Cocaine | | | 3.3    4.2 |
| | | | Meth-amphetamine | | | 4.1    6.7 |

**Japanese**

| | | |
|---|---|---|
| Alcohol | 46.8 | 63.8 |
| Cigarettes | 29.3 | 44.7 |
| Marijuana | 14.4 | 27.6 |
| Cocaine | 2.7 | 2.7 |
| Meth-amphetamine | 3.2 | 3.8 |

**White**

| | | |
|---|---|---|
| Alcohol | 62.7 | 76.0 |
| Cigarettes | 43.9 | 58.9 |
| Marijuana | 26.5 | 45.8 |
| Cocaine | 4.2 | 6.7 |
| Meth-amphetamine | 5.4 | 7.0 |

Price (2002)

Add Health Wave I-1995/Grades 7–12

Lifetime rates of substance use (%)

**Chinese**

| | |
|---|---|
| Drank (2–3 times ever) | 41.1 |
| Smoked cigarettes (past year) | 21.7 |
| Marijuana (ever) | 19.3 |
| Other illicit (ever) | 7.6 |

**Filipino**

| | |
|---|---|
| Drank (2–3 times ever) | 52.7 |
| Smoked cigarettes (past year) | 36.0 |
| Marijuana (ever) | 28.6 |
| Other illicit (ever) | 6.4 |

**Table 27.11** *(Continued)*

| Author (Year) | Data Source/ Age or Grade of Population | Measurement | Ethnicity | Male | Female | Combined |
|---|---|---|---|---|---|---|
| | | | **Japanese** | | | |
| | | | Drank (2–3 times ever) | | | 56.4 |
| | | | Smoked cigarettes (past year) | | | 36.0 |
| | | | Marijuana (ever) | | | 31.6 |
| | | | Other illicit (ever) | | | 12.0 |
| | | | **Korean** | | | |
| | | | Drank (2–3 times ever) | | | 48.0 |
| | | | Smoked cigarettes (past year) | | | 31.6 |
| | | | Marijuana (ever) | | | 11.1 |
| | | | Other illicit (ever) | | | 2.6 |
| | | | **Vietnamese** | | | |
| | | | Drank (2–3 times ever) | | | 35.8 |
| | | | Smoked cigarettes (past year) | | | 23.4 |
| | | | Marijuana (ever) | | | 4.7 |
| | | | Other illicit (ever) | | | 2.2 |

| | | | |
|---|---|---|---|
| Kim (2006) | 2000–2001 **California Healthy Kids Survey (CHKS)** 2000–2001 **California Basic Educational Data System (CBEDS)/ Grades 7, 9, 11** | | |
| | Individual- and school-level predictors of tobacco and alcohol use for Asian American adolescents | | |
| | Relative risk ratios (RRR) and confidence intervals (CI) | | |
| | | **White** | |
| | | Drank (2–3 times ever) | 58.1 |
| | | Smoked cigarettes (past year) | 39.1 |
| | | Marijuana (ever) | 25.9 |
| | | Other illicit (ever) | 9.4 |
| | | **Asian** | |
| | | 1.22 (1.15,1.30) | reference |
| | Risk behaviors (%) | **Asian** | |
| | | 30-day smoking | 9.2** | 6.1 |
| | | 30-day drinking | 14.0** | 11.8 |
| | | Depressiveness | 27.1** | 29.7 |
| | | **PI** | |
| | | 30-day smoking | 18.0 | 16.2 |
| | | 30-day drinking | 26.3 | 26.2 |
| | | Depressiveness | 31.6 | 42.2 |

Significance of differences between Asians and Pacific Islanders (gender-combined) based on a $\chi 2$-test.
** $p < 0.001$.

**Table 27.11** (Continued)

| Author or (Year) | Data Source/ Age or Grade of Population | Measurement | Ethnicity | Male | Female | Combined |
|---|---|---|---|---|---|---|
| Hahm (2003) | Add Health (Wave II-1996 and Wave II-1996)/ Grades 7–12 | Alcohol use adjusting for parental attachment as a continuous scale (Adjusted odds ratio (95% CI) ** $p < 0.01$. | **Asian** | | | |
| | | | English, U.S.-born | | | 3.17** |
| | | | | | | (1.34–7.43) |
| | | | English, foreign-born | | | 1.82 |
| | | | | | | (.67–.98) |
| | | | No English, U.S.-born | | | .53 |
| | | | | | | (.22–2.34) |
| | | | No English, foreign-born | | | Reference |
| | | | Group 1,* parental attachment | | | .85 |
| | | | | | | (.77–.94)** |
| | | | Group 2,* parental attachment | | | .91 |
| | | | | | | (.81–1.04) |
| | | | Group 3,* parental attachment | | | .91 |
| | | | | | | (.75–1.09) |

**Hahm (2003)**

National Youth Risk Behavior Survey 1991, 1993, 1995, and 1997 (Centers for Disease Control and Prevention)/Grades 9–12

Prevalence of tobacco, alcohol, marijuana, and cocaine use by gender and race/ethnicity, youth risk Behavior surveys, 1991–1997

| **AAPI** | | | |
|---|---|---|---|
| Current cigarette use | 21.8 | 18.1 | 20.2 |
| Current alcohol use | 27.6 | 24.5 | 26.3 |
| Current marijuana | 12.0 | 6.5 | 9.6 |
| Current cocaine use | 2.7 | 1.6 | 2.1 |
| **non-Hispanic whites** | | | |
| Current cigarette use | 34.8 | 36.5 | 35.6 |
| Current alcohol use | 53.9 | 50.9 | 52.5 |
| Current marijuana use | 22.8 | 17.4 | 20.3 |
| Current cocaine use | 2.9 | 1.5 | 2.3 |

**Table 27.11** *(Continued)*

| Author or (Year) | Data Source/ Age or Grade of Population | Measurement | Ethnicity | Male | Female | Combined |
|---|---|---|---|---|---|---|
| Wallace (2002) | Monitoring the Future Study (University of Michigan 1996–1998/ Grade 12) | Annual prevalence of selected drugs (past 12 months) | **Asian** | | | |
| | | | Alcohol | | | 57.0 |
| | | | Marijuana | | | 21.7 |
| | | | Cocaine | | | 2.8 |
| | | | Any illicit | | | 24.5 |
| | | | **non-Hispanic white** | | | |
| | | | Alcohol | | | 77.1 |
| | | | Marijuana | | | 38.6 |
| | | | Cocaine | | | 5.9 |
| | | | Any illicit | | | 42.8 |

falling in between (Chen et al. 1999). The hazard of smoking (the rate of smoking initiation at any given age) before the age of twelve was highest among Filipino youth and lowest among Chinese youth, until the age of fourteen, when Korean and Japanese youth had the highest hazard of smoking (Chen and Unger 1999). APIs initiate regular smoking later in life with a peak at ages eighteen to twenty-one years, compared to a peak for non-Hispanic whites from fourteen to seventeen years (Trinidad et al. 2004). Therefore, smoking prevention efforts should focus on young adolescent Asian Americans.

Smoking prevalence also varies according to gender. Kim and McCarthy found that Asian American males show significantly higher thirty-day smoking prevalence rates (9.2) compared to Asian American females (6.1; $p < .001$) (2006). However, among Asian American subgroups, this does not always hold. Chen et al. found that Chinese and Korean adolescents' smoking prevalence rates have been found to be significantly higher among males compared to females, but for Japanese and "Other" Asians, smoking prevalence rates were higher among female youth (1999). Filipino gender smoking prevalence was similar for males and females.

## Alcohol Use and Substance Abuse

Among Asian Americans, acculturation has been associated with alcohol consumption. Asian American adolescents with the highest level of acculturation (English use at home, born in the United States) were identified as the group at highest risk for alcohol consumption (Hahm et al. 2003). However, after adjusting for parental attachment, highly acculturated adolescents with moderate or high parental attachment had no greater risk than adolescents with the same levels of parental attachment who were less acculturated. In fact, for every unit increase in parental attachment, those who were born in the United States and spoke English at home, the odds reduced by a factor of .85 (Hahm et al. 2003). This suggests that interventions fostering parental attachment may play a role in preventing adolescent substance use among Asian Americans.

Numerous studies aggregating Asian Americans and APIs find that Asian Americans are less likely to report alcohol use. Grunbaum et al. reported that API youth were significantly less likely to be current alcohol users and current episodic heavy drinkers (≥ 5 alcoholic drinks on ≥ 1 occasion within the past thirty days) compared to non-Hispanic whites (2000). Annual prevalence data for high school seniors from 1996 to 2000 showed that Asian Americans had lower rates of alcohol consumption rates within the past year compared to non-Hispanic whites (Wallace et al. 2002). Wong et al. showed similar results among California and Hawaii youth, with Asian Americans overall reporting lower lifetime alcohol consumption rates (2004). When compared with Pacific Islanders or Hawaiian Natives, Asian

Americans also have lower alcohol consumption rates (Wong et al. 2004; Kim and McCarthy 2006).

However, certain subgroups are at increased risk for alcohol abuse. For example, Price et al. reported that Vietnamese (35.8%), Chinese (41.1%), and Korean (48%) adolescents were significantly less likely than Japanese (56.4%) and Filipinos (52.7%) to report drinking during their lifetime (two to three alcoholic drinks, ever) (2002). Wong et al. reported lifetime percentage rates of alcohol consumption to be highest among Filipino adolescents, followed by Japanese and Chinese in both California and in Hawaii (2004).

Asian Americans and APIs as a whole report using marijuana and other illicit drugs less than non-Hispanic whites, excluding cocaine (Grunbaum et al. 2000; Price et al. 2002; Wallace et al. 2002). However, among Asian American subgroups, Japanese adolescents have higher usage rates of some illicit drugs compared to other Asian American groups and non-Hispanic whites although their rates of using inhalants were similar to Chinese; cocaine usage was higher among Filipinos; and Koreans and Vietnamese use significantly less marijuana and cocaine than Japanese adolescents (Price et al. 2002). Filipinos have substance use rates that more closely reflect those of non-Hispanic whites (see Table 27.11) (Javier et al. 2007).

Asian American adolescents of mixed heritage show higher substance abuse rates (alcohol, smoking, and illicit drugs) compared to non-mixed heritage adolescents, with the greatest differences found among Chinese and Vietnamese adolescents (Price et al. 2002). Mixed-heritage Chinese and Vietnamese adolescents were 4.3 times as likely and 3.8 times as likely, respectively, to use substances compared to non-mixed Chinese and Vietnamese counterparts. Asian American adolescents who are older and depressed are at increased risk for substance use, including alcohol (Kim and McCarthy 2006). It is possible that being of mixed heritage poses more complicated family dynamics and thus may put these adolescents at greater risk for substance abuse.

## STDS AND SEXUAL ACTIVITY

### Prevalence of STDs

Data from the National Longitudinal Study of Adolescent Health is commonly used to assess the prevalence and risk factors of sexually transmitted diseases and sexual behaviors. Between 1995 and 1996 all races reported a higher percentage of STDs (p < 0.001), except for Asian Americans (Crosby et al. 2002). This study did not disaggregate Asian American subgroups.

AIDS surveillance data for APIs from 1983 (the earliest AIDS case report among APIs) and 1998 revealed that the forty-six child cases resulted from perinatal exposure to HIV (66%) or in the exposure categories of transfusion or hemophilia/coagulation disorder (28%). The majority of the thirty adolescents cases (aged thirteen to nineteen years) also reported exposure due to either transfusion or hemophilia/coagulation disorder category (63%) (Wortley et al. 2002). Surveillance data from 1985 to 2002 for HIV/AIDS (adults, adolescents, and children) reported that 39.6 percent of APIs who received diagnoses of AIDS were born in the United States, 16 percent were born in the Philippines, 6.9 percent were born in Vietnam, and 4.9 percent were born in India, with lower percentages from other countries. Rates among APIs increased slightly from 1999 to 2002 from 3.2 percent to 3.8 percent, with similar trends among African Americans and American Indian/Alaska Natives (Zaidi et al. 2005).

### Sexual Behavior and Risk Factors

Asian American youth typically report lower prevalence rates of sexual activity. In Los Angeles County, among students enrolled in grades nine through twelve, API students (73%) were more likely to report virginity, compared to all other ethnic groups (Schuster et al. 1998). API adolescents also reported having less participation in almost all other genital sexual activities, with no differences between gender (see Table 27.12).

While the above studies show that Asian Americans are less likely to be sexually active, the following studies reveal that risk factors for contracting STDs are no less than those of non-Hispanic whites. According to the 1991 National School Based Youth Behavior Survey, among those currently sexually active, API students were more likely to have multiple sex partners within the past three months compared to non-Hispanic whites (P = .002) (Hou and Basen-Engquist 1997). This suggests that API students are not at lower risk for exposure to sexually transmitted diseases. Two separate studies conducted in San Francisco, California, found that Asian American adolescents and young adult females used no method of contraception more than non-Hispanic white adolescents (14% versus 9%), and when contraception was used barrier methods (condoms) were more

**Table 27.12** Sexual Risk Behavior—Key Point Summary

---
- Currently sexually active API students may be more likely than non-Hispanic whites to have multiple partners
- Asian American female adolescents are more likely than non-Hispanic white females to use no method of contraception
- Foreign-born youth who speak English at home have the highest rates of sexual activity
- Asian youth are less likely to discuss AIDS/HIV with their parents
- The cultural gap between parents and youth may impede discussion about sexually related topics
---

common than hormonal alternatives (i.e., oral or injectable) (Raine et al. 2002, 2003).

Acculturation and age may play a role in sexual behavior for Asian Americans. Asian Americans who were foreign born and who spoke English at home had the highest rates of sexual intercourse (36.7% female, 34.3% male) compared to those who were born in the United States and spoke English at home (most acculturated; 30.5% females, 18.1% males), those born outside of the United States and spoke no English at home (least acculturated; 14.8% female, 18.7% male), and those born in the United States and spoke no English at home (10% female, 7.7% male) (Hahm et al. 2006). A needs assessment conducted by the Orange County API HIV Task Force in 1992 revealed that among API male and female youth (aged fifteen to twenty-four years), younger respondents were most confident communicating about safe sex (65% very sure) and least confident about refusing sex with someone they knew well (55% very sure). Overall, those who were female and more acculturated were 2.78 times more likely to be sure that they could refuse sex with someone they knew well (Takahashi et al. 2006). These findings suggesting that further studies need to explore acculturation and sexual behavior in Asian Americans.

Parental influence also appears to play a large role in sexual behavior for Asian Americans. API adolescents are more likely to report that their mothers and fathers would disapprove if they had vaginal intercourse, compared to all other ethnic groups (Schuster et al. 1998), and are less likely to discuss AIDS/HIV with their parents compared to non-Hispanic white counterparts (Hou and Basen-Engquist 1997). This suggests parental expectations and parental communication about sex may play a role in sexual behavior and related risk factors. For example, Chung et al. found that acculturation (measured by disagreement with traditional Asian American values and preferential use of English) influences Filipino parent-adolescent communication about sex and thus can affect Filipino adolescent sexual health (2007). Interventions addressing this gap in communication to address teen pregnancy prevention have been developed using community-based participatory research methods (Javier et al. 2006b).

## CONCLUSION

Three overarching themes emerge from this chapter. First, data collection is needed to monitor the health status of Asian American children. As mentioned in multiple examples throughout this chapter, aggregating Asian Americans into one group masks key variations within subgroups. National datasets and states datasets should include detailed information on subgroups, especially in states that are home to large Asian American populations. Data then should be analyzed to document disparities in child health among specific Asian American subgroups. For example, Javier and Mendoza completed a review of the literature that summarized and identified health and health-care disparities in Filipino children in the United States (2007b).

Next, given the diversity of the Asian American child population, health providers serving these children need to be culturally sensitive to the beliefs of an individual patient and his or her family. This requires knowledge of cultural factors that may be present in particular subgroups and the ability to elicit individual patient and family beliefs in order to avoid assuming and stereotyping. The current focus on culturally competent health care will require policy makers at every level to commit to serving the needs of culturally diverse populations.

Finally, more research is needed to improve our knowledge about Asian American children in the United States. Specifically, more research is needed in the above topics discussed, in addition to other topics that were not covered (i.e., behavioral and developmental disabilities, use of alternative therapies in the API population, access and quality of care for Asian American subgroups, injury and prevention, oral health, gay and lesbian youth, etc). Research from a multidisciplinary approach with ongoing input from the community will best serve the needs of Asian American children and their families. Addressing these three arenas through policy changes and culturally appropriate interventions will improve the quality of life for Asian American children in the United States.

## REFERENCES

Adair, L.S. and B.M. Popkin. Are child eating patterns being transformed globally? *Obes Res* 2005. 13(7): 1281–1299.

Agency for Healthcare Research and Quality. 2007 National Healthcare Disparities Report. Rockville, MD. U.S. Department of Health and Human Services, Agency for Healthcare Research and Quality; February 2008, AHRQ Pub. No. 08-0041.

Ahmed, S.M. and J.P. Lemkau, Cultural issues in the primary care of South Asians. 2000. 2(2). *Journal of Immigrant Health.*

Allen, M.L., et al., Adolescent participation in preventive health behaviors, physical activity, and nutrition: differences across immigrant generations for Asians and Latinos compared with whites. *American Journal of Public Health* 2007. 97(2): 337–343.

APIOPA. Alliance *Obesity among Asians & Pacific Islanders: Fact Sheet.* 2005. Asian Pacific Islander Obesity Prevention. Little Tokyo, Los Angeles, CA.

Baker, L.C., et al. Differences in neonatal mortality among whites and Asian American subgroups: evidence from California. *Archives of Pediatric & Adolescent Medicine* 2007. 161(1): 69–76.

Barbes, C., et al. Appropriate body-mass index for Asian populations and its implications for policy and intervention strategies. *The Lancet* 2004. 363.

Bates, L.M., et al. Immigration and generational trends in body mass index and obesity in the United States: results of the National Latino and Asian American Survey, 2002–2003. *American Journal of Public Health* 2008. 98(1): 70–77.

Beets, M.W. and K.H. Pitetti. One-mile run/walk and body mass index of an ethnically diverse sample of youth. *Medicine and Science in Sports and Exercise* 2004. 36(10): 1796–1803.

Boneva, R.S., et al. Mortality associated with congenital heart defects in the United States: Trends and racial disparities, 1979–1997. 2001. 2376–2381.

Brahan, D. and H. Bauchner. Changes in reporting of race/ethnicity, socioeconomic status, gender, and age over 10 years. *Pediatrics* 2005. 115(2): e163–166.

Bronner, Y.L. Nutritional status outcomes for children: ethnic, cultural, and environmental contexts. *Journal of the American Dietetics Association* 1996. 96(9): 891–903.

Brown, E.R. et al. Community-based participatory research in the California Health Interview Survey. *Prevention of Chronic Disease.* 2005 Oct; 2(4): A03. Epub 2005 Sep 15.

Bui, K.V. and D.T. Takeuchi. Ethnic minority adolescents and the use of community mental health care services. *American Journal of Community Psychology* 1992. 20(4): 403–417.

Calmes, D., Leake B.D., and C. D.M, Adverse asthma outcomes among children hospitalized with asthma in California. *Pediatrics* 1998 101(5): 845–850.

Centers for Disease Control and Prevention. Hepatitis B vaccination coverage among Asian and Pacific Islander children: United States, 1998. *MMWR Morbidity and Mortality Weekly Report* 2000. 49: 616–619.

Centers for Disease Control and Prevention. Vaccination coverage by race/ethnicity and poverty level among children aged 19–35 months: United States 1997. *MMWR Morbidity and Mortality Weekly Report* 1998. 47: 956–959.

Chabra, A., G.F. Chavez, and E.S. Harris. Mental illness in elementary-school-aged children. *The Western Journal of Medicine* 1999. 170(1): 28–34.

Chang, R.-K.R., A.Y. Chen, and T.S. Klitzner. Factors associated with age at operation for children with congenital heart disease. *Pediatrics* 2000. 105(5): 1073–1081.

Chen, C., Stevenson, H.W. Motivation and mathematics achievement: A comparative study of Asian-American, Caucasian-American, and East Asian high school students. *Child Development* 1995. 66: 1215–1234.

Chen, I.G., R.E. Roberts, and L.A. Aday. Ethnicity and adolescent depression: the case of Chinese Americans. *The Journal of Nervous and Mental Disease.* 1998. 186(10).

Chen, X. and J.B. Unger. Hazards of smoking initiation among Asian American and non-Asian adolescents in California: a survival model analysis. *Preventive Medicine.* 1999. 28(6).

Chen, X., et al. Smoking patterns of Asian-American youth in California and their relationship with acculturation. *The Journal of Adolescent Health* 1999. 24(5).

Choi, H. Understanding adolescent depression in ethnocultural context. *ANS Advances In Nursing Science* 2002. 25(2): 71–85.

Choi, H., et al. Psychometric properties of the DSM scale for depression (DSD) with Korean-American youths. *Issues in Mental Health Nursing* 2002. 23(8): 735–756.

Chow, J.C., K. Jaffee, and L. Snowden. Racial/ethnic disparities in the use of mental health services in poverty areas. *American Journal of Public Health.* 2003. 93(5).

Chung, P.J., Travis, R. Jr, Kilpatrick S.A., Elliott M.N., Lui C., Schuster M.A. Acculturation and parent-adolescent communication about sex in Filipino-American families: a community-based participatory research study. *The Journal of Adolescent Health* 2007. 40(6): 543–550.

Coll, C.G. and Szalacha L.A. Children of Immigrant Families: The Multiple Contexts of Middle Childhood. *The Future of Children* 2004. 14(2): 81–97.

Committee to Study the Prevention of Low Birthweight. Preventing low birthweight. National Academy Press, Editor. 1985, National Academy of Sciences: Washington, DC.

Conrad, M.M. and D.F. Pacquiao, Manifestation, attribution, and coping with depression among Asian Indians from the perspectives of health care practitioners. *Journal of Transcultural Nursing* 2005. 16(1): 32–40.

Crosby, R., J.S. Leichliter, and R. Brackbill. Longitudinal prediction of sexually transmitted diseases among adolescents: results from a national survey. *American Journal Preventive Medicine* 2000. 18(4): 312–317.

Daida, Y., et al. Ethnicity and nutrition of adolescent girls in Hawaii. *Journal of the American Dietetics Association* 2006. 106(2): 221–226.

Davis, A.M., et al. Asthma prevalence in Hispanic and Asian American ethnic subgroups: results from the California Healthy Kids Survey. *Pediatrics* 2006. 118(2).

Edman, J.L., et al. Factor structure of the CES-D (Center for Epidemiologic Studies Depression Scale) among Filipino-American adolescents. *Social Psychiatry and Psychiatric Epidemiology* 1999. 34(4): 211–215.

Edman, J.L., et al. Depressive symptoms among Filipino American adolescents. *Cultural Diversity and Mental Health* 1998. 4(1): 45–54.

Flores, G.L., et al. Errors in medical interpretation and their potential clinical consequences in pediatric encounters. *Pediatrics* 2003. 111(1): 6–14.

Fuentes-Afflick, E. Obesity among Latino Preschoolers: Do Children Outgrow the "Epidemiologic Paradox"? *Archives of Pediatric & Adolescent Medicine 2006.* 160(6): 656–657.

Fuentes-Afflick, E. and N.A. Hessol. Impact of Asian ethnicity and national origin on infant birth weight. *American Journal of Epidemiology* 1997. 145(2).

Fuler GL. The epidemiology of hepatitis B vaccination catch-up among AAPI children in the United States. *Asian American Pacific Islander Journal of Health.* 2001. 9(2):154-61

Garland, A.F., et al. Racial and ethnic differences in utilization of mental health services among high-risk youths. *American Journal of Psychiatry* 2005. 162(7): 1336–1343.

Giammattei, J., et al. Television watching and soft drink consumption: associations with obesity in 11- to 13-year-old schoolchildren. *Archives of Pediatric & Adolescent Medicine* 2003. 157(9): 882–886.

Gordon-Larsen, P., et al. Five-year obesity incidence in the transition period between adolescence and adulthood: the National Longitudinal Study of Adolescent Health. *The American Journal of Clinical Nutrition* 2004. 80(3).

Gordon-Larsen, P., L.S. Adair, and B.M. Popkin, The relationship of ethnicity, socioeconomic factors, and overweight in US adolescents. Obesity Research 2003. 11(1): 121–129. *The Health of Asian American Children in the United States* 495

Gordon-Larsen, P., L.S. Adair, and B.M. Popkin. Ethnic differences in physical activity and inactivity patterns and overweight status. *Obesity Research* 2002. 10(3): 141–149.

Gordon-Larsen, P., R.G. McMurray, and B.M. Popkin, Adolescent physical activity and inactivity vary by ethnicity: The National Longitudinal Study of Adolescent Health. *The Journal of Pediatrics* 1999. 135(3): 301–306.

Grunbaum, J.A., et al. Prevalence of health risk behaviors among Asian American/Pacific Islander high school students. *The Journal of Adolescent Health* 2000. 27(5).

Guagliardo, M.F., et al. Racial and ethnic disparities in pediatric appendicitis rupture rate. *Acad Emerg Med* 2003. 10(11): 1218–1227.

Guendelman, S., et al. Birth outcomes of immigrant women in the United States, France, and Belgium. *Maternal and Child Health Journal* 1999. 3(4): 177–187.

Hahm, H.C., M. Lahiff, and R.M. Barreto. Asian American adolescents' first sexual intercourse: gender and acculturation differences. *Perspectives on Sexual and Reproductive Health [erratum Perspect Sex Reprod Health.* 2006 Jun; 38(2): 75] 2006. 38(1).

Hahm, H.C., M. Lahiff, and N.B. Guterman, Acculturation and parental attachment in Asian-American adolescents' alcohol use. *The Journal of Adolescent Health* 2003. 33(2): 119–129.

Harris, K.M. The health status and risk behaviors of adolescents in immigrant families in children of immigrants. In *Children of immigrants: Health, adjustment, and public assistance*, Hernandez D.J., Editor. 1999, National Academy Press: Washington DC.

Harris, K.M., et al. Longitudinal trends in race/ethnic disparities in leading health indicators from adolescence to young adulthood. *Archives of Pediatric & Adolescent Medicine* 2006. 160(1): 74–81.

Hastert, T.A., et al. More California teens consume soda and fast food each day than five servings of fruits and vegetables. Policy Brief UCLA Cent Health Policy Res, 2005(PB2005-8): 1–7.

Hernandez, D.J., Denton, N.S., Macartney S.E. Indicators of Characteristics and Circumstances of Children Ages 0-17 in Immigrant Families by Country of Origin and in Native-Born Families by Race-Ethnicity based on Census 2000. Downloaded from www.albany.edu/csda/children on March 10, 2008. 2007a [cited].

Hernandez, D.J., Denton, N.S., Macartney S.E. Children in Immigrant Families-The U.S. and 50 States: National Origins, Language, and Early Education, in Children in America's Newcomer Families: Child Trends and the Center for Social and Demographic Analysis. *2007 Research Brief Series.* University at Albany, SUNY. 2007b.

Hernandez, D.J., Denton, N.S., Macartney S.E. Family circumstances of children in immigrant families. In *Immigrant Families in Contemporary Society,* Lansford J.E., Deater-Deckard K, and Bornstein M.H., Editors. 2007c, Guilford Press: New York, NY. 9–29.

Ho, J., Community violence exposure of Southeast Asian American adolescents. *Journal of Interpersonal Violence* 2008. 23(1): 136–146.

Hou, S.I. and K. Basen-Engquist, Human immunodeficiency virus risk behavior among white and Asian/Pacific Islander high school students in the United

Hsu, E., C.A. Davies, and D.J. Hansen. Understanding mental health needs of Southeast Asian refugees: historical, cultural, and contextual challenges. *Clinical Psychology Review* 2004. 24(2): 193–213.

Hwang, W.C. and H.F. Myers. Major depression in Chinese Americans: the roles of stress, vulnerability, and acculturation. *Social Psychiatry and Psychiatric Epidemiology* 2007. 42(3).

Jablonski, K.A. and Guagliardo M.F. Pediatric appendicitis rupture rate: a national indicator of disparities in healthcare access. *Population Health Metrics* 2005. 3(1): 4.

Javier, J.R., Wise, P.H., Mendoza F.S. The relationship of immigrant status with access, utilization, and health status for children with asthma. *Ambulatory Pediatrics* 2007. 7(6): 421–430.

Javier, J.R., L.C. Huffman, and F.S. Mendoza. Filipino child health in the United States: do health and health care disparities exist? *Preventing Chronic Disease* 2007. 4(2): A36.

Javier, J.R., Chamberlain.L., Huffman L., Mendoza F. Letter to the editor (In response to Parent-Adolescent Communication About Sex in Filipino American Families: A Demonstration of Community-Based Participatory Research). *Ambulatory Pediatrics* 2006a. 6(2): 120.

Javier, J.R., et al. Filipino American families and intergenerational communication about sex. *Ambulatory Pediatrics* 2006b. 6(2): 120.

Johnson, C.A., et al. Socio-demographic and cultural comparison of overweight and obesity risk and prevalence in adolescents in Southern California and Wuhan, China. *The Journal of Adolescent Medicine* 2006. 39(6).

Johnson, S.B., et al. Prevalence of overweight in north Florida elementary and middle school children: effects of age, sex, ethnicity, and socioeconomic status. *J Sch Health* 2007. 77(9): 630–636.

Kataoka-Yahiro, M.R., Ceria,C., Yoder M. Grandparent caregiving role in Filipino American families. *Journal of Cultural Diversity* 2004. 11(3): 110–117.

Kim, J. and W.J. McCarthy. School-level contextual influences on smoking and drinking among Asian and Pacific Islander adolescents. *Drug and Alcohol Dependence* 2006. 84(1).

Kozuki, Y. and M.G. Kennedy. Cultural incommensurability in psychodynamic psychotherapy in Western and Japanese traditions. *Journal of Nursing Scholarship*, see Comments in: *J Nurs Scholarsh* 2004; 36(3): 190; author reply 190; PMID: 15495484, 2004. 36(1).

Lai, E., Arguelles D., and eds. *The New Face of Asian Pacific America: Numbers, Diversity, and Change in the 21st Century.* 2003, San Francisco: Asian Week.

Larson, N.I., et al. Food preparation and purchasing roles among adolescents: associations with sociodemographic characteristics and diet quality. *Journal of the American Dietetics Association* 2006. 106(2): 211–218.

Lavarreda, S., B.E., Ponce N. Insurance Rates of Asian American and Pacific Islander Children Vary Widely. 2005, UCLA Center for Health Policy Research: Los Angeles, CA.

Leal, C.C. Stigmatization of Hispanic children, pre-adolescents, and adolescents with mental illness: exploration using a national database. *Issues in Mental Health Nursings* 2005. 26(10): 1025–1041.

Lee, A.C., et al. A comparison of knowledge about asthma between Asians and non-Asians at two pediatric clinics. *Journal Immigrant and Minority Health* 2007. 9(4): 245–254.

Lorenzo, M.K., Frost A.K., and Reinherz H.Z. Social and emotional functioning of older Asian American adolescents. *Child & Adolescent Social Work Journal* 2000. 17: 289–304.

Lu, F.G., et al. A psychiatric residency curriculum about Asian-American issues. *Academic Psychiatry* 2002. 26(4): 225–236.

Madan, A., et al. Racial differences in birth weight of term infants in a northern California population. *Journal of Perinatology* 2002. 22(3): 230–235.

Mangione-Smith, R., et al. Racial/ethnic variation in parent expectations for antibiotics: Implications for public health campaigns. *Pediatrics* 2004. 113(5): e385–394.

Martin, J.A., et al. Births: final data for 2002. *National Vital Statistics Report* 2003. 52(10): 1–113.

Mathews, T.J., Menacker F., and MacDorma M.F. Infant mortality statistics from the 2003 period linked birth/infant death data set (Center for Disease Control) California data from 1991–2001. *NVSR* 2004. 53(10).

Mendoza, F.S., Javier,J.R., Burgos A.E. Health of children in immigrant families. In *Immigrant Families in Contemporary Society*, Lansford J.E., Deater-Deckard K., and Bornstein M.H., Editors. 2007, Guilford Press: New York, NY.

Mendoza, J.A., et al. Dietary energy density is associated with selected predictors of obesity in U.S. children. *The Journal of Nutrition* 2006. 136(5): 1318–1322.

Meng, Y.Y., et al. California's racial and ethnic minorities more adversely affected by asthma. Policy Brief (*UCLA Center for Health Policy Research* 2007(PB2007-3)).

Meurer, J.R., et al. Asthma severity among children hospitalized in 1990 and 1995. *Archives of Pediatric & Adolescent Medicine* 2000. 154(2): 143–149.

Mossakowski, K.N. Coping with perceived discrimination: does ethnic identity protect mental health? *Journal of Health and Social Behavior* 2003. 44(3): 318–331.

Newacheck, P.W. and Halfon N. Prevalence and impact of disabling chronic conditions in childhood. *American Journal of Public Health* 1998. 88(4): 610–617.

NIDA. *Drug and Addiction: One of America's Most Challenging Public Health Problems*. 2008 Jan 2

Novotny, R., et al. Calcium intake of Asian, Hispanic and white youth. *Journal of American College of Nutrition* 2003. 22(1): 64–70.

Ozer, E.J. and K.L. McDonald. Exposure to violence and mental health among Chinese American urban adolescents. *Journal Adolescent Health* 2006. 39(1): 73–79.

Park, S.Y. and K.S. Bernstein. Depression and Korean American immigrants. *Archives of Psychiatric Nursing* 2008. 22(1): 12–19. Table18c, C.M.S.B. California Department of Health Services, Editor.

Phinney, J.S., Ong.A.. Ethnic identity development in immigrant families. In *Immigrant Families in Contemporary Society*, Lansford J.E., Deater-Deckard K., and B. M.H., Editors. 2007, Guilford Press: New York, NY.

Polhamus, B., et al. Pediatric Nutrition Surveillance 2006 Report, C.D.C. U.S. Department of Health and Human Services, Editor. 2007a.

Polhamus, B., et al. Summary of Trends in Growth and Anemia Indicators by Race/Ethnicity. Table18c, in Pediatric Nutrition Surveillance 2006 Report, C.D.C.. U.S. Department of Health and Human Services, Editor. 2007b.

Ponce, N.A., Lavarreda S.A., Yen W., Brown E.R., DiSogra C., Satter D.E., The California Health Interview Survey 2001: translation of a major survey for California's multiethnic population. *Public Health Reports* 2004. 119(4): 388–395.

Popkin, B.M. and J.R. Udry. Adolescent obesity increases significantly in second and third generation U.S. immigrants: the National Longitudinal Study of Adolescent Health. *The Journal of Nutrition* 1998. 128(4): 701–706.

Price, R.K., et al. Substance use and abuse by Asian Americans and Pacific Islanders: preliminary results from four national epidemiologic studies. *Public Health Reports* 2002. 117(Suppl 1).

Raine, T., A.M. Minnis, and N.S. Padian. Determinants of contraceptive method among young women at risk for unintended pregnancy and sexually transmitted infections. *Contraception* 2003. 68(1): 19–25.

Raine, T., et al. Race, adolescent contraceptive choice, and pregnancy at presentation to a family planning clinic. *Obstetrics and Gynecology*. Comment in: *Obstetrics and Gynecology*. 2002 Jul; 100(1): 174; author reply 174–175; PMID: 12100823, 2002. 99(2).

Rappaport, E.B. and J.M. Robbins. Overweight in Southeastern Pennsylvania children: 2002 household health survey data. *Public Health Reports* 2005. 120(5): 525–531.

Reynolds, K.D., et al. Patterns in child and adolescent consumption of fruit and vegetables: effects of gender and ethnicity across four sites. *Journal of the American College of Nutrition* 1999. 18(3): 248–254.

Richardson, L.P., DiGiuseppe, .D., Garrison M., Christakis D.A. Depression in Medicaid-covered youth: Differences by race and ethnicity. *Archives of Pediatric & Adolescent Medicine* 2003. 157(10): 984–989.

Robinson, T.N., Killen, J.D., Litt I.F., Hammer L.D., Wilson D.M., Haydel K.F., Hayward C., Taylor C.B. Ethnicity and body dissatisfaction: are Hispanic and Asian girls at increased risk for eating disorders? *The Journal of Adolescent Health* 1996. 19(6): 384–393.

Ray, G.T., et al. Attention-deficit/hyperactivity disorder in children: excess costs before and after initial diagnosis and treatment cost differences by ethnicity. *Archives of Pediatric & Adolescent Medicine* 2006. 160(10): 1063–1069.

Sanchez, F. and A. Gaw. Mental health care of Filipino Americans. *Psychiatric Services* 2007. 58(6): 810–815.

Schuster, M.A., et al. The sexual practices of Asian and Pacific Islander high school students. *The Journal of Adolescent Health* 1998. 23(4).

Shen, B.J. and D.T. Takeuchi. A structural model of acculturation and mental health status among Chinese Americans. American *Journal of Community Psychology* 2001. 29(3): 387–418.

Smith, S.C., Jr., et al. Discovering the full spectrum of cardiovascular disease: Minority Health Summit 2003: report of the Obesity, Metabolic Syndrome, and Hypertension Writing Group. *Circulation* 2005. 111(10): e134–139.

Snowden, L.R., et al., Racial/ethnic minority children's use of psychiatric emergency care in California's Public Mental Health System. American *Journal of Public Health* 2008. 98(1): 118–124.

Sorof, J.M., et al. Overweight, ethnicity, and the prevalence of hypertension in school-aged children. *Pediatrics* 2004. 113(3 Pt 1): 475–482.

Stettler, N., et al. High prevalence of overweight among pediatric users of community health centers. *Pediatrics* 2005. 116(3): e381–8.

Stevens, G.D. and L. Shi. Racial and ethnic disparities in the primary care experiences of children: A review of the literature. *Medical Care Research and Review* 2003. 60(1): 3–30.

Stoddard, J.J., Back, M.R., and Brotherton, S.E. The respective racial and ethnic diversity of US pediatricians and American children. *Pediatrics* 2000. 105(1): 27–31.

Su, S. Stress and coping as a conceptual framework for studying alcohol and drug use among Asian American adolescents. *Drugs and Society* 1999. 14: 37–56.

Taira, D., Safran D.G., Seto T.B., Rogers W.H., Kosinski M., Ware J.E., Lieberman N., Tarlov A.R. Asian-American patient ratings of physician primary care performance. *Journal of General Internal Medicine* 1997. 12: 237–242.

Takahashi, L.M., et al. HIV and AIDS in suburban Asian and Pacific Islander communities: factors influencing self-efficacy in HIV risk reduction. *AIDS Education Prevention* 2006. 18(6): 529–545.

Thorpe, L.E., et al. Childhood obesity in New York City elementary school students. *American Journal of Public Health* 2004. 94(9).

Trinidad, D.R., et al. Do the majority of Asian-American and African-American smokers start as adults? *American Journal of Preventive Medicine* 2004. 26(2).

Unger, J.B., et al. Acculturation, physical activity, and fast-food consumption among Asian-American and Hispanic adolescents. *Journal of Community Health* 2004. 29(6): 467–481.

U.S. Census Bureau. *We the people: Asians in the United States.* 2004, U.S. Department of Commerce: Washington (DC).

Von Behren, J., R. Kreutzer, and D. Smith. Asthma hospitalization trends in California, 1983–1996. *The Journal of Asthma* 1999. 36(7).

Wallace, J.M., Jr., et al. Tobacco, alcohol, and illicit drug use: racial and ethnic differences among U.S. high school seniors, 1976–2000. *Public Health Reports.* 117(Suppl 1).

Weech-Maldonado, R., Morales, L.S., Spritzer K., Elliott M., Hays R.D. Racial and ethnic differences in parents' assessments of pediatric care in Medicaid managed care. *Health Services Researchs* 2001. 36(3): 575–594.

Weigers, M, Weinick, R., Cohen J. Children's Health, 1996. 1998, *Agency for Healthcare Research and Quality*, US Dept of Health and Human Services Rockville, MD.

Weitz, T., Harper C., and Mohllajee A. Teen pregnancy among Asians and Pacific Islanders in California: final report. 2001, University of California, San Francisco Center for Reproductive Health Research and Policy: San Francisco.

Wiecha, J.M., et al. Differences in dietary patterns of Vietnamese, white, African-American, and Hispanic adolescents in Worcester, Mass. *Journal of the American Dietetics Association* 2001, 101(2): 248–251.

Willgerodt, M.A. and E.A. Thompson. Ethnic and generational influences on emotional distress and risk behaviors among Chinese and Filipino American adolescents. *Research in Nursing Health* 2006. 29(4): 311–324.

Wise, P.H. The transformation of child health in the United States. *Health Affairs* 2004. 23(5): 9–25.

Wolf, A.M., et al. Activity, inactivity, and obesity: racial, ethnic, and age differences among schoolgirls. *American Journal of Public Health* 1993. 83(11): 1625–1627.

Wong, M.M., R.S. Klingle, and R.K. Price. Alcohol, tobacco, and other drug use among Asian American and Pacific Islander Adolescents in California and Hawaii. *Addictive Behaviors* 2004. 29(1).

Wortley, P.M., et al. AIDS among Asians and Pacific Islanders in the United States. *American Journal of Preventive Medicine* 2000. 18(3).

Yeh, M., et al. Racial/ethnic differences in parental endorsement of barriers to mental health services for youth. *Mental Health Services Research* 2003. 5(2): 65–77.

Yu, S.M., et al. Parent's language of interview and access to care for children with special health care needs. *Ambulatory Pediatrics* 2004a. 4(2).

Yu, S.M., Z.J. Huang, and G.K. Singh. Health status and health services utilization among US Chinese, Asian Indian, Filipino, and other sian/Pacific Islander Children. *Pediatrics* 2004b. 113(1 Pt 1).

Zaidi, I.F., et al. Epidemiology of HIV/AIDS among Asians and Pacific Islanders in the United States. *AIDS Education and Prevention* 2005. 17(5).

# Chapter 28

# Asian Pacific American Families and the Child Welfare System

*Wayne Ho*

As the Asian Pacific American population continues to grow and diversify throughout the United States, an increasing number of Asian Pacific American children and families will come into contact with the child welfare system. The goal of the child welfare system is to protect the safety and well-being of children. Similar to other communities, child abuse and neglect do occur in Asian Pacific American families. While Asian Pacific Americans are generally underrepresented in the child welfare system, the challenges faced by Asian Pacific American families in this system are exacerbated because it is not well structured to serve this diverse community. The limited—yet growing—body of research on child welfare issues in the Asian Pacific American community reveals that families from this predominantly immigrant community become unnecessarily caught up in this system because of cultural differences, language barriers, or limited financial resources, not necessarily because of intentional harm to their child. This chapter will provide an overview of the research on Asian Pacific American families and the child welfare system, taking into account the diverse ethnic, cultural, and immigrant backgrounds. This chapter will also examine the implications of the diversity within the Asian Pacific American community on child welfare policies and practices.

## OVERVIEW OF LITERATURE

The child welfare system is responsible for safeguarding children from child abuse and neglect. According to the Child Abuse Prevention and

Treatment Act of 1974, child abuse and neglect are defined as "the physical or mental injury, sexual abuse or exploitation, negligent treatment, or maltreatment of a child by a person who is responsible for the child's welfare, under circumstances which indicate that the child's health or welfare is harmed or threatened" (Wells 1995, 347).

Although there has been an increased interest in understanding racial and ethnic disparities in the child welfare system, relatively little research has been conducted on the experiences of Asian Pacific American children and families who come into contact with the child welfare system. Three factors may contribute to the lack of attention given to the interaction of Asian Pacific American families with the child welfare system: (1) the underrepresentation in reported cases of child abuse and neglect, (2) the model minority stereotype, and (3) the perceived homogeneity of Asian Pacific Americans (Pelczarski and Kemp 2006).

First, Asian Pacific American families are considered underrepresented in the child welfare system. While there are several definitions of *underrepresentation*, research on child welfare generally defines *underrepresentation* as the comparison between the representation of a particular group in the general population to the representation of that group in the child welfare system (McCabe et al. 1999). The percentage of Asian Pacific Americans in the child welfare system, therefore, is less than their percentage in the United States. For example, a forty-state study conducted in 1997 by the National Center on Child Abuse and Neglect found that only 1.2 percent of the victims of all types of child abuse were Asian Pacific American children, although the Asian Pacific American community makes up 4.5 percent of the total population of the United States (Pelczarski and Kemp 2006).

Second, Asian Pacific Americans face the model minority stereotype. There is a pervasive assumption that all Asian Pacific Americans are highly educated and financially successful (Coalition for Asian American Children and Families 2001). The model minority stereotype positions Asian Pacific Americans as the racial group that has fewer needs than other communities of color. Research has shown that the model minority stereotype is as prevalent in child welfare services as throughout the United States (Mass and Geaga-Rosenthal 2000). This stereotype renders invisible the needs of some Asian Pacific American families, including struggles with limited English proficiency and poverty.

Third, Asian Pacific Americans are often viewed as a monolithic racial group. The 2000 census had over forty ethnic categories for the two racial groups of Asians and Native Hawaiians/Pacific Islanders. However, the child welfare system seldom disaggregates data on Asian Pacific Americans to account for the diverse ethnic groups within this racial classification (Pelczarski and Kemp 2006). Disaggregation is essential to understanding the various experiences of Asian Pacific American families involved with the child welfare system (Yoshihama 2001).

**Table 28.1**  Reasons Why Asian Pacific American Families Can Become Involved in the Child Welfare System

| Familial Reasons | Institutional Reasons |
| --- | --- |
| • Childrearing Practices<br>• Health Practices<br>• Challenges Facing Immigrant Families<br>• Lack of Child Welfare System in Native Country<br>• Stigmas Against Utilizing Public Services | • Language Capacity<br>• Cultural Competence<br>• Special Circumstances for Children of Immigrants |

## PRACTICES LEADING TO PERCEPTION OF CHILD ABUSE AND NEGLECT IN ASIAN PACIFIC AMERICAN FAMILIES

### Childrearing Practices

Childrearing practices are culturally determined, meaning that there are few universally accepted standards and practices that cross all cultures and countries around the world. Asian Pacific American families are far from monolithic in the ways that they raise and discipline their children. Nevertheless, a few generalizations can be made, even though they cannot be uniformly applied to every single family of this diverse community (Coalition for Asian American Children and Families 2001).

Corporal punishment is common in Asian Pacific American families. Corporal punishment is defined as "physical contact by a parent with the intent of modifying the behavior of the child by producing an unpleasant and painful sensation" (Maldonado 2008). Traditional child disciplinary practices include spanking a child with hands, chopsticks, slippers, belts, or sticks; having a child kneel on uncooked rice; or forcing a child to hold one position for an extended period of time. In fact, many schools in Asia, as well as other countries, actively use corporal punishment as a means of discipline. Because Asian parents view teachers as authority figures, parents give teachers permission to discipline their children with corporal punishment. Similarly, in observing teachers use corporal punishment, Asian parents themselves may be encouraged to use corporal punishment in their homes (Coalition for Asian American Children and Families 2001).

For Koreans, physical punishment is not usually considered child maltreatment. In an adult-centered culture that has largely ignored children's opinions and perceptions, physical punishment has been accepted as a disciplinary action often employed by parents and teachers. For example, a study showed that teachers in Korea were less likely than the general public to perceive physical punishment as child maltreatment (Doe 2000). A 1997 national telephone survey of nearly 1300 families in Korea showed

that mothers (91.8%) were more likely than fathers (82.9%) to have positive attitudes about using physical punishment on their children, reflecting the traditional role of the mother as the primary parent responsible for
raising children in Korean families (Doe 2000).

For Samoans, physical discipline is used quite readily with children of all
ages, both to train and to punish (Gray and Cosgrove 1985). A preschooler
may have a hand slapped for touching a valued object, or a teenager may
be spanked until the buttocks are bruised for being disobedient. According
to one study, beatings that fall just short of requiring medical attention are
acceptable and appropriate behaviors for the Samoan community. The
Samoan Americans interviewed for this study explained that children
accept these childrearing practices and that parents care enough to guide
their children's development. They explained that rewards for good behavior and corporal punishment for bad behavior communicates the parents'
love and appreciation for their children (Gray and Cosgrove 1985).

For Vietnamese, physical discipline is also used on children as a form of
punishment (Gray and Cosgrove 1985). According to one study, Vietnamese
Americans view physical discipline as a deliberate method to train and to
punish. They believe that the punishment should not be conducted in anger
and that the child should understand the reasons for it. Vietnamese
Americans described physical punishment as a way for parents to show that
they care about their children. In fact, the Vietnamese have a saying: "When
you hate them, give them sweetness; and when you love them, give them
punishment" (Gray and Cosgrove 1985, 393).

Besides physical punishment, other childrearing practices by Asian
Pacific American parents can be considered child maltreatment. According to one study, Japanese American children are expected to use most, if
not all, of their free time studying. Japanese American children also have
little say in decisions regarding their lives until they become adults and
leave home. Japanese American parents also intentionally do not praise
their children. These practices can be misconstrued as emotional harm in
the United States (Gray and Cosgrove 1985).

Filipinos also have childrearing practices that can be misconstrued as
emotional harm. According to one study, Filipino American parents are
overprotective to the point of being emotionally abusive to their children.
For example, the parents interviewed for the study gave examples of children not being allowed to be frustrated, perspire, climb trees, sit on the
floor, or climb stairs without assistance. Filipino American parents also
have childrearing practices that can be misconstrued as neglectful. For
example, many parents interviewed for the study said that they have
allowed their one-year-old and two-year-old children to be naked at
home (Gray and Cosgrove 1985).

For South Asians, however, one study suggests that they do not differ
significantly from the general population in the United States about
socially acceptable childrearing practices (Maiter et. al. 2004). The study

with twenty-nine South Asian parents found that persistent and excessive use of physical discipline was considered to be unacceptable. Several parents did condone, nevertheless, physical discipline if it did not result in marks or injuries. In regards to emotional harm, the South Asian parents acknowledged that childrearing practices leading to negative emotional consequences for children were recognized to be inappropriate. The parents also identified parental conflict in front of children as potentially harmful to their child's development. In regards to child neglect, the South Asian parents said that being too busy to be home or asking older siblings (at ten years old) to care for younger siblings as examples of inappropriate parenting (Maiter et. al. 2004).

Another study showed that Cambodians also do not approve of physical discipline. In 1994, a small study found that Cambodians were not tolerant of physical punishment (Pelczarski and Kemp 2006). In response to a small vignette in which a nine-year-old son was being disciplined by being hit on the hand with a wooden rod, over 75 percent of Cambodians in the study did not approve of this practice. Almost all of the Cambodian respondents viewed a bruise from spanking as physical abuse. Because these studies suggest that immigrant Asian Pacific American parents do understand the difference between appropriate and inappropriate childrearing practices in the United States, it is important to analyze other factors that lead to their involvement with the child welfare system.

As a predominantly immigrant community, Asian Pacific Americans are raising their children through one set of standards and practices that may not be acceptable according to American society. They often do not know which childrearing practices are considered unacceptable, dangerous, abusive, and neglectful according to federal and state laws. Due to insufficient knowledge, many Asian Pacific American parents are introduced to the child welfare system when they first receive notice that they are being investigated for child abuse or neglect (Coalition for Asian American Children and Families 2001).

When Asian Pacific American parents do learn about the child welfare system, they are unclear as to how to determine exactly which childrearing and child disciplinary methods are allowed. Child welfare laws allow for a spectrum of behaviors that are not completely defined. Asian Pacific American parents are often unsure where local laws consider discipline to end and abuse to start. For example, Asian Pacific American parents are told they cannot be verbally abusive of their children, but a parent might then perceive this as meaning they can never scold their child (Coalition for Asian American Children and Families 2001).

## Health Practices

Many Asian Pacific American parents may seek health care from traditional medicine or traditional clinics prior to seeking treatment from mainstream clinics or emergency rooms. Traditional treatments can include herbs, poultices, and special food and drinks (Coalition for Asian American Children and Families 2001). Asian Pacific American families often believe that traditional clinics and medicines are sufficient for treating mild maladies, while mainstream clinics are generally believed to provide better care for more severe illnesses. Thus, if parents mistakenly believe that a malady is mild, their failure to immediately take the child to an emergency room may be misconstrued as medical neglect (Coalition for Asian American Children and Families 2001).

In fact, some Asian traditional medical treatments that leave marks on the skin have been misconstrued as child abuse. For example, the practice of *cao gio* is a Vietnamese dermabrasion therapy, which is also used extensively by Chinese and other Southeast Asians. Aiming to release negative energy, *cao gio* consists of applying an ointment on the skin and rubbing the ointment firmly into the skin with a coin or spoon. (*Cao gio* is commonly referred to as coining and spooning.) This procedure takes about twenty minutes and is judged to be effective if the rubbing produces a red mark (Davis 2000). Another example is the practice of cupping, which involves placing heated glass cups on the skin to release negative energy or illness. This treatment leaves red marks on the skin from the heat of the glass cups and can also be mistaken for child abuse (Coalition for Asian American Children and Families 2001).

While *cao gio* is considered an effective treatment, Asian Pacific Americans living in the United States are willing to seek mainstream health care. If a condition does not improve with *cao gio*, Asian Pacific Americans will turn to mainstream health care, but only if it is financially available. For example, many Southeast Asians view mainstream health care as a luxury that they cannot afford. *Cao gio* is a simple remedy that can be performed at home for free (Davis 2000). Many immigrant Asian Pacific Americans work in the service and manufacturing industries or in small businesses that do not provide health insurance. With low wages, immigrant Asian Pacific American parents cannot afford private health insurance (Coalition for Asian American Children and Families 2001). Children whose immigrant parents do not have health insurance are less likely to receive health care, even if the children themselves have health insurance (Ku and Matani 2000). Immigrant Asian Pacific American parents therefore delay seeking medical treatment for themselves and for their children. If a child's health problems become exacerbated, Asian Pacific American parents can be investigated for medical neglect.

## Challenges Facing Immigrant Asian Pacific American Families

Over 60 percent of Asian Pacific Americans are foreign born, and their backgrounds as immigrants or refugees affect their experiences as parents. Parenting is a demanding task, which can become more difficult due to highly disruptive relocation circumstances. Studies of immigrant families have shown that the immigration process can significantly disrupt parent-child relations, increase high-risk adolescent behavior, and intensify intergenerational conflict (Maiter et. al. 2004).

The process of acculturation also places enormous pressures on Asian Pacific American family systems (Maiter et. al. 2004). The stress of leaving behind family, friends, homes, and jobs and recreating them in a new country with different cultural practices can have adverse affects on families and parenting practices (Committee for Hispanic Children and Families 1999). Immigrant families must balance the maintenance of their ethnic identity and the adaptation to the dominant American culture, which can be emotionally, psychologically, socially, and physically demanding (Maiter et. al. 2004).

Intergenerational conflict in immigrant Asian Pacific American families can be exacerbated because of the role reversal between parent and child in the United States. Traditional Asian Pacific American families are more hierarchical in nature, where parents are in charge. However, Asian Pacific American children and adolescents can find themselves in the parental role because they often assist their parents in negotiating daily tasks caused by cultural and language barriers (Maiter et. al. 2004). Children of immigrants often play the role of "language broker" for their families. Language brokers translate and interpret for their parents, family members, teachers, doctors, neighbors, and other adults (McQuillan and Tse 1995). Acting as a language broker may negatively affect the parent-child relationship because children become the decision maker for the family.

Language brokering can also get Asian Pacific American families involved with the child welfare system. Because immigrant Asian Pacific American parents may be unfamiliar with school attendance laws, they may pull their children out of school to help the family with tasks. For example, children may stay home to help care for younger siblings. Children may also accompany parents and grandparents on daily tasks in order to facilitate translation and interpretation (Coalition for Asian American Children and Families 2007). While unintentional, Asian Pacific American parents can be investigated for educational neglect due to their children's excessive absences from school.

Immigrant Asian Pacific American families also face economic challenges, as a sizable part of the community struggles with poverty. Consequently, many immigrant Asian Pacific American parents cannot afford quality child care. Some parents may leave their children at home alone, employ uncertified or untrained babysitters, or resort to bringing their children to potentially dangerous workplaces, such as factories (Coalition for Asian American Children and Families 2001). Due to cultural and language barriers, immigrant parents are not familiar with licensing requirements or subsidized vouchers for child care.

Because child care is expensive and parents work long hours, some families believe that having an older sibling care for a younger sibling is acceptable (Center for Law and Social Policy 2007). In Asia, children under the age of twelve are regularly left home alone or to babysit younger siblings, especially in rural and less developed regions. While parents are used to having relatives or neighbors care for their children, these supportive relationships may not be readily available when the family immigrates to the United States (Coalition for Asian American Children and Families 2001). These practices could be misconstrued as child neglect.

Immigration status is another potential barrier for Asian Pacific American families. It is not uncommon for Asian Pacific American families to be mixed-status families, meaning that one or more parents is a noncitizen and one or more children is a citizen. Mixed-status families are themselves complex, as they may be made up of any combination of documented immigrants, undocumented immigrants, and naturalized citizens. Their composition also changes frequently, as undocumented family members legalize their status and as documented immigrants become naturalized citizens (Urban Institute 1999). Many Asian Pacific Americans do not report incidents of child abuse and neglect because they fear disclosing their immigration status. Documented Asian Pacific American parents also believe that getting involved in the child welfare system or accessing support services may jeopardize their residency status, citizenship applications, or ability to sponsor relatives (Coalition for Asian American Children and Families 2001).

## Lack of Child Welfare System in Native Country

Most Asian Pacific American immigrants or refugees who live in the United States come from countries that do not have an institutionalized child welfare system. Asian Pacific American parents may be unfamiliar with socially acceptable childrearing practices because their former governments did not have such laws and regulations (Coalition for Asian American Children and Families 2001). For example, China's system of child protection focuses on three groups of children. The first group consists of orphaned and abandoned children, who are often disabled. The second group consists of children of prisoners who have received a long-term or death sentence. The third group consists of street children, of whom many belong to the aforementioned two groups or who are victims of criminal activities like kidnapping and trafficking. In 2002, approximately 50,000 Chinese children were in the care of state-run urban children's welfare institutions or collectively owned rural children's welfare institutions (Shang et. al. 2005). While China's child welfare system provides for these three groups of vulnerable children, its system does not enforce laws and regulations on childrearing or child disciplinary practices.

This means that the child welfare system of China does not focus on protecting children against child abuse and neglect, which occurs within the family.

Similarly, Japan and Singapore seldom develop and enforce public policies dealing with family's affairs. One research found that China, Japan, and Singapore largely presume family's affairs to be a private family matter, not a public policy matter (Lin and Rantalaiho 2003). The research revealed that children are regarded as private assets or as future protectors of family interests, not as individual citizens of the state. Parents make efforts to get their children closely attached to the family, reflecting the ethos of family reliance nourished by the governments of China, Japan, and Singapore. Public policies, therefore, tend to promote family stability and to put the burden of children's welfare on the families, not on the government (Lin and Rantalaiho 2003).

In Korea, children's rights have tended to be ignored because of the traditional social norm that values parents' rights to discipline their own children. Findings suggest that Korean society, except for some professional groups, such as doctors and social workers, seems to be reluctant to consider all physical punishment as child maltreatment (Doe 2000). Given that corporal punishment has been widely accepted as a disciplinary action, the Korean government does not have a child welfare system to investigate intentional and unintentional cases of child maltreatment.

While the examples have focused on East Asian countries, it should not be surprising that most immigrants may be unfamiliar with the United States' child welfare system. Recently immigrated Asian Pacific Americans may not understand all the government laws and social practices of appropriate childrearing in the United States (Coalition for Asian American Children and Families 2001). In fact, many Asian Pacific American immigrants come from countries with a strong distrust of the government. If police arrive in the middle of the night to remove a family member, it is possible that the family member may never be seen again (Coalition for Asian American Children and Families 2001). Ignorance of the child welfare system, combined with a distrust of government intervention, exacerbates the challenges faced by Asian Pacific American parents in disciplining their children.

## Stigmas against Utilizing Public Services

While Asian Pacific Americans have lower rates of child maltreatment than the general population of the United States, the National Center on Child Abuse and Neglect acknowledges that these statistics are documented through reports to child protective services. In other words, low reports of child maltreatment are not equal to low incidents of child maltreatment. The literature reveals that Asian Pacific Americans are hesitant to disclose and report abuse to both family members and authorities

(Pelczarski and Kemp 2006). Asian Pacific Americans generally have a stigma against revealing problems to family members, friends, and authorities (Maker et. al. 2005). When Asian Pacific American families do seek help, they typically seek support from members of their informal network and less frequently from professional service systems (Lu et. al. 2004). For example, a study with twenty-nine South Asian parents revealed that they most frequently suggested obtaining help from relatives or friends and less frequently from professionals in addressing child welfare issues (Maiter et. al. 2004). This stigma most likely leads to underreporting of child abuse and neglect in Asian Pacific American families. For example, one study found that compared to other racial groups, Chinese parents were more tolerant of maltreatment by parents and were less likely to ask for investigation by protective agencies in potential cases of child abuse and neglect (Lu et. al. 2004).

Underreporting is an occurrence that is restricted not only to parents but also to children of Asian Pacific American backgrounds. In a small yet detailed study conducted in 2000, Segal interviewed twenty-eight Vietnamese families in St. Louis. All of the families were refugees, and half of the families were living below the poverty line. Many of the families were coping with high levels of stress. Although the parents' responses to the Child Abuse Potential Inventory (CAPI) indicated a high tendency for physical abuse, most of the Vietnamese parents denied the use of corporal punishment. When the children of those parents were interviewed separately, they also denied being hit by their parents. Segal speculates that the discrepancy between the CAPI results and the parent and child interviews is a reflection of the Asian value of saving face. Asian Pacific Americans prefer not to disclose problems to outsiders and not to discuss family issues with strangers (Pelczarski and Kemp 2006). Disclosure may have negative implications for Asian Pacific American families, such as breaking up the family unit and forcing family members to choose sides.

While Asian Pacific American children are hesitant to acknowledge child maltreatment, the same cannot necessarily be said for Asian Pacific American adolescents. A study of nearly 4000 children and adolescents in San Diego's child welfare system from 1990 to 1991 found that of all racial groups, Asian Pacific American cases were most frequently opened in the eleven- to seventeen-year-old age group. This finding verified earlier research that Asian Pacific American adolescents are self-reporting their child abuse experiences. With proficiency in English and knowledge of child abuse laws, Asian Pacific American adolescents often report their own parents to the child welfare system when they encounter cultural conflicts or parent-child power struggles (Lu et. al. 2004). This finding is similar to the finding of a study of nearly 1300 Asian Pacific American families reported to child protective services in Washington State for suspected child abuse and neglect from 1995 to 1997. The average age of

Asian Pacific American children in this sample was older than children in national samples. Specifically, two-thirds of the Asian Pacific American children were ten or older in Washington State's child maltreatment reports, in contrast to less than one-third of children of other racial groups from forty-two states (Pelczarski and Kemp 2006).

## LIMITATIONS OF THE CHILD WELFARE SYSTEM

### Language Capacity

The lack of translation and interpretation throughout the child welfare system increases the barriers that Asian Pacific American families must overcome. For example, New York City's child welfare system is not fully equipped to meet the language needs of Asian Pacific American families due to the lack of bilingual staff. Families who are investigated for reported child abuse or neglect rarely come in contact with child welfare staff who can communicate with them in their preferred language (Coalition for Asian American Children and Families 2006). A 1998 study found that 3.6 percent of New York City's child welfare employees were Asian Pacific American, with seventy-eight women and sixty-four men out of a total of 3950 caseworkers and supervisors (White et. al. 1998). A recent study of this system found that 82 percent of staff cited language barriers to serving Asian Pacific American families (Coalition for Asian American Children and Families 2007).

Although there is a lack of bilingual caseworkers, home investigations are usually conducted without an interpreter. In these instances, Asian Pacific American children and other family members often act as the interpreters. This practice is inappropriate and in violation of professional standards. It is especially unsuitable for children to play the role of interpreter, as children may sometimes lie to protect their parents or to get their parents in trouble (Coalition for Asian American Children and Families 2007). For New York City's child welfare system, six of the top ten language requests for translation and interpretation are for Asian languages. When interpreters are available, the quality of interpretation is usually poor. Interpreters sometimes use a literal translation and fail to convey the nuances and context of a situation, resulting in miscommunication between families and caseworkers (Coalition for Asian American Children and Families 2006).

Additionally, New York City's child welfare system does not contract with enough agencies that can adequately meet the language needs of Asian Pacific American families. To achieve its mission of keeping children safe, it contracts with seventy-five agencies to provide child abuse preventive services and with sixty agencies to provide foster care services (Coalition for Asian American Children and Families 2006). However, there are only five contracted preventive services agencies that can provide language accessible services to Asian Pacific American families. Unfortunately, these contracted agencies largely serve Chinese-speaking families, leaving an enormous gap in services for families of other Asian Pacific American ethnic groups. Because of the demand, many Chinese-speaking families also experience long delays in accessing these services (Coalition for Asian American Children and Families 2006).

New York City's child welfare system also does not translate its publications, such as *The Parents' Handbook: A Guidebook for Parents with Children in Foster Care, The Parents' Guidebook to New York State Child Welfare Laws,* and *The Children's Rights Pamphlet* into Asian languages. Asian Pacific American parents who are limited English proficient therefore do not understand their rights and cannot advocate for the well-being of their children or themselves (Coalition for Asian American Children and Families 2007). For example, there have been instances in which language barriers have prevented parents from knowing how to locate their children after they were removed from the home (Coalition for Asian American Children and Families 2006).

In 2003, New York City passed a local law to improve language access for residents seeking social services (Office of the City Clerk 2003). While the local law represents an improvement in the language assistance services available to limited English proficient residents, the law is significantly limited in its reach. Specifically, the law does not require New York City's child welfare system to provide language assistance services to limited English proficient individuals. Rather, the law only requires the child welfare system to create a strategic plan to provide translation and interpretation services and to keep records on the number of limited English proficient individuals seeking services from the agency (Coalition for Asian American Children and Families 2006).

## Cultural Competence

While hiring bilingual caseworkers is key for the child welfare system to support Asian Pacific American families, it is equally important to hire culturally competent caseworkers. Fluency in an Asian language does not necessarily mean knowledge of and ability to respect the culture of the speaker of that language. A caseworker can be bilingual but at the same time be insensitive to the culture of a family, particularly if one is from a different country or region, socioeconomic status, or generation (Coalition for Asian American Children and Families 2001).

According to the Office of Minority Health, culture is the "integrated patterns of human behavior that include the language, thoughts, communications, actions, customs, beliefs, values, and institutions of racial, ethnic, religious, or social groups." Competence is defined as "having the capacity to function effectively as an individual and an organization within the context of the cultural beliefs, behaviors, and needs presented by consumers and their communities" (2000, 1).

In child welfare, cultural competence requires consideration for three areas: (1) parenting practices that may be acceptable in one culture but not in another, (2) limits within a culture to identify practices that are out of the range of acceptability and are considered abuse, and (3) societal factors such as poverty, poor health care, lack of housing, and similar issues that are beyond the control of parents (Korbin 1991). While it is important for caseworkers to be competent in working with families from another culture, care must be taken not to uniformly ascribe childrearing characteristics based on generalizations or stereotypes (Maiter et al. 2004).

One strategy to ensure that child welfare professionals are using linguistically and culturally appropriate practices is to provide cultural competency training. Unfortunately, many cultural competency trainings in the child welfare field omit Asian Pacific Americans (Coalition for Asian American Children and Families 2001). For example, a recent study of caseworkers in New York City showed that 69 percent lack understanding of Asian Pacific American cultures and that 78 percent would like support in better serving Asian Pacific American families (Coalition for Asian American Children and Families 2007). In addition to child welfare professionals, other professionals who are mandated to report child abuse and neglect cases may benefit from cultural competency training. School personnel, social services personnel, health-care providers, and law enforcement are the source of two-thirds of child abuse and neglect reports (Citizens' Committee for Children of New York 2002).

Another strategy to promote cultural competence in the child welfare system is the racial and ethnic matching of caseworkers and families. This strategy entails matching clients with human service professionals of the same racial or ethnic background. In order to overcome cultural barriers and to enhance the working relationship, racial and ethnic matching assumes that human service professionals of the same race or ethnicity as their clients are more likely to share similar life experiences and have fewer language differences than individuals of different racial or ethnic backgrounds. Human service professionals would have an easier time establishing a rapport with clients and facilitating client participation in treatment. Racial/ethnic matching may be possible if supported by hiring policies of child welfare agencies that encourage staff diversity to be consistent with client diversity. A 2004 study of child welfare professionals in California found that racial and ethnic matching does occur throughout the state. In fact, Asian Pacific American caseworkers are almost two and half times more likely than caseworkers from another race or ethnicity to have caseloads with a high percentage of clients who match their race or ethnicity (Perry and Limb 2004). Some recent research, however, has shown that better outcomes for Asian Pacific American families are directly related to an increase in culturally competent caseworkers, not to racial and ethnic matching alone (Lu et. al. 2004).

## Special Circumstances for Children of Immigrants

Improving language access and cultural competence to the child welfare system should lead to better outcomes for Asian Pacific American children and families. However, the child welfare system itself may fail to effectively serve Asian Pacific American families because of constraints placed on immigrants. Under federal law, any abused or neglected child is eligible for short-term emergency medical care, shelter, or other services necessary to address an emergency—regardless of immigration status. This includes services provided in the child welfare system (Court Appointed Special Advocates 2006).

Unfortunately, immigrant children and families face a host of unique barriers once they are in the child welfare system. Some immigrant parents cannot meet service plan requirements because they are ineligible for necessary services, such as mental health or substance abuse treatment. Only "qualified" immigrants—such as legal permanent residents, refugees, or asylees—are eligible to access Temporary Assistance to Needy Families (TANF), Medicaid, and the Child Health Insurance programs. In some cases, immigrant parents may be ordered to become a citizen before having their child returned to them because it is assumed that they can only provide a stable home if they are able to work legally (Court Appointed Special Advocates 2006).

There is another issue with kinship care, in which children are placed with relatives. Although a child can legally be placed with undocumented relatives, negotiating the requirements for kinship care can often be insurmountable because of immigration status. For example, undocumented relatives interested in providing kinship care must provide income verification documents (Court Appointed Special Advocates 2006) and may be asked to provide their social security numbers or to be fingerprinted (Coalition for Asian American Children and Families 2001). Family members are afraid to step forward to provide kinship care because of fears of being deported. Immigrant status alone therefore can lead to a child's permanent separation from family, even if that family could provide a stable and loving environment (Court Appointed Special Advocates 2006). In 2000, homes that qualify for kinship care expanded to include distant kin and nonkin homes with significant family relationships. This expanded definition is helpful to Asian Pacific American immigrants who may not have extended family in the United States (Coalition for Asian American Children and Families 2001).

Limited English proficient children are rarely placed with foster parents who speak their native language. The child's stress and anxiety at being separated from their family may be exacerbated by their inability to communicate with their foster parents (Court Appointed Special Advocates 2006). In long-term placements, immigrant foster children may learn English and lose their ability to speak their native language, causing major problems when the children return to their birth parents, who are limited English proficient. Recruiting and training Asian Pacific American families to be foster families can be difficult. Foster families must have the time and English skills to be trained and certified (Coalition for Asian American Children and Families 2001).

Undocumented immigrant children in foster care face additional barriers. While in foster care, undocumented children will usually receive all of their necessary services, but they lose all benefits once they age out of the system at eighteen. Even if they have lived in the United States for most of their lives, they cannot live permanently in the United States, travel freely, get financial aid for college, or be legally employed because they are considered undocumented immigrant adults. The threat of deportation can be traumatic for a young adult who may not remember living in his or her native country or who may not be familiar with that country's language and culture (Court Appointed Special Advocates 2006).

There are steps that caseworkers can take to assist undocumented children in foster care. Caseworkers can submit an application for special immigrant juvenile status (SIJS) if they can show that it is in the best interest of the child to remain in the United States. In 1990, SIJS legislation was passed as a way for immigrant children in long-term foster care to become legal permanent residents. Children who age out of the foster care system at eighteen have until the end of their twentieth year to apply for SIJS. However, the process is costly and complicated and can take up to thirty-six months. Caseworkers may have difficulties in securing resources to help with the SIJS process, so it is important to begin the process well before the undocumented child leaves foster care (Court Appointed Special Advocates 2006).

## IMPLICATIONS

Asian Pacific American families face challenges with the child welfare system because of their own childrearing and health practices, immigration experiences, unfamiliarity with the child welfare system, and cultural stigmas. The child welfare system also faces challenges in serving Asian Pacific American families because of its own limitations (e.g., language capacity and cultural competence) and institutional policies toward immigrant families.

To determine the consequences of these challenges, it is important to analyze if there is a disproportionate representation of Asian Pacific American families in the child welfare system. Disproportionality refers to the differences in the percentage of families of a certain racial or ethnic group in the country as compared to the percentage of the families of the same group in the child welfare system. This means that Asian Pacific American families may be overrepresented or underrepresented in the child welfare system relative to their proportion in the census population. Research shows that parents of all racial and ethnic groups are equally likely to abuse or neglect their children, but research also shows that there is an overrepresentation of communities of color in the child welfare system (Hill 2006). It is vital to examine this research for the Asian Pacific American community to comprehend the full picture.

**Table 28.2**   Racial and Ethnic Representation in San Diego Country's Child Welfare System, 1996–1997 (N = 4,272)

| Racial/Ethnic Group | Number in Child Welfare System | Proportion in Child Welfare System | Proportion in Census Estimates |
|---|---|---|---|
| African American | 1,230 | 29% | 7% |
| Asian Pacific American | 107 | 3% | 9% |
| White | 1,759 | 41% | 49% |
| Latino | 1,064 | 25% | 32% |
| Other | 112 | 2% | 3% |
| Total | 4,272 | 100% | 100% |

*Source:* McCabe, Kristen, May Yeh, Richard L. Hough, John Landsverk, Michael S. Hurlburt, Shirley Wells Culver, and Beth Reynolds. "Racial/Ethnic Representation Across Five Public Sectors of Care for Youth." *Journal of Emotional and Behavioral Disorders.* Summer 1999, p. 77.

According to the National Center on Child Abuse and Neglect, Asian Pacific American ethnic groups had relatively lower rates of child maltreatment than in the population at large in 1999 (Pelczarski and Kemp 2006). Similarly, a study of San Diego's child welfare system from 1990 to 1991 found that Asian Pacific Americans are underrepresented, as they are represented at approximately two-thirds (67 percent) of their census proportion (Garland et. al. 1998). Another study of San Diego's child welfare system from 1996 to 1997 had a similar finding that Asian Pacific American families are underrepresented, as they made up 9 percent of the county's population but only 3 percent of the child welfare system (McCabe et. al. 1999).

Reports for child maltreatment usually consist of the following six categories: physical abuse, sexual abuse, physical neglect, medical neglect, emotional abuse, and educational neglect. Compared to the general population, Asian Pacific American families have a higher incidence of physical abuse and a lower incidence of sexual abuse and physical neglect (Pelczarski and Kemp 2006). The rates, however, are captured by reports to child protective services, and there is an underreporting of all forms of family violence in the Asian Pacific American community.

These rates are similar to a study of Asian Pacific American families reported to child protective services in Washington State for suspected child abuse and neglect. In 1995, Asian Pacific American families made up 2.9 percent of the 2438 substantiated referrals for child abuse and neglect, which was the lowest rate of substantiated referrals of all racial groups. Of the substantiated referrals for Asian Pacific American families, 55.6 percent were for physical abuse, 33.3 percent for physical neglect, and 11.1 percent for sexual abuse (Pelczarski and Kemp 2006). In another study of Asian Pacific American families reported to child protective services in

**Table 28.3** Types of Abuse in Washington State by Asian and Pacific Islander Ethnic Group, 1995–1997 (N = 993)

| Ethnicity | Number and Percentage of Cases | | | | | | | | | |
|---|---|---|---|---|---|---|---|---|---|---|
| | Sexual | % | Physical | % | Physical | % | Medical | % | Emotional | % |
| Asian Indian | 7 | 15.2 | 22 | 47.8 | 15 | 32.6 | 1 | 2.2 | 1 | 2.2 |
| Cambodian | 16 | 11.3 | 67 | 47.2 | 38 | 26.8 | 16 | 11.3 | 5 | 3.5 |
| Chinese | 4 | 8.7 | 24 | 52.2 | 14 | 30.4 | — | — | 4 | 8.7 |
| Filipino | 17 | 11.3 | 76 | 50.7 | 47 | 31.3 | 5 | 3.3 | 5 | 3.3 |
| Japanese | 4 | 12.1 | 14 | 42.4 | 12 | 36.4 | 3 | 9.1 | — | — |
| Korean | 6 | 7.0 | 46 | 53.5 | 30 | 34.9 | — | — | 4 | 4.7 |
| Lao | 7 | 15.6 | 24 | 53.3 | 9 | 20.0 | 4 | 8.9 | 1 | 2.2 |
| Thai | 3 | 13.6 | 7 | 31.8 | 11 | 50.0 | 1 | 4.5 | — | — |
| Vietnamese | 8 | 5.5 | 81 | 55.9 | 40 | 27.6 | 8 | 5.5 | 8 | 5.5 |
| Hawaiian | 7 | 14.9 | 21 | 44.7 | 17 | 36.2 | 2 | 4.3 | — | — |
| Samoan | 10 | 11.2 | 57 | 64.0 | 15 | 16.9 | 6 | 6.7 | 1 | 1.1 |
| Guamanian | 2 | 15.4 | 6 | 46.2 | 3 | 23.1 | 1 | 7.7 | 1 | 7.7 |
| Other Asian | 19 | 14.7 | 59 | 45.7 | 44 | 34.1 | 1 | 0.8 | 6 | 4.7 |
| Total | 110 | 11.1 | 504 | 50.8 | 295 | 29.7 | 48 | 4.8 | 36 | 3.6 |

*Source:* Division of Child and Family Services. *Case and Management Information System.* July 1995 to June 1997. As cited in Pelczarski and Kemp 2006, 19.

**Table 28.4**  Reports to Washington State's Child Protective Services by Asian and Pacific Islander Ethnic Group, 1995–1997 (N = 1,263)

| Ethnicity | Number of of Reports | Percentage of Reports | Population in Washington State | Percentage of Population |
|---|---|---|---|---|
| Asian Indian | 62 | 4.9 | 7,965 | 3.9 |
| Cambodian | 172 | 13.6 | 10,757 | 5.2 |
| Chinese | 57 | 4.5 | 34,114 | 16.6 |
| Filipino | 203 | 16.1 | 45,705 | 22.2 |
| Japanese | 38 | 3.0 | 34,989 | 17.0 |
| Korean | 109 | 8.6 | 30,292 | 15.0 |
| Lao | 62 | 4.9 | 5,878 | 2.9 |
| Thai | 28 | 2.2 | 2,606 | 1.3 |
| Vietnamese | 182 | 14.4 | 18,248 | 8.9 |
| Hawaiian | 52 | 4.1 | 5,047 | 2.4 |
| Samoan | 126 | 10.0 | 3,589 | 1.7 |
| Guamanian | 14 | 1.1 | 3,816 | 1.8 |
| Other Asian | 158 | 12.5 | 2,334 | 1.1 |
| Total | 1,263 | 100.0 | 205,338 | 100.0 |

*Source:* Division of Child and Family Services. *Case and Management Information System.* July 1995 to June 1997. As cited in Pelczarski and Kemp 2006, 16.

Washington State from 1995 to 1997, the overall rate of physical abuse (50.8%) was more than twice the rate of physical abuse (21.3%) in a fifty-state national sample of child maltreatment reports gathered by the U.S. Department of Health and Human Services (Pelczarski and Kemp 2006).

When child maltreatment rates are disaggregated by ethnicity for the Asian Pacific American community, there is an overrepresentation of some ethnic groups and an underrepresentation of others. For example,

**Table 28.5**  Reported Cases of Child Abuse and Neglect in Hawaii by Ethnicity of Child, 1996–1998 (N = 2,268)

| Ethnicity | 1996 | 1997 | 1998 |
|---|---|---|---|
| Hawaiian | 779 | 988 | 843 |
| Mixed | 462 | 446 | 456 |
| White | 297 | 318 | 263 |
| Filipino | 124 | 202 | 109 |
| Samoan | 46 | 75 | 78 |
| Unknown | 321 | 299 | 322 |
| Other | 239 | 203 | 171 |
| Total | 2,268 | 2,531 | 2,242 |

*Source:* State of Hawaii Department of Human Services. Child Abuse and Neglect in Hawaii. Honolulu Department of Human Services. 1998, p. 18. As cited in Mokuau 2002, 583.

the Washington State study of Asian Pacific American families involved in the child welfare system from 1995 to 1997 examined the extent to which an ethnic group's level of child maltreatment reports is similar to or different from its representation in the state's population. Samoan families had the largest proportion of child protective services referrals relative to their representation in the general population. Constituting 1.7 percent of the state's Asian Pacific American population, Samoan families made up 10 percent of the Asian Pacific American referrals to the child welfare system. Similarly, Cambodian families were overrepresented, as their proportion (13.6%) of child maltreatment referrals was nearly three times greater than their proportion (5.2%) of the state's Asian Pacific American population (Pelczarski and Kemp 2006). Thai, Lao, and Vietnamese families were also overrepresented in child maltreatment reports.

In contrast, the study found several Asian Pacific American ethnic groups to be underrepresented in Washington State's child welfare system. Filipino families, who represent the largest group in terms of child maltreatment reports (16.1%), were underrepresented relative to their proportion (22.2%) of the state's Asian Pacific American population. Similarly, Korean families were underrepresented in the child welfare system, as they represented 15 percent of the state's Asian Pacific American population but only made up 8.6 percent of the child maltreatment reports. Underrepresentation is particularly marked for Chinese and Japanese families (4.5% and 3%, respectively) compared with their representation in the Washington State's Asian Pacific American population (16.6% and 17%, respectively) (Pelczarski and Kemp 2006).

Another study showed that Native Hawaiians are overrepresented in the child welfare system in Hawaii. From 1996 to 1998, Native Hawaiians accounted for the largest number of child abuse and neglect cases. People with Native Hawaiian ancestry represented 23 percent of the state's population but accounted for 34 percent of child abuse and neglect cases in 1996, 39 percent in 1997, and 38 percent in 1998 (Mokua, 2002). Another study of Hawaii's child welfare system in 1995 showed that Native Hawaiians and Samoans were overrepresented while Japanese were underrepresented (Pelczarski and Kemp 2006).

## CONCLUSION

Keeping children safe is of utmost importance not only for the child welfare system but also for society as a whole. Yet the decision to remove a child from a home may be made without fully assessing the context of Asian Pacific American families or acknowledging the constraints of the child welfare system. On average, Asian Pacific Americans are underrepresented in the child welfare system. For any family suspected of child abuse and neglect, navigating the child welfare system and accessing support services can be challenging. However, these challenges are exacerbated for Asian Pacific American families due to their own childrearing practices as well as institutional barriers.

There is a need to conduct more research on Asian Pacific American families and their involvement with the child welfare system. Much of the research cited for this chapter was conducted in the 1990s or on the West Coast. Given the growth of the Asian Pacific American community in the Midwest, South, and Northeast, additional research in these areas of the United States would provide a comprehensive perspective on these communities' experiences with the child welfare system.

It is also important to ensure that disaggregated data are available from agencies providing child welfare services as well as research on Asian Pacific American families. Because of the diversity of this community, disaggregated data are necessary to evaluate the similarities and differences of experiences for Asian Pacific American ethnic groups involved with the child welfare system. Data should be disaggregated according not only to ethnicity but also to gender, socioeconomic status, immigration status, language proficiency, and generation. Without these data, it will be difficult to develop child welfare policies, practices, and services to effectively address the diverse Asian Pacific American community.

The existing research does show that meaningful child welfare policies, practices, and services must account for the unique backgrounds and experiences of Asian Pacific American families. Child welfare professionals must recognize the effects that different childrearing and health practices, immigration experiences, unfamiliarity with the child welfare system, and cultural stigmas may have on Asian Pacific American children and families. At the same time, child welfare professionals must address the systemic constraints in serving Asian Pacific American families because of the child welfare system's own language, cultural, and immigrant barriers. It is therefore important to examine not only child welfare policies and practices but also immigration and social policies.

The struggles of immigrant communities and the barriers of the child welfare system can have devastating consequences for Asian Pacific American families. Families new to the United States can become reported for child abuse and neglect. Families mandated to receive child welfare services can have difficulty in fulfilling their requirements. Families in preventive services can have their children removed. Families with children in foster care can have their parental rights terminated. Additional research, disaggregated data, community education, and accessible child welfare systems may help to keep Asian Pacific American children safe and families together.

## REFERENCES

Center for Law and Social Policy. *The Challenges of Change: Learning from the Child Care and Early Education Experiences of Immigrant Families.* 2007.

Citizens' Committee for Children of New York. *Keeping Track of New York City's Children.* 2002.

Coalition for Asian American Children and Families. *Building Bridges: Increasing Language Access for the Asian Pacific American Community of New York City.* 2006.

Coalition for Asian American Children and Families. *Crossing the Divide: Asian American Families and the Child Welfare System.* 2001.

Coalition for Asian American Children and Families. *Connecting the Dots: Improving Neighborhood-Based Child Welfare Services for Asian Pacific American Families.* 2007.

Committee for Hispanic Children and Families and Coalition for Asian American Children and Families. *Opening the Door: A Survey of the Cultural Competence of Preventive Services to Asian and Latino Families in New York City.* 1999.

Court Appointed Special Advocates. Immigrant Children and Families in the Foster Care System. *The Connection.* Vol. 22. No. 3. Summer 2006. p. 6–13.

Davis, Ruth E. Cultural Health Care or Child Abuse? The Southeast Asian Practice of Cao Gio. *Journal of the American Academy of Nurse Practitioners.* Vol. 12. No. 3. March 2000. p. 89–95.

Doe, Sondra SeungJa. Cultural Factors in Child Maltreatment and Domestic Violence in Korea. *Children and Youth Services Review.* Vol. 22. 2000. p. 231–236.

Garland, Ann, Elissa Ellis-Macleod, John A. Landsverk, William Ganger, and Ivory Johnson. Minority Populations in the Child Welfare System: The Visibility Hypothesis Reexamined. *American Journal of Orthopsychiatry.* Vol. 68. No. 1. 1998. p. 142–146.

Gray, Ellen and John Cosgrove. Ethnocentric Perception of Childrearing Practices in Protective Services. *Child Abuse & Neglect.* Vol. 9. 1985. p. 389–396.

Hill, Robert B. *Synthesis of Research on Disproportionality in Child Welfare: An Update.* 2006.

Korbin, Jill. Cross-Cultural Perspectives and Research Directions for the 21st Century. *Child Abuse and Neglect.* Vol. 15. No. 1. 1991. p. 67–77.

Ku, Leighton and Sheetal Matani. *Immigrants' Access to Health Care and Insurance on the Cusp of Welfare Reform.* Urban Institute. June 2000.

Lu, Yuhwa Eva, John Landsverk, Elissa Ellis-Macleod, Rae Newton, William Granger, and Ivory Johnson. Race, Ethnicity, and Case Outcomes in Child Protective Services. *Children and Youth Services Review.* Vol. 26. 2004. p. 447–461.

Maiter, Sarah, Ramona Alaggia, and Nico Trocme. Perceptions of Child Maltreatment by Parents from the Indian Subcontinent: Challenging Myths about Culturally Based Abusive Parenting Practices. *Child Maltreatment.* Vol. 9. No. 3. August 2004. p. 309–324.

Maker, Azmaira H., Priti V. Shah, and Zia Agha. Child Physical Abuse: Prevalence, Characteristics, Predictors, and Beliefs about Parent-Child Violence in South Asian, Middle Eastern, East Asian, and Latina Women in the United States. *Journal of Interpersonal Violence.* Vol. 20. 2005. p. 1405–1427.

Maldonado, Martin. Cultural Issues in the Corporal Punishment of Children. Kansas Association for Infant Mental Health. http://www.kaimh.org/corporal.htm. Web site download March 2, 2008.

Mass, Amy and Joselyn Geaga-Rosenthal. Child Welfare: Asian and Pacific Islander Families. *Child Welfare: A Multicultural Focus.* Boston, MA: Allyn and Bacon. 2000. p. 145–164.

McCabe, Kristen, May Yeh, Richard L. Hough, John Landsverk, Michael S. Hurlburt, Shirley Wells Culver, and Beth Reynolds. Racial/Ethnic Representation across Five Public Sectors of Care for Youth. *Journal of Emotional and Behavioral Disorders.* Summer 1999.

McQuillan, Jeff and Lucy Tse. Child Language Brokering in Linguistic Minority Communities: Effects on Cultural Interactions, Cognition, and Literacy. *Language and Education.* Vol. 9. No. 3. 1995. p. 195–215.

Mokuau, Noreen. Culturally Based Interventions for Substance Use and Child Abuse among Native Hawaiians. *Public Health Reports.* Vol. 117. 2002. p. 582–587.

Office of the City Clerk, The City of New York. Local Laws of the City of New York for the Year 2003. No. 73. 2003.

Office of Minority Health. Moving Towards Consensus on Cultural Competency in Health Care. *Closing the Gap: a newsletter of the Office of Minority Health.* Washington, DC: Department of Health and Human Services. 2000.

Pelczarski, Yoshimi and Susan P. Kemp. Patterns of Child Maltreatment Referrals among Asian and Pacific Islander Families. *Child Welfare.* Volume LXXXV. No. 1. January and February 2006.

Perry, Robin and Gordon E. Limb. Ethnic/Racial Matching of Clients and Social Workers in Public Child Welfare. *Children and Youth Services Review.* Vol. 26. 2004. p. 965–979.

Shang, Xiaoyuan, Xiaoming Wu, and Yue Wu. Welfare Provision for Vulnerable Children: The Missing Role of the State. *The China Quarterly.* 2005. p. 122–136.

Urban Institute. *All under One Roof: Mixed-Status Families in an Era of Reform.* 1999.

Wells, S. J. Child Abuse and Neglect Overview. *19th Encyclopedia of Social Work.* Vol. 1. Washington DC: National Association of Social Workers; 1995. p. 346–353. Quotation from the Child Abuse Prevention and Treatment Act of 1974, p. 347.

White, Andrew, John Courtney, and Adam Fifield. Race, Bias and Power in Child Welfare. *Child Welfare Watch.* No. 3. Spring/Summer 1998. p. 1.

Yoshihama, Mieko. Immigrants-in-Context Framework: Understanding the Interactive Influence of Social-Cultural Contexts. *Evaluation and Program Planning.* Vol. 24. No. 3. 2001. p. 307–318.

# Chapter 29

# Voices of the Community
## Coalition for Asian American Children and Families (CACF)

### Vanessa Leung

The Coalition for Asian American Children and Families (CACF) is the nation's only pan-Asian children's advocacy organization. CACF aims to improve the health and well-being of Asian Pacific American children, youth, and families in New York City. CACF challenges stereotypes of the model minority and speaks out on behalf of marginalized families in our community, especially immigrants struggling with poverty and limited English skills. CACF advocates for better policies, funding, and services to ensure that children of all backgrounds have the support they need to thrive. CACF represents the East Asian, South Asian, Southeast Asian, and Pacific Islander communities of New York City. CACF's work in New York City has been used as a model for other metropolitan areas and marginalized communities throughout the United States.

## HISTORY

*1986–1994:* CACF began with a meeting of concerned service providers to address the lack of political presence and the lack of a unified voice for the growing Asian Pacific American community in New York City. In the 1980s, New York City experienced a huge increase in the Asian Pacific American population. However, the model minority myth that all Asian Pacific Americans are successful and the lack of understanding on the part of policy makers and city agencies hid the growing needs of this diverse community. In 1986, a social work intern named Alice Chin was completing her field placement at the Chinese-American Planning Council (CPC), the largest Asian Pacific American community-based organization in New York City. It was while interning at CPC that Ms. Chin became concerned that the needs of the community were not understood and initiated the process of bringing together other providers who shared the same concerns.

The first meeting of providers resulted in the decision to plan a conference to bring attention to the needs of the Asian Pacific American community and to develop a network of individuals concerned about children and family issues. The group soon established itself as the Asian American Coalition for Children and Families Inc., which was fiscally sponsored by the Chinese-American Planning Council. In 1992, the organization became incorporated as a 501(c)3 non-profit organization. CACF operated as a volunteer-run organization for the first ten years. Volunteers worked to involve Asian Pacific Americans in advocating on children's issues, such as participating in the Children's Defense Fund rally, where they brought busloads of Asian Pacific American parents, children, and concerned individuals to Albany, New York, and Washington DC.

*1995–2000:* In 1995, through a three-year seed grant from the New York Foundation, the organization hired its first executive director and renamed itself the Coalition for Asian American Children and Families, emphasizing its focus on children's issues facing this community. With actual staff, CACF began to take a larger role as the policy and advocacy voice of Asian Pacific American children and families, educating policy makers and the public at large about the issues facing the growing and diversifying Asian Pacific American community.

CACF initially focused its advocacy efforts on the child welfare system. The New York City child welfare system lacked understanding of the challenges and strengths of Asian Pacific American families, placing families who came into contact with the system at risk. Being in the system can be very stressful for the entire family unit, and for Asian Pacific American families who lack access to culturally competent and linguistically appropriate services, being in the system can be even more traumatic. CACF developed reports and resource lists, educated elected and city officials, and trained child welfare workers to improve the outcomes for Asian Pacific American and immigrant families in the child welfare system.

*2001–2004:* CACF's budget experienced a substantial increase following September 11th. This catastrophic event in 2001 left many communities in New York City vulnerable. The Asian Pacific American community was greatly affected, especially those living in Manhattan's Chinatown. CACF filled an immediate need by training mental health professionals on culturally competent services for Asian Pacific American families and by educating service providers already working with the Asian Pacific American community on more child friendly approaches to delivering mental health services. CACF also partnered with organizations to directly help families regain a sense of safety and community through the development of family-centered programming. With this growth in budget, CACF was able to attract additional funding to sustain and expand its work.

*2005–2008:* As of 2008, CACF is still the nation's only children's advocacy organization focused on the Asian Pacific American community. In 2005, CACF completed its strategic plan, deciding to prioritize policy advocacy as the main strategy to bring about systemic change. CACF also reinvigorated its membership of community-based organizations led by or serving Asian Pacific Americans, forming a collective voice to advocate for better policies, services, and funding for children and families.

Since 2005, CACF has been recognized by the U.S. Office of Minority Health, New York State Legislature, New York City Mayor, New York City Council, New York City Comptroller, *Newsday*, and several community-based organizations as a vital advocacy partner for community leaders from all racial and ethnic groups.

## VISION, MISSION, AND GOALS

CACF is committed to ensuring that Asian Pacific American children and their families have the resources, supports, and opportunities that they need to lead safe and healthy lives. CACF currently focuses its policy advocacy initiatives on five issue areas that have great impact on the lives of children and families: child welfare, early childhood education, education, health, and youth services.

CACF values representing a pan-Asian perspective and involving the community in our work. By ensuring that its board of directors, staff, volunteers, and membership represent different Asian Pacific American ethnic groups, CACF is committed to being fully inclusive of the diverse Asian Pacific American community. Additionally, the Asian Pacific American community helps in identifying the concerns and needs of families, and CACF works to empower individuals—such as youth, parents, and service providers—to be involved in advocating for policy change.

CACF believes that working with individuals and the community will lead to an improved unity of voices and leadership for the Asian Pacific American community. In turn, the increased visibility of the Asian Pacific American community will influence decision makers to improve policies, resources, and services that every child and family in New York City needs to thrive. Ultimately, CACF aims to increase the capacity of every community to provide safe, supportive environments for children and families.

## STRATEGIES

*Policy Advocacy:* CACF employs a variety of strategies to bring about positive change for the community. Policy advocacy forms the foundation of its work. Strategies include lobbying city and state officials, analyzing policies, identifying gaps in services, and educating the community and the media. While direct service organizations are meeting the immediate needs of individuals in the Asian Pacific American community, there is a need for broader, systemic approaches to improving the situation for children and families. The lack of representation of Asian Pacific American perspectives in policy making necessitates the existence of an organization like CACF to be the policy voice to ensure that there are better policies, more funding, and improved services to meet the critical needs of underserved Asian Pacific American children and families.

*Research:* Data is important to document and understand the needs of populations and gaps in services. Unfortunately, quantitative and qualitative data on Asian Pacific Americans in New York City is limited, inaccessible, or nonexistent. Often times, Asian Pacific Americans are relegated to the category of "Other," or, if data is disaggregated by race, the diversity of the Asian Pacific American community gets lost. In addition, research studies rarely have sizable Asian Pacific American samples. These limitations make it difficult to demonstrate the needs in the Asian Pacific American community of New York City and to support the development of programs targeting specific communities. CACF has conducted its original research to help inform policy advocacy efforts, educate decision makers, and support community-based organizations. CACF's first report, *Half-Full or Half-Empty,* was the first major report that offered comprehensive data on Asian Pacific American children and families in New York City and documented gaps in services, issues, and trends in health care, child care, and youth programs. CACF followed this landmark report with others examining the child welfare system, public schools, and language access to public services. CACF continues to disseminate research on the needs of the community and on policies and practices to effectively address these needs.

*Youth and Parent Mobilizing:* Community involvement in advocacy is necessary to represent a collective voice and the needs of the diverse Asian Pacific American community. When individuals are part of the process to bring about positive change, they can speak directly on the impact of policies and the gaps in services. CACF believes that it has a role in developing the next generation of advocates. Through its youth leadership program, the Asian American Student Advocacy Project (ASAP), CACF is supporting the development of advocacy skills and instilling the importance of being a voice for the community in young people. ASAP participants have met with high-ranking officials at the Department of Education and the Department of Health and Mental Hygiene to present their research finding and recommendations.

In addition, CACF currently engages Asian Pacific American parents by training them on their rights and their children's rights to various public systems and on actions they can take if challenges arise. Through this initial engagement, CACF aims to mobilize diverse Asian Pacific American parents, through which they can develop their advocacy skills and can share their concerns with decision makers.

*Capacity Building:* To meet the needs of the growing and diverse Asian Pacific American community, there has to be culturally competent and language-accessible services. CACF works to ensure not only better services for the diverse Asian Pacific American community but also the sustainability of community-based organizations offering those services in New York City. Community-based organizations serving the Asian Pacific American community are faced with a high demand for their services, and city agencies are working to make their services more language accessible and culturally competent. To help ensure that services are effective and available, CACF creates opportunities for learning, capacity building, and information sharing among our stakeholders, such as member organizations, service providers, schools, and city agencies. For example, CACF hosted a meeting on how organizations can access city funds to help them diversify their funding streams. On another occasion, CACF brought together service providers and the chancellor of New York City's public schools to discuss the current needs of Asian Pacific American students. It is through these meetings that stakeholders learn about current and emerging community needs and effective approaches to meet and resolve those needs.

*Coalition Building:* CACF views coalition building as integral to strengthening the advocacy voice for Asian Pacific American children and families in New York City. CACF works to develop pan-Asian unity, because strength in numbers has proven to be an effective strategy in bringing about policy change. Through its twenty-two-year history, CACF has seen the diversity and growth in the number of community-based organizations serving Asian Pacific American children and families. Their knowledge of the needs of the children and families whom they serve makes them important partners in CACF's advocacy efforts. CACF also recognizes that it is important to develop strategic partnerships with advocates representing immigrant communities and communities of color as well as with advocates working on specific issue areas, such as education, child welfare, and health. CACF works to ensure that an active, effective, and knowledgeable coalition of community-based and advocacy organizations become dedicated to addressing issues facing Asian Pacific American children and families.

## ACCOMPLISHMENTS

While policy change is a long-term struggle, CACF has had several key victories in the past few years. In 2002, CACF achieved a noteworthy win when it successfully advocated for the New York State Department of Social Services to change its ethnicity data category from the derogatory term "Oriental" to the acceptable term "Asian."

Since then, CACF has achieved other budget, legislative, and administrative victories. In 2004, CACF worked with a broad coalition to advocate for the New York City Council to pass the Dignity in All Schools Act (DASA), an anti-bullying legislation. In 2005, CACF worked with advocates and the city council to create chancellor's regulations on providing translation and interpretation services in schools and to allocate $12 million to launch the New York City Department of Education's Translation and Interpretation Unit. In 2006, CACF worked with child welfare advocates to allocate $4.2 million to community-based preventive service programs to bring on 240 more staff to keep caseloads to the national standard that would better ensure children are safe. In 2007, CACF worked with immigrant education advocates to get $700 million over four years in New York State funding for English Language Learner students.

CACF has grown to be seen as an important advocate, knowledgeable not only on the Asian Pacific American community but also on children and family issues. For example, CACF Executive Director Wayne Ho was appointed to the Governor's Children's Cabinet Advisory Board in December 2007 and has been advising on how to expand universal prekindergarten programs and increase health insurance coverage for underserved children in New York State. In 2007, CACF Deputy Director Vanessa Leung was selected as one of twenty representatives to participate in the city council's Middle School Task Force to improve the performance of the city's middle schools.

## CHALLENGES

CACF faces external and internal factors that challenge its success as a policy advocacy organization. Systemic change, in and of itself, is a long-term struggle that requires persistent efforts. Our partnerships with community-based organizations support our advocacy efforts. However, it can be difficult to keep these direct service providers at the table because of the time commitment necessary. The priority of direct service providers is to utilize their time to serve their clients. CACF also recognizes that being politically savvy and developing relationships with policy makers is essential. Yet the challenge arises when changes in power occur and relationships have to be redeveloped. Negotiating the oftentimes capricious dynamics between the governor, mayor, and city council can prove challenging to even the most seasoned advocate.

CACF also faces challenges because of its small staff. CACF realizes that it does not have capacity to work on all issues facing the community because of its staff size. While CACF has been successful in increasing our staff and budget over the years, identifying funding for policy advocacy is difficult because most funders and donors prefer to support services that have a direct and immediate impact on society. Cultivating new funders and individual donors is necessary to sustain and grow CACF's capacity as an influential advocate.

Tension between immigrant rights and racial justice can result in issues becoming divisive and, therefore, a barrier to achieving CACF's goals. Many immigrant rights advocates and immigrants themselves do not frame their interests in terms of racial justice, and racial justice work often is not inclusive of immigrants. The Asian Pacific American community is predominantly an immigrant population, as the vast majority of children are children of immigrants or immigrants themselves. CACF's advocacy initiatives take an immigrant rights perspective on certain issues, but CACF also sees the totality of our work as part of the movement for racial justice.

The Asian Pacific American community spans the socioeconomic spectrum, concentrating at the extreme ends, resulting in the Asian Pacific American community often missing in discussions of both racial justice and social justice. As part of the larger social justice movement, CACF brings attention to how poverty and lack of access are challenges to the health and well-being of Asian Pacific American families. The model minority myth that the Asian Pacific American community is uniformly successful and faces few difficulties poses a great challenge when working to end injustices. People, including some Asian Pacific Americans themselves, do not see the need for a specific Asian Pacific American voice in the fight for justice. What results is a continuous need for CACF to educate the society at large of the diversity of the community and the challenges that face it.

As a policy advocacy organization, CACF must decide the best way to achieve the desired outcomes, whether through legislative, administrative, or budget changes. Achieving a win through any of these does not necessarily result in improvements for Asian Pacific American children and families. Real success means actual improvements in the lives of children and families. Barriers to real success can be due to a change in administration, lack of institutional support, and lack of funding. Therefore, CACF's advocacy efforts do not end with simply achieving a legislative, administrative, or budget change. CACF continues its work by monitoring the implementation and evaluation of the changes, ensuring that positive changes that improve the lives of children and families are actually happening.

## REFERENCES

All CACF reports can be downloaded from www.cacf.org.

*Breaking Down Barriers: Immigrant Families and Early Childhood Education in New York City;* May 2008.

*Building Bridges: Increasing Language Access for the Asian Pacific American Community of New York City;* January 2006.

*Connecting the Dots: Improving the Neighborhood-Based Child Welfare Services for Asian Pacific American Families;* March 2007.

*Crossing the Divide: Asian American Families and The Child Welfare System;* January 2002.

*Half-Full or Half-Empty? Health Care, Child Care, and Youth Programs for Asian American Children in New York City;* April 1999.

*Hidden in Plain View: An Overview of the Needs of Asian American Students in the Public School System;* May 2004.

*Opening the Door: A Survey of the Cultural Competence of Foster Care Preventive Services to Asian and Latino Families in New York City;* August 1999.

*A Seat at the Table: Toward a National Agenda for Asian Pacific American Children;* 2000.

# PART VI

---

# Migration and Social Context

# Chapter 30

# Diaspora and Settlement

## Gem P. Daus

The diversity of Asian Americans[1] can hardly be overstated. As documented elsewhere in this text, this population varies widely by such health indicators as utilization of mental health care services, access to cancer screening, and prevalence of certain infectious diseases. And contrary to the persistent characterization as a model minority that is successfully assimilating by its own bootstraps, the population experiences wide disparities in educational attainment, income, career advancement, and other socioeconomic indicators (Danico and Ng 2004). With such diversity, one may question whether the term *Asian American* is even a useful unit of analysis. However, while specific identity groups, scholars, and others debate the utility of the term, its legitimacy is rooted in self-determination: it was U.S.-born Chinese, Filipino, and Japanese college students and organizations that first coined the term in the 1960s (Wei 1993). Its staying power seems assured as evidenced by the growing number of ethnic media, community-based organizations, and funders that use the term in their names and programs. And as the term continues to apply to an ever growing number of people and organizations, it is useful to be reminded of the diverse histories and experiences of those who are called Asian American. This chapter provides a basic history of the migration and settlement patterns of specific Asian American groups, particularly as those patterns impact their health and adaptation to U.S. health care systems. The chapter also includes a discussion of the consequent building of Asian American communities, organizations, and movements as a context for future health planning. Finally, a few recommendations for further study are included.

## HISTORICAL CENSUSES

The U.S. census provides a rough outline of the size of specific Asian ethnic groups in the United States over time. As shown in Table 30.1, the U.S. Census Bureau has listed seven Asian subcategories on its forms (Asian Indian, Chinese, Filipino, Japanese, Korean, Vietnamese, and Other Asian) and reported data for as many as seventeen ethnic groups since 2000 (Barnes and Bennett 2002). In addition, census forms have check boxes for "Native Hawaiian," "Guamanian or Chamorro," "Samoan," and "Other Pacific Islander," resulting in the ability to report as many as twelve or more ethnic groups (Grieco 2001).

This level of detail was not always the case as shown in Table 30.2. Asians were first identified in the 1860 census. The 34,933 individuals counted were Chinese living in California. Japanese were identified separately for the 1870 census, which counted 55 Japanese and nearly twice as many Chinese compared to 1860 (63,199). Both groups have been identified separately ever since. The 1910 census added categories for Filipino, Hindu, Korean, and Maori. The Filipino category has been used for every census since 1910; however, Maori was used only one more time, in 1920; Hindu was used from 1910 to 1940; and Korean was used from 1910 to

**Table 30.1** Asian, Native Hawaiian, and Other Pacific Islander Categories Reported by Census 2000

| Asian | Native Hawaiian, and Other Pacific Islander |
|---|---|
| **Asian Indian** | Polynesian: |
| Bangladeshi | **Native Hawaiian** |
| Cambodian | **Samoan** |
| **Chinese, except Taiwanese*** | Tongan |
| **Filipino** | Other Polynesian |
| Hmong | Micronesian: |
| Indonesian | **Guamanian or Chamorro** |
| **Japanese** | Other Micronesian |
| **Korean** | Melanesian: |
| Laotian | Fijian |
| Malaysian | Other Melanesian |
| Pakistani | **Other Pacific Islander** |
| Sri Lankan | Other Pacific Islander, not specified |
| Taiwanese | |
| Thai | |
| **Vietnamese** | |
| **Other Asian** | |
| Other Asian, not specified | |

The items in bold are listed on census forms.
*Only the word *Chinese* is on the forms.

1940 and again from 1970 to the present. After brief attempts to count Hawaiians and other groups from 1920 to 1940, the 1950 census only counted Chinese, Japanese, and Filipinos. Hawaiian and Part-Hawaiian were added in 1960, but subsequent censuses used only the Hawaiian category. Since 1970 no categories have been deleted, only added. As previously mentioned, the Korean category was restored in 1970. In 1980, categories were added for Asian Indian, Vietnamese, Guamanian, and Samoan. In 1990, new categories included Cambodian, Hmong, Laotian, Thai, Other Asian, and Other Pacific Islander (Gibson and Jung 2002).

In all of these censuses, the categories were totaled into one race category called "Asian" or "Asian and Pacific Islander." In 2000, that category was split into two ("Asian" and "Native Hawaiian and Other Pacific Islander"; hereafter NHPI), which, after the count was over, allowed the census to report totals for the aforementioned seventeen Asian ethnic groups and twelve NHPI groups. The 2000 census was unique also because it allowed individuals, for the first time, to check off all race categories that applied, rather than forcing them to choose only one race (Grieco and Cassidy 2001). This revealed significant differences in counts for some groups depending on whether one chose to use the single-race count (i.e., "Asian Alone") or the multirace count (i.e., "Asian Alone or in any Combination"). For example, Native Hawaiians numbered 140,652, if one counted only those who checked "Native Hawaiian"; but when one counted those who checked "Native Hawaiian" and any other category, the number of Native Hawaiians almost tripled to 401,162 (Grieco 2001). Similarly, Japanese numbered 796,700 when only those who checked "Japanese" were counted; but "Japanese alone or in any combination" numbered 1,148,932, meaning that 30 percent of Japanese are multiracial (Barnes and Bennett 2002). The difference is also significant when one considers that the 1990 count for Japanese was 847,562 (U.S. Census Bureau 1990). One could be misled into believing that the Japanese population was shrinking.

In fact, all categories of Asians and Pacific Islanders are growing. In 1860, Asians accounted for only 0.1 percent of the U.S. population. By 1970, the proportion had grown to just 0.8 percent, but nearly doubled to 1.5 percent in 1980, and nearly doubled again to 2.9 percent in 1990 (Gibson and Jung 2002). According to the 2000 census, Asians (including multiracial Asians) were 4.2 percent of the population, and NHPI (again including multiracial) were 0.3 percent of the population (Grieco and Cassidy 2001). The counts for any category are not directly comparable from census to census for a number of methodological reasons (Martin and Gerber 2003). For example, mixed-race individuals have been treated differently by different censuses; sometimes several states were left out, as was the case for the Filipino count in 1950; and methods differed for tabulating write-in data for Asian and Pacific Islander groups not specifically

**Table 30.2** Historical Census Asian Categories and Counts (1860–1990)

| Census | Total | Groups Enumerated | | | | | | | | | |
|---|---|---|---|---|---|---|---|---|---|---|---|
| 1860 | Total 34,933 | | | | | | | | | | |
| 1870 | Total 63,254 | Chinese 63,199 | Japanese 55 | | | | | | | | |
| 1880 | Total 105,613 | Chinese 105,465 | Japanese 148 | | | | | | | | |
| 1890 | Total 109,527 | Chinese 107,488 | Japanese 2,039 | | | | | | | | |
| 1900 | Total 114,189 | Chinese 89,863 | Japanese 24,326 | | | | | | | | |
| 1910 | Total 146,863 | Chinese 71,531 | Japanese 72,157 | Filipino 160 | Hindu 2,545 | Korean 462 | Maori 8 | | | | |
| 1920 | Total 182,137 | Chinese 61,639 | Japanese 111,010 | Filipino 5,603 | Hindu 2,507 | Korean 1,224 | Hawaiian 110 | Malay 19 | Siamese 17 | Samoan 6 | |
| 1930 | Total 264,766 | Chinese 74,954 | Japanese 138,834 | Filipino 45,208 | Hindu 3,130 | Korean 1,860 | Hawaiian 660 | Malay 96 | Siamese 18 | Samoan 6 | Maori 2 |
| 1940 | Total 254,918 | Chinese 77,504 | Japanese 126,947 | Filipino 45,563 | Hindu 2,405 | Korean 1,711 | All other[2] 788 | | | | |
| 1950 | Total 321,033 | Chinese 117,629 | Japanese 141,768 | Filipino 61,636 | | | | | | | |
| 1960 | Total 980,337 | Chinese 237,292 | Japanese 464,332 | Filipino 176,310 | Hawaiian 11,294 | Part Hawaiian 91,109 | | | | | |

|  | | | | | | | | | | | | |
|---|---|---|---|---|---|---|---|---|---|---|---|---|
| 1970 | Total 1,538,721 | Chinese 435,062 | Japanese 591,290 | Filipino 343,060 | Korean 69,130 | Hawaiian 100,179 | | | | | | |
| 1980 | Total 3,500,439 | Chinese 806,040 | Japanese 700,974 | Filipino 774,652 | Korean 354,593 | Asian Indian 361,531 | Vietnamese 261,729 | Hawaiian 166,814 | Guamanian 32,158 | Samoan 41,948 | | |
| 1990 | Total Asian 6,908,638 | Chinese 1,645,472 | Japanese 847,562 | Filipino 1,406,770 | Korean 798,849 | Asian Indian 815,447 | Vietnamese 614,547 | Cambodian 147,411 | Hmong 90,082 | Laotian 149,014 | Thai 91,275 | Other Asian 302,209 |
| 1990 | Total Pacific Islander 365,024 | Hawaiian 211,014 | Samoan 62,964 | Guamanian 49,345 | Other Pacific Islander 41,701 | | | | | | | |

listed on the census questionnaire (Gibson and Jung 2002). Nevertheless, there is a clear pattern of growth in terms of number and proportion.

## PRE-1965 IMMIGRATION PATTERNS

Even though the census only started counting Asians in 1860, there is evidence of migration and settlement much earlier. For example, Filipinos were part of a Spanish expedition that landed in what is now Morro Bay, California, in 1587 (Borah 1995). In 1763, Filipinos settled near New Orleans, Louisiana. Known as Manilamen, they had escaped servitude aboard Spanish galleon trading ships and established shrimp fisheries (Espina 1988).

The regular migration of larger numbers of Asians was motivated by America's thirst for cheap labor, labor required by westward expansion, industrial revolution, and abolition. The timing of specific ethnic waves of migrations coincided with the exclusion of previous groups, exclusion that was officially sanctioned and motivated by economic competition and "yellow peril" racism despite the need for more workers (Zia 2000). To illustrate, more than 275,000 Chinese entered the United States from 1849 to 1882 to work in gold mines and farms, and to help build the transcontinental railroad (Zane et al. 1994). But the passage of the Chinese Exclusion Act in 1882 legally barred any more Chinese from immigrating to the United States (Kitano and Daniels 2000). Within six years, severe labor shortages in Hawaii and California prompted recruitment of laborers from Japan. Koreans started arriving in Hawaii in 1903, and Asian Indian laborers were being recruited to work in California by 1907. That year the Gentlemen's Agreement between the United States and Japan effectively barred further immigration of Japanese "laborers," but not of the parents, wives, and children of those already here (Takaki 1998). By then, the Philippines was a U.S. territory, so the Hawaii Sugar Plantation Association started recruiting Filipino workers. The National Origins Act of 1924 officially barred immigration from Japan and other Asian countries (Zane et al. 1994). But as residents of a U.S. territory, Filipinos could not be barred from immigrating. Tens of thousands sailed to the mainland from the Philippines and Hawaii to work in agricultural jobs in California, Oregon, and Washington, and in salmon canneries in Alaska. The Tydings-McDuffie Act of 1934 put the Philippines on the road to independence, allowing immigration to be limited to fifty Filipinos per year and classifying Filipinos already in the United States as "aliens." The law did not apply to Hawaii, so sugar plantations could continue to import Filipinos; however, Filipinos could not remigrate to the U.S. mainland from Hawaii (Takaki 1998).

These exclusionary immigration acts, along with other discriminatory laws and practices, severely limited the ability of early Asian immigrants to form families and communities. Plantation owners and other employers overwhelmingly recruited men; therefore, at least 90 percent of immigrants from China, Korea, India, and the Philippines were male. Even without these labor practices or exclusionary immigration laws, the migration of women was discouraged by cultural attitudes about single women traveling, or the laborer's belief that he would eventually return home (Takaki 1998). The Japanese were an exception: they were able to immigrate and work as families (Lott 1997). Anti-miscegenation laws, which forbade white women from marrying nonwhite men, further conspired to keep immigrants from marrying and starting families in those states where such laws were enforced. Nevertheless, interracial marriages and interracial children happened. The trend continues today in varying degrees by ethnic group (Qian et al. 2001). Finally, Asian political empowerment was limited by a 1790 law that restricted naturalization to whites. Although some exceptions were made at various times for various groups such as Hindus (because they were once classified as Caucasian) and Filipinos (who volunteered to fight in World War II), Asian immigrants were denied citizenship (Takaki 1998).

The period from World War II to the 1960s is characterized by a thaw in immigration and naturalization policies toward Asians, even though

**Table 30.3** Immigration and Naturalization Laws (including Asian exclusion acts)

| Year | Name/Event | Provisions |
| --- | --- | --- |
| 1790 | Naturalization Law | Restricted naturalized citizenship to whites |
| 1860 | Census | First enumeration of Asians |
| 1882 | Chinese Exclusion Act | Stopped immigration from China |
| 1898 | Treaty of Paris | Ended the Spanish-American War; United States purchases the Philippines for $20 million |
| 1907 | Gentleman's Agreement | Limited immigration from Japan |
| 1924 | National Origins Act | Excluded immigration from Asia |
| 1934 | Philippine Independence Act (a.k.a. Tydings-McDuffie Act) | Granted independence to the Philippines; limited Filipino immigration to 50 per year |
| 1952 | Immigration and Naturalization Act (a.k.a. McCarran-Walter Act) | Did away with racial restrictions on naturalization; established immigration quotas by country |
| 1965 | Immigration and Nationality Act | Did away with country quotas; established system of family preference |
| 1990 | Immigration Act | Substantially increased the number of professional category visas |

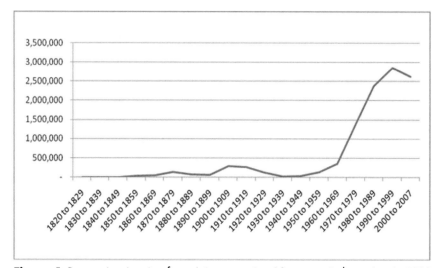

**Figure 1** Persons immigrating from Asian countries, 10-year periods starting in 1820
*Source:* Yearbook of Immigration Statistics 2007, Table 2 (U.S. Department of Homeland Security 2008).

the policies still preserved a preference for Europeans. Chinese exclusion was repealed in 1943, but immigration was limited to an annual quota of 105. The quota for Filipinos was similarly raised to 100 after World War II, and Filipinos and Asian Indians were allowed to become citizens. In 1952, the McCarran-Walter Act did away with the 1790 whites-only naturalization law, but it still enforced racism by allowing the unequal country quotas to continue. For example, the quota set in 1924 for Great Britain and Northern Ireland was 65,000, but that for Italy was only 6000 (Takaki 1998; Kitano and Daniels 2000). The quotas, however, did not apply to immediate relatives of U.S. citizens, so Asian Americans were able to sponsor family members. Other laws allowed for the entry of nonquota immigrants for work and study (Kitano and Daniels 2000). Thus, immigration from China, India, Korea, and the Philippines slowly and steadily increased until 1965, though immigration from Japan stabilized (U.S. Department of Homeland Security 2007). After 1965, immigration rates increased exponentially.

## POST-1965 IMMIGRATION PATTERNS

Considered in aggregate, the pre-1965 migrations comprise the first wave of Asian immigrants. The second wave was triggered by the unintentional pull of the Immigration and Nationality Act of 1965 and the unexpected push of refugees from Southeast Asia after 1975 (Takaki 1998; Ludden 2006; Zane et al. 1994). Whereas the first wave consisted mostly of men who thought they would eventually return to their home country, the second wave arrived as families with the intention of making America their new home. Employment-based immigrants were part of the second wave as well, but not as prominently as before. Immigrants in the second wave usually emigrated from cities rather than rural areas, and they had more education and skills than immigrants from the first wave (Takaki 1998). In contrast, the nature of forced migration meant that Southeast Asian refugees were more diverse, representing the gamut of educational attainment, occupations, and urban/rural experiences when they emigrated, and occupying lower socioeconomic status upon resettlement. Although the flow of Southeast Asian refugees has subsided, the second wave of Asian immigration continues unabated today because of the pull and push of subsequent amendments to the 1965 Immigration Act and complex global economic and political factors (Lobo and Salvo 1998; Skop and Li 2005).

## The Pull of Family

The 1965 Immigration Act changed the face of America (Ludden 2006). It did away with unequal quotas that favored European countries and instituted a standard annual quota of 20,000 immigrants per country, with a cap on annual admissions from the Eastern Hemisphere of 170,000, and 120,000 from the Western Hemisphere. The law established a preference for family reunification, allowing for 125,800 new immigrants annually under family categories compared to 34,000 under employment categories—a significant departure from the previous practice of prioritizing labor needs (Lobo and Salvo 1998). Thus, Asians who were already settled in the United States were able to petition for family members (Takaki 1998). Moreover, spouses, minor children, and parents of U.S. citizens were exempt from the country quota. Consequently, the actual number of annual immigrants was significantly higher for some countries, in some cases more than double: for example, more than 40,000 Chinese immigrants obtained legal permanent residence in Fiscal Year 2000. The administration did not anticipate that these provisions would result in such an extraordinary increase in the flow of immigrants from Asia and Latin America (Ludden 2006; Daniels 2007). More than 358,000 immigrants from Asian countries obtained legal permanent residence from 1960 to 1969. That number almost quadrupled in the next decade, to 1.4 million. It increased to 2.4 million from 1980 to 1989, then 2.8 million from 1990 to 1999. The number of immigrants from 2000 to 2007 has already reached 2.6 million (U.S. Department of Homeland Security 2008).

## Refugees Pushed Out of Southeast Asia

Refugees are considered a special class of immigrants, characterized by involuntary and forced migration due to war, persecution, or political unrest in their home country. Despite this special status, the United States has, at times, been as exclusionary toward refugees as toward other immigrants. For example, before World War II, the United States refused to accept 20,000 mostly Jewish children from Germany, children who might have been saved from the concentration camps. By the 1970s, the political consensus was that the United States had "failed the test of civilization" (Daniels 2007). So starting with the U.S. withdrawal from Vietnam in 1975 until 1993, the United States accepted more than one million refugees from the Southeast Asian countries of Vietnam, Cambodia, and Laos (Niedzwiecki and Duong 2003). More than 130,000 arrived in the first year alone (see Table 30.4).

**Table 30.4** Southeast Asian Refugee Arrivals to the United States, Fiscal Years 1975–2002 (SEARAC 2003)

| Fiscal Year | Cambodia | Laos | Vietnam | Annual Total | Cumulative Total |
|---|---|---|---|---|---|
| 1975 | 4,600 | 800 | 125,000 | 130,400 | 130,400 |
| 1976 | 1,100 | 10,200 | 3,200 | 14,500 | 144,900 |
| 1977 | 300 | 400 | 1,900 | 2,600 | 147,500 |
| 1978 | 1,300 | 8,000 | 11,100 | 20,400 | 167,900 |
| 1979 | 6,000 | 30,200 | 44,500 | 80,700 | 248,600 |
| 1980 | 16,000 | 55,500 | 95,200 | 166,700 | 415,300 |
| 1981 | 38,194 | 19,777 | 65,279 | 123,250 | 538,550 |
| 1982 | 6,246 | 3,616 | 27,396 | 37,258 | 575,808 |
| 1983 | 13,041 | 2,907 | 22,819 | 38,767 | 614,575 |
| 1984 | 19,727 | 7,218 | 24,856 | 51,801 | 666,376 |
| 1985 | 19,175 | 5,195 | 25,222 | 49,592 | 715,968 |
| 1986 | 9,845 | 12,313 | 21,700 | 43,858 | 759,826 |
| 1987 | 1,786 | 13,394 | 19,656 | 34,836 | 794,662 |
| 1988 | 2,897 | 14,597 | 17,571 | 35,065 | 829,727 |
| 1989 | 2,162 | 12,560 | 21,924 | 36,646 | 866,373 |
| 1990 | 2,329 | 8,715 | 27,797 | 38,841 | 905,214 |
| 1991 | 179 | 9,232 | 28,396 | 37,807 | 943,021 |
| 1992 | 163 | 7,285 | 26,795 | 34,243 | 977,264 |
| 1993 | 63 | 6,944 | 31,401 | 38,408 | 1,015,672 |
| 1994 | 15 | 6,211 | 34,110 | 40,336 | 1,056,008 |
| 1995 | 6 | 3,682 | 32,250 | 35,938 | 1,091,946 |
| 1996 | 5 | 2,203 | 16,107 | 18,315 | 1,110,261 |
| 1997 | 9 | 915 | 6,612 | 7,536 | 1,117,797 |
| 1998 | 7 | 9 | 10,266 | 10,282 | 1,128,079 |
| 1999 | – | 19 | 9,622 | 9,641 | 1,137,720 |
| 2000 | – | 64 | 2,839 | 2,903 | 1,140,623 |
| 2001 | 23 | 22 | 3,109 | 3,154 | 1,143,777 |
| 2002 | – | 18 | 2,855 | 2,873 | 1,146,650 |
| Totals | 145,172 | 241,996 | 759,482 | 1,146,650 | |

The refugees literally changed the face of America as they were resettled throughout the United States, including places where few other Asian Americans lived. In fact, the face of *Asian* America also changed as there were not many Southeast Asians in the United States at the time. From 1951 to 1974, less than 20,000 Southeast Asians entered the United States, mostly from Vietnam. However, they were mostly sojourners who had come to the United States to study and return home. There were only 603 Vietnamese living in the United States in 1964 as students and diplomats (Takaki 1998). Therefore, whereas post-1965 immigrants from China and the Philippines, for example, were joining families and communities, the refugees had no family or ethnic enclaves to rely on. As the tide of refugees steadily declined, starting in the mid-1980s, immigration through family reunification and other preferences increased. The annual number of Southeast Asians coming in as immigrants has surpassed the number coming as refugees since 1997 (Niedzwiecki and Duong 2003). Nevertheless, the initial lack of family networks and community infrastructure made refugee adjustment to the United States materially different from immigrant adjustment, not to mention the trauma of war, famine, and persecution.

## Geographic Settlement Patterns

As stated previously, the need for cheap labor and westward expansion was primarily responsible for the first wave of Asian immigrants. Hence, Asian immigrants settled primarily in the western states and in immigrant gateway cities such as New York City. After 1965, the preference for family reunification meant that new immigrants would settle initially in those areas where Asians were already living. According to the 2000 census, just over half (51 percent) of Asians lived in three states: California, New York, and Hawaii. The ten states with the largest Asian populations represented 75 percent of the Asian population (California, New York, Hawaii, Texas, New Jersey, Illinois, Washington, Florida, Virginia, and Massachusetts). By comparison, the total population of these ten states comprised only 47 percent of the total population of the United States (Barnes and Bennett 2002). Moreover, Asians are concentrated in metropolitan areas in these states, in the suburbs as well as urban centers (Skop and Li 2005).

Nevertheless, Asian populations are growing in other states and rural areas. The proportion of Asians living in California, New York, and Hawaii in 2000 was less than in 1990, when those three states comprised 58 percent of the Asian population (U.S. Census Bureau 1990). The Association of Asian Pacific Community Health Organizations (AAPCHO 2004) analyzed the 2000 census data for sixteen states and found significant growth in many Asian ethnic groups. To illustrate, Georgia's Asian Indian, Pakistani, and Vietnamese populations each more than tripled between 1990 and 2000. Similarly, Nevada's Filipino, Asian Indian, and Pakistani populations each tripled. North Carolina's Hmong population in 2000 was ten times larger than in 1990; its Vietnamese population increased by 199.3 percent, and its Laotian and Cambodian population increased by 120.9 percent. The Chinese population more than doubled in these three states; and the Korean population almost doubled in these states.

This trend toward dispersion is fueled by both new immigrants as well as migration from other states (Skop and Li 2005). For example, the Hmong, an ethnic group from Laos, arrived as refugees and were resettled throughout the United States. Soon after arriving, they began to relocate in large numbers to be closer to family and job opportunities. By the mid-1980s, this secondary migration made California home to more than half of the Hmong in the United States, concentrated in Fresno, a town in the rural central valley region. In the mid-1990s, Hmong started moving out of Fresno to Minnesota, Wisconsin, and other midwestern states to escape high unemployment and poor economic conditions (Yang 2001). California still has the largest number of Hmong (71,741; 40 percent of all Hmong Americans) followed by Minnesota (45,443; 24.4 percent), Wisconsin (36,809; 19.8 percent), North Carolina (7982; 4.3 percent), and Michigan (5998; 3.2 percent) (Niedzwiecki and Duong 2003).

## Complexities of Immigration Categories

The pathways to immigration today are exceedingly complex. Visas, the documents that represent one's immigration status, are one level of complexity. It is possible for one family to have members with different

**Table 30.5** Pathways to Legal Permanent Resident (LPR) Status (U.S. Department of Homeland Security 2008)

**Family-sponsored preferences (as amended in 1990):**
1. unmarried sons and daughters of U.S. citizens;
2. spouses, children, and unmarried sons and daughters of permanent resident aliens;
3. married sons and daughters of U.S. citizens;
4. brothers and sisters of U.S. citizens.

**Employment-based preferences are (as amended in 1990):**
1. priority workers (persons of extraordinary ability, outstanding professors and researchers, and certain multinational executives and managers);
2. professionals with advanced degrees or aliens with exceptional ability;
3. skilled workers, professionals (without advanced degrees), and needed unskilled workers;
4. special immigrants; and
5. employment creation immigrants (investors).

visas and for those members to be in the process of obtaining a different status. Therefore, it is likely that health care providers and community-based organizations will serve immigrants of all categories.

Legal permanent residents (LPRs), commonly known as green card holders, come in through family or employment preferences as listed in Table 30.5. Also referred to as legal resident aliens, they are able to petition family members to also become LPRs (Table 30.5, second family preference). Refugees and asylees constitute another category, with an annual cap set by the president. Nonimmigrant admissions applies to those individuals who come in as visitors for business or pleasure, temporary workers, foreign government officials and their families, or other purposes for a limited period of time: Their visas expire, though the period can vary from a few weeks to a few years, with renewals. Those who enter with nonimmigrant visas can also apply for legal permanent residence (U.S. Department of Homeland Security 2008). However, sometimes the application process goes well beyond the expiration date on their nonimmigrant visa, thus converting them into unauthorized immigrants, more commonly known as undocumented immigrants or illegal aliens, if they choose to remain in the country and "overstay their visa." Other unauthorized immigrants never had documents in the first place; however, there are legal processes available to some of them to legalize their status (Hoefer et al. 2007).

The Office of Immigration Statistics (OIS) annually reports numbers of immigrants by category. According to the OIS, more than 1.2 million people became LPRs in 2006, of which 65 percent were already living in the United States when they became LPRs. More than 422,000, or 33.4 percent, were born in an Asian country. Of the top ten source countries, four are in Asia: People's Republic of China (second with 87,345 LPRs), Philippines (third: 74,607), India (fourth: 61,369), and Vietnam (ninth: 30,695). Korea ranks eleventh with 24,386 LPRs, and Pakistan ranks eighteenth with 17,418 LPRs. Approximately 62 percent of those coming from Asian countries came through family connections, and 19 percent through employment-based preferences. Almost 16 percent were refugees and asylees from Asia who became eligible for LPR status after one year of U.S. residence (Jefferys 2007).

The OIS estimated the unauthorized immigrant population in 2006 at 11.6 million, an increase of 4.2 million since 2000. Approximately 1.4 million, or 12 percent, were born in Asia: of that, 95 percent were born in the Philippines, India, Korea, China, or Vietnam (Hoefer et al. 2007).

The preference for family reunification still exists as of this writing. However, subsequent amendments to the 1965 Immigration Act and more recent proposals from Congress and the White House may signal a shift toward prioritizing employment-based immigration over family reunification. Congress did away with the hemispheric caps in 1978, establishing one worldwide annual cap of 270,000 immigrants, with 216,000 allotted for family preferences and 54,000 for employment preferences—a ratio of 4 to 1. The Immigration Act of 1990 increased the worldwide annual cap to 461,000, but the allotment for family preferences was only increased by 10,000, to 226,000, while the allotment for employment preferences increased by more than 250 percent, to 140,000—a ratio of 1.6 to 1 (Lobo and Salvo 1998). This represents a significant change in policy, though the previously mentioned OIS data suggest that family preferences still predominate for Asian countries of origin. In 2007, the White House sought to limit family categories to nuclear family and parents, and add new employment visa categories (The White House 2007). Congress has not considered these proposals as of this writing; however, considerable opposition to them exists among Asian American advocacy organizations (Asian American Justice Center 2007).

## IMMIGRATION AND HEALTH

Being an immigrant has a significant impact on the health of Asian Americans. Immigration influences demographic characteristics such as nativity, English language proficiency, and citizenship status, as well as socioeconomic status (SES) variables such as educational attainment, income, poverty, and occupation. All of these factors are part of the ecosystem impacting the health status of Asian Americans. However, research has only just begun to show the extent to which these factors influence health, in what direction, and how they are related to one another (i.e., dependent or independent variables). More research is needed to document trends and to discover their underlying causes. Furthermore, researchers must be able to differentiate among specific Asian ethnic populations and/or immigrant cohorts, given their diverse cultures, demographics, socioeconomic positions, immigration histories, and acculturation experiences. What follows is a brief discussion of some of the research to date. The findings from this research strongly suggest that the health care needs of foreign-born Asian Americans are different from U.S.-born Asian Americans, which should be considered in developing health interventions (Dhooper 2003). Additionally, Asian Americans regardless of immigration status are underserved in health care in comparison to the general population. This can be attributed to the extraordinary population growth of the past 40 years, lack of health data, and the assumption that Asian Americans are a healthy model minority (Chen and Hawks 1995).

### Nativity and Acculturation

The net effect of continuous and increasing immigration since 1965 is that a significant portion of Asian Americans, as a whole and by specific ethnic group, is foreign born. As shown in Table 30.6, approximately 13 percent of U.S. residents are foreign born compared to two-thirds of

**Table 30.6** Proportion of Native- and Foreign-born by Asian Subgroup, and Proportion of Foreign-born by Date of Entry

| | Total Population | Native | % | Foreign Born | % | Foreign born | | |
| --- | --- | --- | --- | --- | --- | --- | --- | --- |
| | | | | | | Entered 2000 or Later | Entered 1990 to 1999 | Entered Before 1990 |
| Total | 299,398,485 | 261,851,170 | 87.5% | 37,547,315 | 12.5% | 25.3% | 30.5% | 44.1% |
| Asian alone | 13,100,095 | 4,295,286 | 33% | 8,804,809 | 67% | 24.5% | 30.7% | 44.8% |
| Asian Indian alone | 2,482,141 | 642,002 | 26% | 1,840,139 | 74% | 32.7% | 35.2% | 32.1% |
| Cambodian alone | 212,157 | 78,545 | 37% | 133,612 | 63% | 11.7% | 13.1% | 75.1% |
| Chinese alone | 3,090,453 | 937,415 | 30% | 2,153,038 | 70% | 23.3% | 31.2% | 45.5% |
| Filipino alone | 2,328,097 | 782,883 | 34% | 1,545,214 | 66% | 21.1% | 28.0% | 50.9% |
| Hmong alone | 205,101 | 113,703 | 55% | 91,398 | 45% | 11.7% | 28.9% | 59.4% |
| Indonesian alone | 66,431 | 16,482 | 25% | 49,949 | 75% | 36.8% | 36.0% | 27.1% |
| Japanese alone | 829,767 | 500,175 | 60% | 329,592 | 40% | 40.3% | 20.0% | 39.7% |
| Korean alone | 1,335,075 | 332,975 | 25% | 1,002,100 | 75% | 24.0% | 23.6% | 52.4% |
| Laotian alone | 194,320 | 72,873 | 38% | 121,447 | 62% | 4.1% | 14.3% | 81.6% |
| Pakistani alone | 194,462 | 56,760 | 29% | 137,702 | 71% | 28.0% | 41.1% | 30.9% |
| Thai alone | 150,414 | 35,088 | 23% | 115,326 | 77% | 23.0% | 20.1% | 56.8% |
| Vietnamese alone | 1,475,798 | 485,902 | 33% | 989,896 | 67% | 14.8% | 39.5% | 45.7% |

*Source:* U.S. Census Bureau, 2006; American Community Survey, 2007.

Asians. More than two-thirds of Thai, Indonesians, Koreans, Asian Indians, Pakistani, and Chinese are foreign born. Moreover, one-quarter of foreign-born Asians arrived in 2000 or later, with Pakistanis, Asian Indians, Indonesians, and surprisingly, Japanese, exceeding that rate (U.S. Census Bureau 2007).

The connection between immigration and health rests on two hypotheses: first, foreign-born individuals are generally healthier than native-born individuals because migration tends to select for healthier individuals; second, this "immigrant advantage" fades with time spent in the United States (duration) as immigrants acculturate or adopt behaviors of the dominant culture. Asian and Pacific Islander (API) respondents to two large national surveys—the National Health Interview Survey (NHIS) and the National Longitudinal Mortality Study (NLMS)—seem to conform to the immigrant advantage and acculturation hypotheses (Frisbie et al. 2001; Singh and Siahpush 2002). Paradoxically, better health among newer immigrants seems to exist despite the fact that APIs who have been in the United States for less than ten years are three to four times more likely to have *no* regular source of care (Frisbie et al. 2001). Furthermore, socioeconomic and demographic variables such as education, income, marital status, and place of residence do not seem to contribute to the differences between foreign-born and U.S.-born APIs (Singh and Siahpush 2002). This does not mean socioeconomic status has no effect, only that its effects remain undiscovered.

The National Health Interview Survey (NHIS) is an annual survey of U.S. households that collects data on socioeconomic status, demographics, health behavior, morbidity, and health care utilization. Frisbie et al. (2001) analyzed data from the 1992–1995 NHIS, which yielded a sample of 8249 APIs. Enough data were available to analyze eight groups separately: Chinese, Filipino, Asian Indian, Japanese, Korean, Vietnamese, Pacific Islander, and Other Asians. Additionally, the sample was segmented into four cohorts by nativity and duration: immigrant, 0–4 years in the United States; immigrant, 5–9 years; immigrant, 10 or more years; and U.S.-born. In general, health outcomes were better for the "immigrant, 0–4 years" groups, rating their health as good or better,[2] reporting fewer limitations to daily activities and fewer days in bed due to illness. Analyzing a smaller sample of the NHIS (1993–1994), Singh et al. (2002) found foreign-born APIs to have substantially lower risks of smoking, obesity, hypertension, and chronic conditions than U.S.-born APIs; but, consistent with the acculturation hypothesis, these risks increased with duration in the United States. This study did not disaggregate the Asian population by ethnicity.

The National Longitudinal Mortality Study (NLMS) tracked the causes of death of a fixed sample of individuals from 1979 to 1989, in association with socioeconomic, occupational, and demographic factors. Singh et al. (2002) showed that in comparison to U.S.-born whites with equivalent socioeconomic and demographic characteristics, U.S.-born APIs had 32 percent lower mortality risk, and foreign-born APIs had 43 percent lower mortality risk. The same trend held for both males and females, and for specific causes of death. For example, U.S.-born APIs and foreign-born APIs had 29 percent and 58 percent, respectively, of lower cardiovascular disease mortality risk than U.S.-born whites of equivalent background. Although these trends in mortality and the aforementioned trends in morbidity have been observed, it is not known exactly why they exist. The ways in which such variables as health behavior, social support, conditions in the country of origin, and acculturation impact the differences between foreign born and U.S. born have yet to be described.

When comparing Asian ethnic groups to one another (as opposed to native born versus foreign born), a seemingly opposite consequence of duration has been observed: the longer duration of an immigrant *group* in the United States translates into positive social, economic, and political adaptations, which in turn confers health advantages. In the NHIS sample studied by Frisbie et al. (2001), 88.6 percent of the Chinese and 91.8 percent of the Japanese reported their health as good, very good, or excellent, while only 75.8 percent of the Vietnamese did. As documented by the Census Bureau, the Chinese and the Japanese are the two groups with the longest duration in the United States, and Southeast Asian refugees have the shortest duration.

However, there is significant variation between groups and between different health measures. A larger proportion of Asian Indians than of Vietnamese is new immigrants, having arrived in 2000 or later (24.5 percent versus 14.8 percent, from Table 30.6), yet 85.6 percent of Asian Indians reported their health as good or better. This particular finding may reflect the continuing impact of refugee trauma (Frisbie et al. 2001; Kandula et al. 2007). Other variations between groups may be explained by diversity of cultural norms or other factors that are not included in statistical models. For example, low self-reported ratings of health could be a reflection of more holistic concepts of health among many traditional Asian cultures. Thus, Asians may rate their health lower even in the absence of physical ailments or medical disease because they are also considering emotional or spiritual well-being (Kandula et al. 2007). Also, the National Health Interview Survey, like most national surveys, is administered in English, thus biasing the sample toward those who already show some level of acculturation. A study of Asian respondents to the California Health Interview Survey (CHIS), which is administered in several Asian languages, showed that individuals with limited English proficiency rated their health lower than those who were English proficient (Kandula et al. 2007).

The existence of health advantages conferred by positive social, economic, and political adaptations argues for the importance of community organizing as a means to attaining better health outcomes for the

**Table 30.7** Citizenship and Naturalization

| | Population of Naturalized U.S. Citizens | Population of Foreign-born | Naturalization Rate |
|---|---|---|---|
| Total population | 15,767,731 | 37,547,789 | 42.0% |
| Asian alone | 4,894,046 | 8,804,809 | 55.6% |
| Asian Indian alone | 829,393 | 1,840,139 | 45.1% |
| Cambodian alone | 77,037 | 133,612 | 57.7% |
| Chinese alone | 1,264,837 | 2,153,038 | 58.7% |
| Filipino alone | 965,403 | 1,545,214 | 62.5% |
| Hmong alone | 53,803 | 91,398 | 58.9% |
| Indonesian alone | 15,371 | 49,949 | 30.8% |
| Japanese alone | 86,180 | 329,592 | 26.1% |
| Korean alone | 542,243 | 1,002,100 | 54.1% |
| Laotian alone | 72,611 | 121,447 | 59.8% |
| Pakistani alone | 76,403 | 137,702 | 55.5% |
| Thai alone | 61,350 | 115,326 | 53.2% |
| Vietnamese alone | 709,049 | 989,896 | 71.6% |

*Source:* U.S. Census Bureau, 2006; American Community Survey, 2007.

population. Specific examples of such organizing are discussed at the end of the chapter.

## Citizenship

Most LPRs are eligible to be naturalized (become citizens) after five years of residence. The naturalization rate for Asian Americans is 55.6 percent. The percentage ranges from 71.6 percent for the Vietnamese to 26.1 percent for the Japanese; however, with the exception of the Japanese, Indonesians (30.8 percent), and Asian Indians (45.1 percent), more than half of all other Asian ethnic groups become citizens. The relatively low rate of Asian Indian naturalization may be due to the significant numbers of recent immigrants (U.S. Census Bureau 2007).

Lack of citizenship can have an adverse impact on an immigrant's ability to get health insurance and receive high-quality care. Citizens are more likely to have jobs that offer private health insurance; noncitizens are more likely to work for employers that do not. Owing to 1996 federal legislation, LPRs who have been lawfully present in the United States for less than five years can be denied Medicaid and other types of public assistance even though their low income level, lack of health insurance, and poor health would otherwise qualify them for assistance (Ku 2007). In practice, this has created a patchwork maze of eligibility qualifications and exceptions depending on other laws, age, health condition, and availability of state funding. Refugees and asylees are exempt from this policy, and they can continue to get insurance for their first seven years of U.S. residence. However, after these initial years, many refugees and asylees will face the inevitable challenge of maintaining health insurance coverage. Almost half of the states have "replacement" programs that provide the coverage that would have been paid for by federal funds. Still, disparities in health insurance coverage between low-income, immigrant children and low-income, native-born citizen children have increased. From 1995 to 2005, the uninsurance rate dropped for low-income, native-born citizen children from 19 percent to 15 percent. In the same time period, the uninsurance rate for low-income, immigrant children including Hispanics and Asians increased from 44 percent to 48 percent (Ku 2007). LPRs can live and work anywhere in the United States and serve in the U.S. armed forces (U.S. Department of Homeland Security 2008). Yet, they are excluded from needed public health insurance that assists other low-income, working people.

## Language

The diversity of languages that Asian Americans speak challenges the nation's health care system. Immigrants from Asia speak more than 100 languages—including English, which is commonly spoken in several Asian countries. Still, about 77 percent of Asian Americans speak a language other than English at home according to the Census Bureau (2007).

**Table 30.8** Language

| | Population 5 Years and Over | English Only | Language Other than English | Speak English Less than "Very Well" (LEP) |
|---|---|---|---|---|
| Total population | 279,012,712 | 80.3% | 19.7% | 8.7% |
| Asian alone | 12,271,573 | 23.3% | 76.7% | 36.0% |
| Asian Indian alone | 2,278,866 | 20.5% | 79.5% | 22.6% |
| Cambodian alone | 199,060 | 17.4% | 82.6% | 44.2% |
| Chinese alone | 2,911,016 | 16.6% | 83.4% | 46.4% |
| Filipino alone | 2,210,104 | 33.4% | 66.6% | 22.1% |
| Hmong alone | 183,020 | 5.6% | 94.4% | 42.6% |
| Indonesian alone | 61,262 | 23.8% | 76.2% | 35.7% |
| Japanese alone | 802,967 | 54.5% | 45.5% | 25.4% |
| Korean alone | 1,265,188 | 19.7% | 80.3% | 47.2% |
| Laotian alone | 181,987 | 11.7% | 88.3% | 45.4% |
| Pakistani alone | 176,086 | 13.5% | 86.5% | 30.6% |
| Thai alone | 147,030 | 22.3% | 77.7% | 42.8% |
| Vietnamese alone | 1,375,962 | 13.9% | 86.1% | 52.9% |

*Source:* U.S. Census Bureau, 2006; American Community Survey, 2007.

This includes 2.5 million people who speak Chinese and more than one million speakers each of Tagalog, Korean, and Vietnamese. A second measure of language use is proficiency in English. The census asks respondents to assess their English language proficiency by choosing one of the following options: "Very well," "Well," "Not well," or "Not at all." Those who speak it less than "Very well" are considered as having limited English proficiency (LEP).[3] In aggregate, 36 percent of Asian Americans are LEP. However, there is wide variation, with a larger proportion of Vietnamese, Korean, and Chinese who are LEP (52.9 percent, 47.2 percent, and 46.4 percent, respectively). Asian Indians and Filipinos, because of their histories of colonization by English-speaking nations, are the least likely to be LEP—22.6 percent and 22.1 percent, respectively (U.S. Census Bureau 2007). The final measure of language use is linguistic isolation, a measure of a household's capacity to communicate in English. In linguistically isolated households, there is no one over the age of 14 who speaks English "very well." Nationally, 27.4 percent of households that speak an Asian or Pacific Islander language are linguistically isolated; and 16.5 percent of households that speak an Indo-European language (not including Spanish, but including South Asian languages) are linguistically isolated (U.S. Census Bureau 2007).

As mentioned previously, research on the health of Asian American populations does not adequately take into account the impact of being LEP. First, most surveys are conducted only in English (and increasingly, Spanish), effectively leaving out linguistically isolated Asian households and LEP individuals. Second, the health status of LEP Asians cannot be assumed to be similar to that of English-proficient Asians. As demonstrated by CHIS and other research that is conducted in an Asian language, their health status is often worse. Finally, how foreign language and culture influence one's interpretation of the questions and possible responses is not fully understood (Kandula et al. 2007).

Even though inclusion in research is important, it is in the access to and actual provision of care that being LEP can have life-threatening consequences. Compared to proficient English speakers, LEP patients are less likely to have health insurance and less likely to receive preventive care. When patients and providers cannot speak the same language (provider-patient language discordance), physicians order unnecessary diagnostic procedures and cannot communicate directions for taking medication correctly; patients miss out on health education, leave unsatisfied with the care, and are likely to miss follow-up care (Green et al. 2005; Ngo-Metzger et al. 2007).

Interpreter services and provider-patient language concordance have been shown to improve health care and satisfaction among LEP Asian patients. A study of four community health centers in Massachusetts revealed that Chinese and Vietnamese LEP patients preferred high-quality, professional interpreters over family members (Ngo-Metzger et al. 2003).

The use of family members as interpreters is rightly discouraged because of concerns about confidentiality, conflict of interest, and competence (their knowledge of medical terminology in either language may be limited). The patients also preferred interpreters to be of the same sex. A much larger study of eleven community health centers nationwide suggests that having a language-concordant provider may be preferable to using an interpreter, at least for Chinese and Vietnamese patients (Green et al. 2005; Ngo-Metzger et al. 2007). Patients using an interpreter were less likely to ask questions, especially about mental health, than those with language-concordant providers. This may be due to the difficulty in establishing rapport with a physician through an interpreter and to perceived time pressures. Similar findings have been reported for patients using Spanish-language interpreters. Despite this communication barrier, patients were equally satisfied with either method of communication (Green et al. 2005). The same preferences may not hold for other ethnic groups. And given the number of LEP Asians, both professional, competent interpreters *and* competently bilingual physicians should be more available. Having an interpreter does facilitate health education as much as a language-concordant provider (Ngo-Metzger et al. 2007).

Although language has been a barrier to accessing quality health care, it is not an excuse for providing poor quality care or denying care altogether. Providing meaningful access to health care regardless of English-language proficiency is a civil rights issue as well as a quality of care issue. The foundation for this was laid even before the influx of immigrants with the passage of the Civil Rights Act of 1964. The act banned discrimination based on race, color, or national origin. Language has been interpreted to be closely related enough to national origin such that discrimination based on inability to speak English is the same thing as discrimination based on national origin (U.S. Department of Health and Human Services 2003). Acts that hinder the meaningful access to health care because of English language proficiency may therefore be deemed discrimination.

## SOCIOENONOMIC STATUS AND THE MODEL MINORITY MYTH

The relatively high socioeconomic status (SES) of Asian Americans, as measured by their educational attainment, income, and other factors, has led to the characterization of Asians as the model minority. The *New York Times Magazine* first used the term "model minority" in 1966 to marvel at the success of Japanese Americans despite the long history of discrimination against them, culminating in their internment during World War II. A similar story touting Chinese American success appeared in *U.S. News and World Report* later that same year. Given the times, this new myth was a rebuke of the landmark civil rights law enacted just a year earlier. The underlying message was that institutional racism of the type that the civil rights movement sought to undo was impossible given the success of

Asian Americans. Working hard and not complaining was enough to achieve success in America (Danico and Ng 2004). As new immigrants began arriving, they were enveloped in this expectation of success no matter the barrier. Even the trauma of war could be overcome: Southeast Asian refugees were profiled as part of "Asian-Americans: A Model Minority" by *Newsweek* in 1982. While acknowledging the socioeconomic extremes occupied by Asians, with Southeast Asians at the low end, the article nonetheless treated Asian American success as the inexorable result of hard work and superior values. The article also acknowledged past discrimination, noting the centennial of the 1882 Chinese Exclusion Act, but made no mention of civil rights. Yet it is reasonable to attribute, though difficult to quantify, some of Asian Americans' supposed success to the civil rights movement, which created opportunities and assured that new immigrants would not be mistreated at work or school like their predecessors were.

So the myth persists. But the reality of how Asian Americans have achieved their socioeconomic status (whether high or low) is not so easily explained. Just as their immigration stories vary, their SES also varies— wildly. And as for how SES affects their health, research is beginning to uncover some unexpected patterns. SES may have a different meaning or impact across different racial and ethnic groups (Kandula et al. 2007).

## Educational Attainment

Census surveys ask for the "highest degree or level of education completed" for those who are 25 years of age and older. Asians, as a whole, have a similar percentage of people with "less than a high school diploma" (14.4 percent) compared to the general U.S. population (15.9 percent). However, there is a wide variation depending on ethnicity. Southeast Asians have significantly higher percentages of people who have not completed high school: 39.3 percent of Hmong, 37.7 percent of Laotians, 35.0 percent of Cambodians, and 27.8 percent of Vietnamese. In addition, 18.4 percent of Chinese do not have a high school diploma. At the other end of the educational spectrum, 49.2 percent of Asians have attained a bachelor's degree or higher, which is a much higher proportion than the general U.S. population of 27.0 percent. Again, however, lower proportions of Southeast Asians have attained a bachelor's degree or higher—lower, even, than the general U.S. population: 10.8 percent of Laotians, 12.7 percent of Hmong, 13.8 percent of Cambodians, and 26.0 percent of Vietnamese. In terms of male and female educational attainment, more Asian men achieve a bachelor's or higher, with the exception of Filipinos (U.S. Census Bureau 2007).

The census does not ask where the education or degree was attained. Therefore, educational attainment is not a measure of achievement in U.S. schools. While many immigrants arrive at a young age and complete all

**Table 30.9** Educational Attainment

| | Population 25 Years and Over | Less than High School Diploma | High school Graduate (Includes Equivalency) | Some College or Associate's Degree | Bachelor's Degree | Graduate or Professional Degree |
|---|---|---|---|---|---|---|
| Total population | 195,932,824 | 15.9% | 30.2% | 26.9% | 17.1% | 9.9% |
| Asian alone | 8,902,052 | 14.4% | 17.4% | 18.9% | 29.6% | 19.6% |
| Asian Indian alone | 1,671,281 | 9.7% | 11.6% | 10.2% | 32.1% | 36.5% |
| Cambodian alone | 120,351 | 35.0% | 29.4% | 21.8% | 11.3% | 2.5% |
| Chinese alone | 2,152,735 | 18.4% | 16.0% | 13.9% | 25.4% | 26.3% |
| Filipino alone | 1,644,266 | 8.3% | 15.7% | 28.7% | 39.1% | 8.2% |
| Hmong alone | 76,631 | 39.3% | 24.4% | 23.6% | 10.5% | 2.2% |
| Indonesian alone | 45,251 | 4.6% | 21.6% | 26.8% | 32.4% | 14.6% |
| Japanese alone | 672,023 | 6.5% | 20.7% | 26.6% | 31.8% | 14.5% |
| Korean alone | 891,547 | 8.8% | 20.5% | 17.9% | 35.0% | 17.8% |
| Laotian alone | 116,800 | 37.7% | 30.3% | 21.2% | 8.9% | 1.9% |
| Pakistani alone | 110,261 | 12.9% | 16.4% | 16.3% | 31.2% | 23.2% |
| Thai alone | 117,639 | 15.9% | 19.3% | 23.7% | 26.3% | 14.8% |
| Vietnamese alone | 983,849 | 27.8% | 24.2% | 22.0% | 18.6% | 7.4% |

*Source:* U.S. Census Bureau, 2006; American Community Survey, 2007.

or part of their schooling in the United States, many others immigrate because they cannot find jobs in their home country that match their level of education. Immigration policy favors educated professionals. For example, more than 4000 Philippine-educated engineers and scientists immigrated to the United States from 1966 to 1970, as did a comparable number of Philippine-educated physicians and nurses (Choy 2003). The flow of nurses has been constant ever since. More recently, U.S. school systems have been filling teacher shortages by recruiting hundreds of teachers from the Philippines (Katigbak 2008).

The distinction of foreign-educated or U.S.-educated is significant for Asian Americans. For the U.S. population in general, those with more education are also healthier on a number of health status measures. More education tends to lead to more and better employment opportunities and higher income which, in turn, leads to better access to health care, lifestyles that promote healthy behavior, and the psychosocial supports for that behavior. However, this "health return on increased education" may be diminished for those who are educated outside of the United States (Walton and Takeuchi 2005). Data from the National Latino & Asian American Survey (NLAAS), the most comprehensive study of Asian Americans to date, show that those educated in the United States were more likely to rate their health as good, whereas foreign-educated Asian Americans were more likely to rate their health as poor (Walton and Takeuchi 2005).

The explanation for the low health return on education is not clear. Those who are educated abroad may also experience lower income and occupational returns, relative to those who are U.S.-educated. For example, many foreign medical graduates do not practice medicine in the United States because equivalency exams are difficult to pass, which may be related to language or financial issues. Consequently, their higher educational attainment does not lead to higher income, which in turn does not lead to higher health status. However, cohort studies that would empirically match location of educational attainment, income level, and health status—and perhaps suggest which variable is a consequence of the other—do not exist. Finally, although self-reported health is accepted as a robust measure of health, it is still just one measure. Therefore, it may be premature to expect other health indicators to be similarly influenced by foreign educational attainment.

## Income and Poverty

Low income and high rates of poverty have been associated with lack of health insurance, lower health care utilization, and worse health outcomes for Asian Americans as well as the general population. For example, a review of NHIS data from 1997 to 2000 showed that Asian children of mothers with high rates of poverty and low educational attainment

**Table 30.10** Income

|  | Households | Median Household Income (Dollars) | Average Household Size | Per Person in Household |
|---|---|---|---|---|
| Total population | 111,617,402 | 48,451 | 2.61 | 18,564 |
| Asian alone | 4,141,995 | 63,642 | 3.03 | 21,004 |
| Asian Indian alone | 815,231 | 78,315 | 3.03 | 25,847 |
| Cambodian alone | 53,655 | 47,743 | 3.92 | 12,179 |
| Chinese alone | 1,029,424 | 62,705 | 2.89 | 21,697 |
| Filipino alone | 664,054 | 72,548 | 3.34 | 21,721 |
| Hmong alone | 37,704 | 44,164 | 5.33 | 8,286 |
| Indonesian alone | 21,323 | 57,594 | 3.06 | 18,822 |
| Japanese alone | 357,649 | 61,276 | 2.29 | 26,758 |
| Korean alone | 446,530 | 50,565 | 2.71 | 18,659 |
| Laotian alone | 47,554 | 54,490 | 4.05 | 13,454 |
| Pakistani alone | 51,303 | 55,908 | 3.75 | 14,909 |
| Thai alone | 49,512 | 48,140 | 2.69 | 17,896 |
| Vietnamese alone | 424,026 | 52,299 | 3.39 | 15,427 |

*Source:* U.S. Census Bureau, 2006; American Community Survey, 2007.

were more likely to rate their health as poor and less likely to have a usual source of care, when compared to children of mothers with a college education and not in poverty (Yu et al. 2004). A study of Chinese in San Francisco showed that poverty (as well as language and citizenship status) was a significant barrier to access and use of health care (Jang et al. 1998).

Measures of income and poverty among various Asian American ethnic groups vary widely, as one should expect by this point in the chapter. It is also important to consider the artifacts of survey design when interpreting these data. Median household income, which tends to be higher for Asians than for the general population, must be considered in relation to average household sizes, which also tend to be larger among Asians. The definition of poverty, which tends to be lower for Asians than for the general population, is based on pretax cash income with no consideration for geography (Asians tend to live in metropolitan areas with a higher cost of living) or for the various types of expenses a household may have (immigrants must pay significant fees for visa and naturalization applications). The threshold for poverty is based on family size and whether children live in the household (U.S. Census Bureau 2007).

As shown in Table 30.10, the median household income for the United States is $48,451, which must provide for the 2.61 people in the average household: this comes out to $18,564 per person. The median household income for Asian Americans is $63,642, which seems significantly higher than the U.S. average until one considers that their average household has

**Table 30.11** Poverty

| | All People | Under 18 Years | 18 to 64 Years | 65 Years and Over | People in Families | Average Family Size | Total Population |
|---|---|---|---|---|---|---|---|
| Total population | 13.3% | 18.3% | 12.0% | 9.9% | 10.8% | 3.2 | 299,398,485 |
| Asian alone | 10.7% | 11.6% | 10.2% | 12.3% | 8.0% | 3.53 | 13,100,095 |
| Asian Indian alone | 8.2% | 8.7% | 8.0% | 7.9% | 6.1% | 3.45 | 2,482,141 |
| Cambodian alone | 18.5% | 24.0% | 16.3% | 16.5% | 16.9% | 4.13 | 212,157 |
| Chinese alone | 12.1% | 10.2% | 11.7% | 17.9% | 8.8% | 3.4 | 3,090,453 |
| Filipino alone | 5.3% | 5.7% | 5.0% | 6.2% | 3.3% | 3.72 | 2,328,097 |
| Hmong alone | 26.6% | 30.9% | 22.5% | 26.9% | 26.1% | 5.49 | 205,101 |
| Indonesian alone | 11.8% | 10.2% | 12.3% | 10.1% | 7.6% | 3.47 | 66,431 |
| Japanese alone | 9.1% | 6.4% | 10.3% | 7.3% | 3.4% | 2.98 | 829,767 |
| Korean alone | 13.7% | 12.6% | 13.6% | 17.8% | 9.8% | 3.28 | 1,335,075 |
| Laotian alone | 11.7% | 16.5% | 9.9% | 11.7% | 9.8% | 4.33 | 194,320 |
| Pakistani alone | 17.2% | 25.2% | 14.0% | 7.6% | 16.9% | 4.26 | 194,462 |
| Thai alone | 13.3% | 20.2% | 12.7% | 5.0% | 7.2% | 3.27 | 150,414 |
| Vietnamese alone | 13.6% | 16.0% | 12.4% | 16.4% | 11.3% | 3.8 | 1,475,798 |

*Source:* U.S. Census Bureau, 2006; American Community Survey, 2007.

3.03 people: this comes out to $21,004 per person. In relation to their average household size, Southeast Asians, Pakistanis, and Thai have lower median household incomes than the general U.S. population.

As for poverty, shown in Table 30.11, 10.7 percent of Asian Americans live in poverty, compared to 13.3 percent of the general population. The variation by ethnicity is extremely wide: the poverty rate of the Hmong is 26.6 percent, which is five times the rate of Filipinos (5.3 percent). Other Southeast Asian groups and Pakistanis also have high rates of poverty.

## Occupational Diversity

Asian immigrants, like immigrants from other continents, tend to cluster in certain jobs or industries. This may be caused by their visa status. Filipino nurses, Asian Indian technology workers, and Chinese scientists are examples of people who immigrate through employment preferences, and therefore they may be more likely to work at a level that is equivalent to their education. For other immigrants, being LEP leads them to service sector jobs where English is not necessary; hence Laotian meatpackers, Korean grocers and dry cleaners, Vietnamese nail salon workers, and South Asian taxi drivers and housekeepers of all ethnicities. Finally, community connections facilitate access to certain industries, thereby reinforcing labor market segmentation, particularly at the low-end of the market (Sanders et al. 2002). However, this is not always the case, as Asian Indians own 46 percent of the economy hotels and motels in the United States (Danico and Ng 2004).

According to Table 30.12, 34 percent of U.S. civilians aged 16 years and over are in "management, professional, and related occupations." This category includes most health care employees. For Asians, the proportion is much higher, at 46.7 percent. However, Southeast Asians are less likely than the general U.S. population to be employed in these occupations: 15.9 percent of Laotians, 19.8 percent of Cambodians, 20.1 percent of Hmong, and 30 percent of Vietnamese. Southeast Asians are more likely to be employed in "production, transportation, and material moving occupations" (39.3 percent of Laotians, 35.0 percent of Hmong, 27.3 of Cambodians, 20.5 percent of Vietnamese) compared to the U.S. population (13.0 percent) and the Asian population in aggregate (10.5 percent). As mentioned previously, many immigrants are not in occupations that match their educational attainment. Whether this improves over time for first generation immigrants is not clear.

Asian Americans may experience health disparities in access and outcomes because of disproportionate representation in some industries. Companies with 100 or more employees are more likely to have employer-sponsored health insurance, compared to companies with 100 or fewer employees. Therefore, people who work for smaller companies, such as ethnic-owned businesses, are more likely to be uninsured. In

**Table 30.12** Occupational Diversity

| | Civilian Employed Population 16 Years and Over | Management, Professional, and Related Occupations | Service Occupations | Sales and Office Occupations | Farming, Fishing, and Forestry Occupations | Construction, Extraction, Maintenance, and Repair Occupations | Production, Transportation, and Material Moving Occupations |
|---|---|---|---|---|---|---|---|
| Total population | 141,501,434 | 34.0% | 16.5% | 25.9% | 0.7% | 10.0% | 13.0% |
| Asian alone | 6,526,309 | 46.7% | 15.6% | 23.3% | 0.2% | 3.7% | 10.5% |
| Asian Indian alone | 1,287,051 | 62.2% | 7.3% | 20.7% | 0.2% | 2.2% | 7.4% |
| Cambodian alone | 94,125 | 19.8% | 19.0% | 27.0% | 0.2% | 6.6% | 27.3% |
| Chinese alone | 1,539,423 | 53.4% | 15.4% | 20.8% | 0.1% | 3.1% | 7.3% |
| Filipino alone | 1,262,010 | 40.6% | 19.0% | 26.8% | 0.4% | 4.1% | 9.2% |
| Hmong alone | 67,402 | 20.1% | 16.2% | 23.6% | 0.8% | 4.3% | 35.0% |
| Indonesian alone | 34,458 | 39.4% | 25.4% | 23.7% | 0.2% | 3.3% | 8.1% |
| Japanese alone | 405,367 | 51.5% | 12.8% | 25.7% | 0.2% | 4.3% | 5.5% |
| Korean alone | 619,453 | 43.9% | 14.6% | 28.9% | 0.1% | 3.7% | 8.8% |
| Laotian alone | 91,086 | 15.9% | 17.2% | 19.8% | 0.7% | 7.1% | 39.3% |
| Pakistani alone | 86,215 | 39.2% | 10.1% | 33.4% | 0.1% | 3.2% | 14.1% |
| Thai alone | 84,585 | 32.4% | 30.7% | 22.5% | 0.1% | 4.2% | 10.1% |
| Vietnamese alone | 715,762 | 30.0% | 24.3% | 18.9% | 0.5% | 5.7% | 20.5% |

*Source:* U.S. Census Bureau, 2006; American Community Survey, 2007.

fact, Koreans are more likely than other Asians to work in these small business (60 percent compared to 40 percent), and they have the highest rate (31 percent) of uninsurance of all Asian groups (Henry J. Kaiser Family Foundation 2008). The extent to which occupation influences health outcomes is less clear. The first peer-reviewed study of the impact of carcinogens and other chemical exposures on nail salon workers in California, the majority of whom are Vietnamese women, revealed that 62 percent said they had developed a health problem after they started working in a salon. The women reported headaches, skin problems, trouble breathing, and chronic pain. The investigators will need to conduct further studies to determine if there is a link to cancer rates (Adams 2008).

## BUILDING COMMUNITIES, BUILDING MOVEMENTS

The Asian American movement, if one can be said to exist, was built upon the organizing experiences and social capital amassed by the first wave of immigrants. Forced into ethnic enclaves, they built organizations for mutual assistance and to organize—often with other racial and ethnic groups—against the racism and discrimination they faced (Takaki 1998; Zia 2000). The mission of the Japanese American Citizens League, founded in 1929, is representative of Asian American activism: "to secure and maintain the civil rights of Japanese Americans and all others who are victimized by injustice and bigotry" (Japanese American Citizen's League 2008). Through its activism, JACL influenced immigration policy in the 1950s, civil rights in the 1960s, and in the 1980s secured an official apology and remuneration for the unjust internment of Japanese Americans during World War II. In similar fashion, Filipino Americans organized against dangerous and discriminatory working conditions in Hawaii, Alaska, and the western United States starting in the 1920s. By the 1960s, their activism and collaboration with Mexican laborers led to the founding of the United Farm Workers union. Finally, Chinese Americans built Chinatowns for economic empowerment and cultural preservation, in turn strengthening the economies and cultural offerings of the cities they inhabited. By the time new Asian immigrants started arriving after the 1965 immigration reform, the country was in the throes of a transformation that yielded civil rights, voting rights, Medicare, Medicaid and, of course, immigrants.

The second wave of Asian immigrants benefited from this prior organizing. Often with the help of the families that sponsored them, they built new organizations and strengthened the community infrastructure to provide an array of services to their communities, while also adjusting to their new homes. The second wave did not experience the same level of discrimination that their predecessors had, but their sheer numbers overwhelmed traditional social service providers. So they had to build their own organizations. As described by Helen Zia in *Asian American Dreams:*

> Still, a dynamic process was set in motion: we were reclaiming our stake in a land and a history that excluded us, transforming a community that was still in the process of becoming. We were following our destinies as Asian Americans. (2000, p. 20)

The multiplicity of identities and issues that emerge from the immigration and settlement experiences of such a diverse population is reflected in the organizations they have formed: cultural, legal, social service, professional, and faith based. Two communities are profiled here to illustrate the community capacity for organizing and advocacy.

## Southeast Asian American Community-Based Organizing

Southeast Asians are the largest group of refugees ever to build new lives in the United States (Southeast Asia Resource Action Center 2008). Unlike other Asian immigrants, there was no established Southeast Asian community to help them adjust to a new country. There were, at least, government-sponsored refugee resettlement programs and religious organizations to provide housing, health screenings, job placement, and other needed services. From these small beginnings, the refugees devoted their energy and limited resources into establishing temples and churches, and into building a network of faith-based organizations (FBOs) and mutual assistance associations (MAAs).

A 2004 survey by the Southeast Asia Resource Action Center (SEARAC, a "national MAA") found hundreds of these grassroots organizations, MAAs, and FBOs, that exist "for the betterment of their communities." Many of them are not formally incorporated. The 188 that are formally incorporated are included in SEARAC's *Directory of Southeast Asian American Community-Based Organizations: Mutual Assistance Associations and Religious Organizations Providing Social Services* (2004). The survey found that most of the incorporated organizations (57 percent) function on budgets of less than $300,000 and provide many necessary services without specific funding. They are located in thirty-two states, but half of the organizations are in just three states: California (30 percent), Wisconsin (11 percent), and Minnesota (11 percent), which correlates with the settlement pattern of Southeast Asian Americans, particularly Hmong in the case of Wisconsin and Minnesota. However, Texas, the state with the second-largest population of Southeast Asians, has only five organizations.

Interpretation and translation was the most commonly reported service (139 organizations), followed by youth services (133). A large percentage also reported advocacy (116) and health education (98) among their services. The two services are not disconnected. In California, MAAs have collaborated to provide health services to continuing streams of refugees, while also visiting the state capitol to advocate for funding and offer testimony on the health needs of Southeast Asians.

## South Asian Americans Organizing

Organizations serving South Asians exhibit similar characteristics. *South Asian* refers to individuals with ancestry from Bangladesh, Bhutan, Pakistan, India, Maldive Islands, Nepal, and Sri Lanka (SAALT 2008). Ten percent of foreign-born Asian Indians (more than 180,000 individuals) were not born in Asia, but rather Latin American (5.4 percent), Africa (2.1 percent), and Europe (1.2 percent), reflecting their history of global migration (U.S. Census Bureau 2007). In addition to their diverse national origins, South Asians speak several languages, with Bengali, Gujurati, Hindi, Punjabi, and Urdu being the most common in the United States. Because several South Asian countries were formerly British colonies, most are English proficient, as mentioned previously. South Asians also practice many different faiths, including Buddhism, Christianity, Hinduism, Islam, and Sikhism (SAALT 2008).

A survey of thirty-one community-based organizations serving South Asians throughout the United States revealed similarities with Southeast Asian organizations. The majority of South Asian organizations have budgets of less than $500,000. The organizations regularly link service provision with advocacy. And most (three-quarters) were founded after 1990. South Asian Americans Leading Together (SAALT), the organization that conducted the survey, describes the thirty-one organizations this way:

> Community-based organizations are the eyes and ears of our country's immigrant communities. The organizations . . . are becoming a visible and integral part of the fabric of community-based groups in the United States. They act as advocates, service providers, information and referral sources, organizers, and opinion leaders. Often the initial point of contact and resource provider for new immigrants, youth, seniors, women, and individuals in need of basic information and services, South Asian organizations play a pivotal role in strengthening and empowering our communities. (2007, p. 6)

## Building Capacity

The creativity and fortitude of South Asian, Southeast Asian, and other community-based organizations is commendable. However, additional skills, infrastructure, and resources will be necessary for them to truly meet the needs of communities that are continuing to grow, diversify, and change. Neither should the burden fall to just Asian American community-based organizations. More established and mainstream public and private organizations must also develop the skills, infrastructure, and resources to serve their diverse constituencies. The community responses to two national calamities illustrate these points.

In the wake of the 9/11 attacks, South Asians became the target of hate crimes, racial profiling, and other bias-related incidents proving that xenophobia is not a relic of pre-1965 immigration reform. The individuals, families, and communities affected found themselves in need of a variety of services, ranging from legal services to mental health care. Southeast Asian refugees were also uniquely traumatized by 9/11: MAAs reported clients were experiencing flashbacks and other post-traumatic stress, thus impairing their mental health and daily functioning. The organizations serving these communities responded by advocating for law enforcement, developing partnerships with government agencies and other CBOs, and forming their own organizations. However, additional resources and community capacity are necessary, particularly in the area of mental health care.

The second calamity was Hurricane Katrina, which affected parts of Louisiana, Mississippi, and Alabama in September 2005. Among the busloads of people who were evacuated to Houston and other destinations were thousands of Vietnamese Americans. In fact, there were approximately 70,000 Asians Americans living in the affected areas according to the 2000 census, including large concentrations of South Asians as well as Vietnamese (SAALT 2005). The Vietnamese had settled in the Gulf Coast and were concentrated in the fishing industry; however, the hurricane destroyed their boats and, with them, their livelihood. So thousands fled to Houston, which also has a large Vietnamese population. However, this second refugee experience overwhelmed the few MAAs and other community-based organizations in Houston. With the help of other Asian CBOs and businesses, volunteers coordinated access to health and other necessary services such as finding housing, food, and jobs. However, making referrals to established hospitals and clinics was challenging because of the lack of interpreters. So community advocates have jump-started the application process for a federally qualified health center to serve Houston-area Asian Americans. Back in the Gulf region, many Southeast Asians chose to stay or returned to rebuild their business and community. They are learning to engage community, faith, and political leaders in the process.

## RECOMMENDATIONS FOR FURTHER STUDY

Thousands of Chinese Americans prospected for gold during the California gold rush of the mid-1800s. Few, if any of them, became rich as a result, but they did lay the foundation for the Chinese American community. Similarly, today we must prospect for new knowledge about Asian American immigration, adaptation, and health, and lay the foundation for a healthy and whole Asian American community. Many new studies are needed to fully understand the impact of the past 40 years of immigration on health and the ecosystems that affect health. Here are just a few recommendations.

## 1. Understand Intra-group Diversity as Variables

To understand the impact of immigration on health, researchers often use country of origin or race as the frame of reference, creating a false impression of homogeneity within such categories. In fact, many countries are ethnically, culturally, and socioeconomically diverse, and these differences endure even many years after immigrating. This within-group diversity may have more relevance to health behavior, risk, and status than country of origin or race (Kagawa-Singer and Pasick 2002). Therefore more studies should define groups according to these dimensions of diversity. Untangling these variables is necessary to understand behavior change and to design effective interventions.

## 2. Differentiate Immigration and Geographic Settlement Patterns

As illustrated by the immigration pattern of South Asians, immigration can take place over generations. Country of last residence does not always correlate to racial and ethnic labels. More than 200,000 Chinese Americans were born in Latin America, as were 50,000 Filipinos, 40,000 Koreans, and 8000 Japanese (U.S. Census Bureau 2007). Further study is needed to understand how multiple migrations affect self-concept, health, and well-being.

South Asians and other Asian groups are also immigrating directly to suburbs, bypassing the urban centers as the traditional place of first residence (Skop and Li 2005). Is this related to the increase in employment-based immigration? If so, are these employed immigrants more likely to be insured and have access to high quality care?

## 3. Multiethnic and Multiracial Families

Interracial and interethnic marriages become more likely as Asians assimilate (Qian et al. 2001). What impact do these marriages have on insurance rates and quality of care for the married partners and their children? Interracial families also result from the adoption of babies from Asian countries such as Korea, China, and the Philippines. As these children grow up, one might hypothesize that their access to health care will be excellent, a sort of selection bias that selects for well-resourced parents. Nonetheless, the children will experience adjustment issues as their self-concept begins to include awareness of differences based on phenotype.

## CONCLUSION

Asian Americans have been in the United States since before the Declaration of Independence, contributing the skills, talent, and wit necessary for the nation to grow and thrive. From various trickles of migrants brought by the need for cheap labor, then legally excluded because of racism, the population hit the one-million mark sometime in the early

1960s. Then the 1965 changes to immigration law and the resettlement of Southeast Asian refugees starting in 1975 caused the population to swell from that mere million to almost 15 million, or 5 percent of the total U.S. population, in 40 years. The next 40 years may not be as dramatic, as the census estimates the population will increase to 33.5 million by 2050, or 8 percent of the population (U.S. Census Bureau 2004). Even though this is slower than the current growth rate, the trend of Asian Americans increasing in number and proportion will continue, fed both by continued immigration and native births. The diversity and complexity of their experiences must continue to be studied.

## NOTES

1. In general, the term *Asian American* as used in this chapter is consistent with the 2000 census definition. Variations such as *Asian and Pacific Islander* (API) are used to be consistent with the study described. Pacific Islanders are included in the history of the census because the separation between the two groups is recent, and, census categories notwithstanding, because their histories are inter-twined (especially in Hawaii). Otherwise, although many Pacific Islanders do have migration experiences that may impact health, they are not technically immi-grants; therefore, the information in this chapter may not apply to them.

2. Self-reported health is accepted as a robust predictor of morbidity, mortal-ity, disability, and health care utilization.

3. In some studies, those who speak English at least "well" are not considered LEP (e.g., Kandula et al. 2007). Given the high level of English literacy necessary to understand health communications, it is reasonable to use the higher threshold of "very well." Nevertheless, using the lower threshold does not change the con-clusion that limited English proficiency adversely impacts health.

## REFERENCES

Adams, Amy. *Survey Takes Health Snapshot of Nail Salon Workers.* May 28, 2008. http://med.stanford.edu/mcr/2008/nailsalon-0528.html (accessed June 3, 2008).

Asian American Justice Center. "Immigration Publication & Materials: Recent Pro-posed Legislation: Statements from Panelists on White House Proposal for Immigration Reform." 2007. http://www.advancingequality.org/en/cms/?193 (accessed April 22, 2008).

Association of Asian Pacific Community Health Centers. 2004. http://www.aapcho.org/site/aapcho/section.php?id=10950 (accessed April 17, 2008).

Barnes, Jessica S., and Claudette E. Bennett. *The Asian Population: 2000.* Census 2000 Brief, Washington: U.S. Census Bureau, 2002.

Borah, Eloisa G. "Filipinos in Unamuno's California Exploration in 1587." *Amerasia Journal* 21, no. 3, (1995): 175–183.

Bureau of the Census. "The Nation's Asian and Pacific Islander Population: 1994 Statistical Brief." Statistical Brief, U.S. Department of Commerce, Washington, 1995. http://www.census.gov/apsd/www/statbrief/sb95_24.pdf.

Carter, Susan B., Scott S. Garner, Michael R. Haines, Alan L. Olmstead, Richard Sutch, and Gavin Wright. *Historial Statistics of the United States.* New York: Cambridge University Press, 2006.

Chen, Moon, and Betty Lee Hawks. "A Debunking of the Myth of the Healthy Asian Americans and Pacific Islanders." *American Journal of Health Promotion* 9, no. 4 (March–April 1995): 261–268.

Choy, Catherine Ceniza. *Empire of Care: Nursing and Migration in Filipino American History.* Durham and London: Duke University Press, 2003.

Danico, Mary Yu, and Franklin Ng. *Asian American Issues.* Westport, CT: Greenwood, 2004.

Daniels, Roger. "Historians on America." *The Immigration Act of 1965: Intended and Unintended Consequences.* September 2007. http://usinfo.state.gov/products/pubs/historians/chapter11.htm (accessed February 28, 2008).

Dhooper, S. S. "Health Care Needs of Foreign-Born Asian Americans." *Health & Social Work* 28, no. 1 (February 2003): 63–73.

Espina, Marina E. *Filipinos in Louisiana.* New Orleans, LA: A.F. Laborde and Sons, 1988.

Frisbie, W. P., Youngtae Cho, and Robert A. Hummer. "Immigration and the Health of Asian and Pacific Islander Adults in the United States." *American Journal of Epidemiology* 153, no. 4 (2001): 372–380.

Gibson, Campbell, and Kay Jung. *Historical Census Statistics on Population Totals by Race, 1790 to 1990, and by Hispanic Origin, 1970 to 1990, for the United States, Regions, Divisions, and States.* Working Paper Series No. 56, Washington: U.S. Census Bureau, 2002.

Green, Alexander R., Quyen Ngo-Metzger, Anna T. R. Legedza, Michael P. Massagli, Russell S. Phillips, and Lisa I. Iezzoni. "Interpreter Services, Language Concordance, and Health Care Quality: Experiences of Asian Americans with Limited English Proficiency." *Journal of General Internal Medicine* 20, no. 11 (November 2005): 1050–1056.

Grieco, Elizabeth M. *The Native Hawaiian and Other Pacific Islander Population: 2000.* Census 2000 Brief, Washington: U.S. Census Bureau, 2001.

Grieco, Elizabeth M., and Rachel C. Cassidy. *Overview of Race and Hispanic Origin: 2000.* Census 2000 Brief, Washington: U.S. Census Bureau, 2001.

Henry J. Kaiser Family Foundation. "Health Coverage and Access to Care among Asian Americans, Native Hawaiians and Pacific Islanders." April 2008. http://kff.org/minorityhealth/7745.cfm (accessed May 28, 2008).

Hoefer, Michael, Nancy Rytina, and Christopher Campbell. "Estimates of the Unauthorized Immigrant Population Residing in the United States: January 2006." Population Estimates, Office of Immigration Statistics, U.S. Department of Homeland Security, Washington, August 2007.

Jang, Michael, Evelyn Lee, and Kent Woo. "Income, Language, Citizenship Status: Factors Affecting Health Care Access and Utilization of Chinese Americans." *Health & Social Work* 23, no. 2 (May 1998): 136–145.

Japanese American Citizen's League. 2008. http://jacl.org/about/about.htm (accessed February 28, 2008).

Jefferys, Kelly. "U.S. Legal Permanent Residents: 2006." Annual Flow Report, Office of Immigration Statistics, U.S. Department of Homeland Security, Washington, 2007.

Kagawa-Singer, Marjorie, and Rena J. Pasick. "Cultural Norms." In *The Encyclopedia of Public Health*. Ed. Lester Beslow. New York: Macmillan Reference USA/Gale Group Thomson Learning 2002, 302–304.

Kandula, Namratha R., Daine S. Lauderdale, and David W. Baker. "Differences in Self-Reported Health among Asians, Latinos and Non-Hispanic Whites: The Role of Language and Nativity." *Annual Epidemiology* 17 (2007): 191–198.

Katigbak, Jose. *ABS-CBN News Online.* January 22, 2008. http://www.abs-cbnnews.com/storypage.aspx?StoryId=106362 (accessed May 29, 2008).

Kitano, Harry H. L., and Roger Daniels. *Asian Americans: Emerging Minorities.* 3rd ed. Upper Saddle River, NJ: Prentice Hall, 2000.

Ku, Leighton. "Reducing Disparities in Health Coverage for Legal Immigrant Children and Pregnant Women." Center on Budget and Policy Priorities, Washington, 2007.

Liu, Jan, and Bari Samad. *Diverse Communities, Diverse Experiences: A Review of Six Socioeconomic Indicators and Their Impact on Health.* San Francisco: Asian and Pacific Islander American Health Forum, 2004.

Lobo, Arun Peter, and Joseph J. Salvo. "Changing U.S. Immigration Law and the Occupational Selectivity of Asian Immigrants." *International Migration Review* 32, no. 3 (Autumn 1998): 737–760.

Lott, Juanita Tamayo. *Asian Americans: From Racial Category to Multiple Identities.* Walnut Creek, CA: AltaMira Press, 1997.

Ludden, Jennifer. "1965 Immigration Law Changed Face of America." *NPR.* May 9, 2006. http://www.npr.org/templates/story/story.php?storyId=5391395 (accessed February 28, 2008).

Martin, Elizabeth, and Eleanor Gerber. "Methodological Influences on Comparability of Race Measurements: Several Cautionary Examples." Proceedings of the American Statistical Association. 2003. 2697–2704.

Ngo-Metzger, Quyen, Michael P. Massagli, Brian R. Clarridge, Michael Manocchia, Roger B. Davis, Lisa Iezzoni, and Russell S. Phillips. "Linguistic and Cultural Barriers to Care: Perspectives of Chinese and Vietnamese Immigrants." *Journal of General Internal Medicine* 18 (2003): 44–52.

———. "Providing High-Quality Care for Limited English Proficient Patients: The Importance of Language Concordance and Interpreter Use." *Journal of General Internal Medine* 22, Supplement 2 (November 2007): 324–330.

Niedzwiecki, Max, and T. C. Duong. "Southeast Asian American Statistical Profile." SEARAC. 2003. http://www.searac.org/refugee_stats_2002.html (accessed February 28, 2008).

Qian, Z. C., S. L. Blair, and S. D. Ruf. "Asian American Interracial and Interethnic Marriages: Differences by Education and Nativity." *International Migration Review* 35, no. 2 (Summer 2001): 557–586.

Sanders, Jimy, Victor Nee, and Scott Sernau. "Asian Immigrants' Reliance on Social Ties in a Multi-ethnic Labor Market." *Social Forces* 81, no. 1 (September 2002): 281–314.

Singh, Gopal K., and Mohammad Siahpush. "Ethnic-Immigrant Differentials in Health Behaviors, Morbidity, and Cause-Specific Mortality in the United States: An Analysis of Two National Data Bases." *Human Biology* 74, no. 1 (2002): 83–109.

Skop, Emily, and Wei Li. "Asians in America's Suburbs: Patterns and Consequences of Settlement." *Geographical Review* 95, no. 2 (April 2005): 167–188.

South Asian Americans Leading Together. 2008. http://www.saalt.org/about community.php (accessed February 28, 2008).

Southeast Asia Resource Action Center. "Definitions: Mutual Assistance Associations (MAAs) and Religious Organizations Providing Social Services." 2004. http://www.searac.org/maa/definitions.html (accessed February 28, 2008).

———. "Refugee Arrivals to the U.S. from Southeast Asia, Fiscal Years 1975–2002." 2003. http://www.searac.org/refugee_stats_2002.html (accessed February 28, 2008).

———. 2008. http://www.searac.org (accessed February 28, 2008).

———. "Survey Findings." October 20, 2004. http://www.searac.org/maa/charts.html (accessed February 28, 2008).

Takaki, Ronald. *Strangers from a Different Shore: A History of Asian Americans.* Revised and updated edition. New York: Back Bay Books, 1998.

The White House. "Fact Sheet: Ending Chain Migration." June 1, 2007. http://www.whitehouse.gov/news/releases/2007/06/20070601-22.html (accessed April 22, 2008).

U.S. Census Bureau. *American Fact Finder, Data Set: 1990 Census, Summary Tape File 1–100 percent data.* 1990. http://www.factfinder.census.gov (accessed May 23, 2008).

———. *American Fact Finder, Data Set: 2006 American Community Survey, Data Profiles.* September 27, 2007. http://www.factfinder.census.gov (accessed February 28, 2008).

———. *American Fact Finder, Data Set: American Community Survey 2006, Table S1602.* 2007. http://www.factfinder.census.gov (accessed May 21, 2008).

———. *American Fact Finder, Data Set: Annual Population Estimates, 2006 Population Estimates, Tables T-1 and T-5.* 2007. http://www.factfinder.census.gov (accessed April 22, 2008).

———. *How the Census Bureau Measures Poverty (Official Measure).* August 28, 2007. http://www.census.gov/hhes/www/poverty/povdef.html (accessed May 22, 2008).

———. "U.S. Interim Projections by Age, Race, Sex, and Hispanic Origin, Table 1a." *Census Bureau.* March 18, 2004. http://www.census.gov/ipc/www/usinterimproj (accessed April 22, 2008).

U.S. Department of Health and Human Services. "LEP Policy Guidance for HHS Recipients." Limited English Proficiency: A Federal Interagency Website. 2003. http://www.lep.gov/guidance/guidance_index.html (accessed April 22, 2008).

U.S. Department of Homeland Security. "2007 Yearbook of Immigration Statistics." Office of Immigration Statistics, Washington, 2008.

———. *Immigration Statistics, Data Standards and Definitions.* 2008. http://www.dhs.gov/ximgtn/statistics/stdfdef.shtm#17 (accessed February 28, 2008).

Walton, Emily C., and David T. Takeuchi. "Contextualizing the Education and Health Status Association: Evidence from a National Study of Asian Americans." American Sociological Association, Annual Meeting. Philadelphia, 2005: 1–24.

Wei, William. *The Asian American Movement.* Philadelphia, PA: Temple University Press, 1993.

Yang, Kou. "The Hmong in America: Twenty Five Years after the U.S. Secret War in Laos." *Journal of Asian American Studies* 4, no. 2 (June 2001): 165–174.

Yu, Stella M., Zhihuan J. Huang, and Gopal K. Singh. "Health Status and Health Services Utilization among U.S. Chinese, Asian Indian, Filipino, and Other Asian/Pacific Islander Children." *Pediatrics* 113, no. 1 (January 2004): 101–107.

Zane, Nolan W. S., David Takeuchi, and Kathleen N. J. Young. *Confronting Critical Health Issues of Asian and Pacific Islander Americans.* Thousand Oaks, CA: Sage Publications, 1994.

Zia, Helen. "Surrogate Slaves to American Dreamers." In *Asian American Dreams.* Ed. Helen Zia. New York: Farrar, Straus and Giroux, 2000, 21–52.

# Chapter 31

# Asian American Health: Discrepancies, Convergence, and Enclave-Specific Trends

## Tom Lun-Nap Chung

Three efforts to improve the health of Asian Americans are at the same time restricting their own scope and effectiveness: the emphasis on diseases more common in Asia; the focusing on problems primarily pertaining to the most recent immigrants; and the reliance on inadequate aggregation units for data collection and analysis. The purpose of this chapter is to draw more attention to the converging trends, particularly those related to chronic diseases, and to propose "the ethnic-enclave complex" as a more inclusive and practical conceptual framework than ethnicity, socioeconomic grouping, and "community" for research and policy development.

The strong emphasis in public health policies and programs on health conditions more common in Asia than in the United States is a natural and proper response to the fact that over 60 percent of the current Asian American population is composed of immigrants. However, as the proportion of U.S.-born Asians expands and earlier immigrants age, the morbidity pattern is shifting from mainly infectious and acute diseases toward one that comprises more chronic conditions. Prevention and treatment of chronic conditions require a lot more long-term adjustments in diet, lifestyle, and the environment than infectious and acute diseases. Although the discrepancy among disease patterns is narrowing, the need for culturally sensitive intervention is increasing. The effort to eliminate health discrepancies therefore could be hampered if "discrepancy elimination" is confined to "targeting foreign diseases" at the expense of "local diseases."

The emphasis on diseases more common in Asia, reinforced by the recognition of socioeconomic, language, and cultural barriers, has led to the focusing on discrepancies in mainly the most recent immigrants who live in poor urban settings. Health care needs of earlier immigrants and U.S.-born Asians who live in middle-income areas, regardless of where they came from, have received inadequate attention. While the poorest segment gets some attention now, it is the middle-income segment, the rapidly increasing and already the largest segment, that is assigned the image of model minority who seems to be self-sufficient.

## ORIGINAL DIFFERENCES

Health conditions and health-related behaviors more common in Asia could be better or worse than those in the United States. For detailed discussions please refer to other chapters in this handbook. This section will only touch on a few points: (1) whereas some conditions and risk behaviors have received some attention, others have not; (2) not all of the differences in Asia are burdensome, the United States actually benefits from the healthy immigrant effect and could benefit more by selectively promoting certain Asian practices; (3) Asia is heterogeneous and changing fast; attributing Asian American problems to original differences in Asia therefore would lead to wrong questions or incomplete answers; and (4) the confluence effect of socioeconomic status.

### Negative Impacts Originating in Asia.

Asian Americans are definitely burdened with certain diseases that are more common in Asia, including tuberculosis; parasitic infestations; and liver, cervical, and other cancers resulting from infection. A few diseases also prevalent in the United States, such as hepatitis B and thalassemia, have been targeted in the public health sector. Diseases less common in other races have yet to receive more attention—such as lower bone mineral density among Chinese elders, which may lead to higher risk for osteoporosis (Lauderdale et al. 2003), and middle teeth bone loss, which is tied to the inadequate control of type 2 diabetes (Leong et al. 2007). Unique conditions confined to a smaller group have difficulty drawing continuous attention, such as Native Hawaiian male-to-female transgenders who are limited to prostitution, drug dealing, and minimum-wage jobs (Odo and Hawelu 2001), and the undocumented Fuzhounese immigrants who have higher rates of hospitalization, lower treatment compliance, and many more social disadvantages than other Chinese mental patients (Law et al., 2003).

Whereas risk behaviors common in both Asia and the United States such as smoking and unhealthy diets are being addressed with public funding, problems affecting mainly Asians have received only sporadic attention. One example is the higher suicide rates among Asian women, which is attributed to the cultural and social bias in Asia against seeking mental health services. Asians with mental illnesses tend to feel embarrassed, guilty, and shameful, and blame themselves (HJ Chen 2005). Other examples include the high acceptance level for physical discipline with children and a high tolerance level for wife beating conducive to family violence in Asia. The taboo to disclose, seek professional help, or leave the abusive system further places the victim in a helpless situation. The experience of physical discipline or abuse, even within families of higher SES, is a more important factor in predicting violence across generations among East and South Asians than the number of years they lived in the United States (Maker et al. 2005).

Quite a few of Asian habits are detrimental to health or are risk factors for chronic diseases. Smoking rates among Asian men, particularly those from Southeast Asian countries, are the highest of any racial/ethnic group (Yu et al. 2002). While 14.2 percent of Asian and Pacific Islanders (APIs) smoke nationally, the rate can exceed 50 percent in some recently arrived groups. A study of restaurant workers in Boston's Chinatown found that 80 percent of the smokers started smoking before entering the United States; some started as early as age seven. Most of these workers were aware that cigarettes are addictive, cause lung cancer, and lead to heart disease; but nearly half believe low tar and low nicotine cigarettes to be safer than standard brands, as the cigarette commercials say (Averback et al. 2002). Another health hazard difficult to solve in Asian families is secondhand smoking, because the smoker is often the oldest male, the one who sets the rules in the family (Ferketich et al., 2004). Many Asians continue to consume foods high in sodium, animal fats, proteins, and refined sugar. As they pick up more unhealthy food habits, they suffer from a higher mortality rate from heart disease compared with U.S.-born Asians. Chinese American women engage in markedly less physical activity than their counterparts in China, thereby losing the protective effects of physical activity on breast cancer risk, following the same course reported for Japanese and Filipino Americans (Yang et al. 2003).

## Positive Impacts Originating in Asia

Like other immigrants, foreign-born Asians are generally healthier than their U.S.-born counterparts (Dey et al. 2006; Frisbie et al. 2001). Except for the relatively small proportion of refugees, the self-selection process and the U.S. immigration policies ensure that those who arrive are younger and healthier. Their advantage in health remains even after taking into account age, nativity, and duration in the United States (Cho and Hummer 2001). Studies show that Asian immigrants are less likely to be obese and hypertensive, and they have fewer risk factors for chronic diseases (Dey et al. 2006). Chinese and Japanese Americans have lower total cholesterol levels and lower incidence of coronary heart disease than Caucasians (Pinnelas et al. 1992). The "Western style cancers"—such as colorectal, prostate, and breast cancer—are less prevalent in Asians (Choe et al. 2005; Mills et al. 2005; Sadler et al. 2003). Asian women nursing-home residents have lower functional limitations and much lower rates of Alzheimer's and other mental disorders, even though they are diagnosed with more conditions (JA Davis, 2005).

The alcoholism rate is lower among Asians. One reason suggested is that they are genetically more susceptible to develop unpleasant symptoms such as flushing, nausea, headache, dizziness, and rapid heartbeat (Price et al. 2002). A study of middle-aged Asian women with college degrees supports earlier findings that Asian women are less likely to experience menopausal symptoms frequently experienced by white women. Many of them did not place any meaning on the symptoms and chose not to manage their symptoms because they perceived them as natural, normal, and part of aging (Im and Chee 2005). A widespread medical condition in the West in this case has become a socio-culturally constructed entity that is a nonissue in a group without the same cultural definition.

## Uncertain Impacts Originating in Asia

Meanwhile, there are quite a few Asian physical and cultural differences, the health impacts of which are hard to judge. Even though many clinical workers are dealing with many of these differences on a daily basis, there has been inadequate research to support the development of corresponding clinical guidelines. For instance, it is suggested that Asians may need a lower medication dosage compared to Caucasians, or may experience more severe side effects (HJ Chen, 2005). The widespread experience (not just impression) of strong adverse effect of Western medicine has led many Asian patients to arbitrarily reduce the prescription dosage, often without the physician's knowledge. Many other Asian values may lead to mixed intervention results, ranging from the role of the family in illness to that of the approach toward teenage independence in inter-generational tension. Although the family provides a patient with reliable support, it may also deprive the patient of professional help and take a toll on the family. Asian students are constantly under pressure to perform well academically. To most Asian parents, academic performance is not just something traditionally valued; it is also the best guarantee of career development and financial stability in the new world. Even highly acculturated Chinese mothers maintain an authoritarian parenting style (Chen and Kennedy 2005). The price to pay is stress and the deprivation of social and recreational activities for both parents and children. Cultural values can sometimes complicate family functioning. The traditional Asian emphasis of interdependence is often at odds with the Western societal advocacy of independence for late adolescence (Lorenzo et al.

2000). Intergenerational conflict in immigrant families is stronger than that in other families because of intergenerational discrepancy in acculturation. Being exposed to competing expectations and norms, Southeast Asian adolescents may be unwilling to abide by their parents' traditional values, thereby setting the stage for the development of intergenerational/intercultural conflict. Differential acculturation reinforces the impact of intergenerational conflict upon depression (Ying and Han 2007). Understanding how culture shapes the course and interpretation of health conditions would inspire the whole society with better ways to conceive and to intervene many mental and physical conditions.

## Why Ethnic Data Alone Is Inadequate

Many attempts to explain intra-Asian difference have been focusing on ethnicity or country of origin. Such original difference is a powerful source to argue against data lumping. However, preoccupation with differences in the past is an endless pursuit that may divert attention to issues here and now. There are twenty-eight countries in Asia; each has a multiethnic composition. South Asians have the widest range of skin-color and religious diversity. Living in the same area of Yanbian, Han and Korean Chinese have different prevalence rates of abnormal blood lipid (Cui et al. 2006). Moreover, Asia is changing fast. The Korean American researcher who found Asian women less likely than white women to experience menopausal symptoms also reported that Korean American women were less likely to experience menopausal symptoms than Korean women in South Korea (Im 2003). Whereas the proportion of women in South Korea who experienced hot flashes was similar to that of white women, the proportion of Korean American women who experienced these symptoms paralleled that of Chinese, Thai, and Japanese women in Asia. One explanation for these unexpected findings is the recent introduction of industries associated with menopause in South Korea, which brought about a reversal in the patterns of cultural transition to menopause. Accepting Western pharmaceutical industries' promotion of hormones as a magical medication for eternal youth, South Korean women began to talk about sexual life and other bodily experiences that were taboo in the past. In contrast, Korean women who immigrated to the United States earlier tend to preserve their traditional values and attitudes toward menopause, in part because they were isolated from the mainstream American society.

## Socioeconomic Status (SES) as a Confounding Variable

The link between Asian Americans' health and original differences is often confounded by SES. Low SES is often seen as a major cause of Southeast Asians' inferior health (Cho and Hummer 2001), and some Chinese patients' depression and anxiety (Lubetkin et al. 2003). On the other hand, higher-risk behaviors among certain Asian groups are sometimes attributed to their higher SES. Substance abuse rates among Japanese Americans are close to or exceeding those of whites. Vietnamese Americans reported the lowest levels of substance use and abuse. Differences are less striking among Filipino, Chinese, and Korean Americans. The ranking of substance use and abuse was consistent with the ranking of acculturation and socioeconomic indicators of these five groups, which is tied to the year of immigration and the number of years living in the United States (Price et al. 2002).

The impact of SES on health measures should not be overemphasized. Despite their lower SES, Vietnamese Americans do not have a higher mortality rate than other Asians (Lauderdale and Kestenbaum 2002). One possible explanation is that in the United States, food, hygiene, and shelter are basically adequate even for the poor. The poorest in the United States still fare much more easily than many better-to-do in Asia.

## CARE DISCREPANCIES

This section presents key evidence for the generally lower utilization rates of health care by Asian Americans, its causes, and the role of traditional Asian medicine as complementary and alternative medicine (CAM).

### Low Utilization

Although Asian Americans vary widely in their health status, their utilization rates of health services are almost uniformly low. After adjustment for health status, foreign-born Asians still lag behind all U.S.-born adults in most aspects of health care access and utilization (Frisbie et al. 2001). They certainly are less likely to be institutionalized, as indicated by their fewer bed days (Dey et al. 2006). Asian women nursing-home residents have more diagnosed conditions (Davis, 2005), and Asian home-care program clients are older (Chung 1986), implying that those who have fewer diagnosed conditions and who are younger are less likely to be enrolled. Asian elders visit their doctors at an annual rate of about 2/3 of the national average, after considering other factors (Yee and Chung 1991). Despite high cervical cancer rates, Asians have very low screening rates (Maxwell et al. 2000). A study in Chicago's Chinatown found that 85 percent of the respondents had never been screened with the fecal occult blood test, compared with 70 percent of the general population, far below the 50 percent target set by the Healthy People 2000 program (Yu et al. 2001b). A majority of Vietnamese Americans never had their cholesterol levels checked, compared to below 40 percent of the general U.S. population (National Diabetes Education Program 1992). From institutionalization and ambulatory care to screening, the pattern of postponed participation or delayed enrollment in the Asian American population is too consistent to dismiss.

## Causes of Lower Utilization

Why do Asians in general use less health care services? There are institutional, socioeconomic, and cultural factors ranging from lack of adequate insurance, provider discrimination, patients' information and attitudes, as well as the role of traditional Asian medicine.

Foreign-born adults are more likely to be uninsured. The proportion of uninsured among foreign-born Asian is 15 percent, compared to 6 percent of U.S.-born Asians (Dey et al. 2006). The 1999 National Nursing Home Survey revealed that Asian women residents had by far the lowest proportion of Medicare coverage: 11 percent versus 31 to 35 percent among other women of color (Davis 2005). Children without a regular source of health care are exposed to higher risk, such as missing needed immunizations. The no-usual-source-of-care rate for Asian children was estimated to be 8.6 percent in 1996, which was lower than that of Hispanics and blacks, but still 43 percent above that of the 6 percent rate for whites (Weinick and Krauss 2000). Disparities are also seen in pain management. Like other minority women, Asian elders in nursing homes were less likely to receive analgesics than whites. Minority Medicaid women during spontaneous vaginal birth were also less likely to receive epidural analgesic than whites. Although researchers cannot agree on what caused the differential treatment, a study found no difference in pain-control expectations among racial groups (Ezenwa et al. 2006).

SES is often found to be significantly related to health care utilization, but like in its relationships with health conditions, other factors affecting utilization are often implicated, especially language and cultural barriers. The low level of knowledge of cancer screening is tied to the low screening rate in Chicago's Chinatown (ESH Yu et al. 2001a). Over 90 percent of the Southeast Asian population in central Ohio did not know what blood pressure was, and 85 percent did know what could be done to prevent heart disease. There were wide spread misconceptions about cancer that act as screening deterrents (e.g., "testing for cancer can cause cancer"). Community members were unfamiliar with clinical trials and would not participate unless they were "sick," and would participate only upon their physicians' recommendation. Their physicians did not see the relevance or value of clinical trials for their patients (Lin et al. 2005).

Knowledge and attitude changes, however, do not guarantee behavior change. Most Chinese smokers know the danger of smoking (Averback et al. 2002). Chinese women's knowledge of mammography screening was insignificant in predicting their screening behavior (M. Yu et al. 2003, 2005). Screening rates of highly educated women from various Asian countries are all below the Healthy People 2010 target rate of 70 percent (Sadler et al. 2003).

Traditional values could block some Asian women from ever performing breast self-exams (Wu et al. 2005). Hmongs are reluctant to have their blood drawn, and they avoid certain screening procedures. The bias against surgery stems mainly from the reluctance of losing blood among people who believe in traditional Chinese medicine, including Koreans, Japanese, Vietnamese, and tens of millions of overseas Chinese.

### Traditional Medicine as Complementary and Alternative Medicine (CAM)

Use of traditional Asian medicine, effective or not, has reduced the utilization level of Western medicine. Traditional medicines are still popular among Asian Americans, regardless of their SES and health status (Kim et al. 2002; Ma 1999; Yee and Chung 1991). The National Institutes of Health's National Center for Complementary and Alternative Medicine 2002 Report found Asians more likely to use CAM (excluding prayer and megavitamins) than whites and blacks (43.1%, 35.9%, and 26.2%, respectively). Asian medical traditions—such as Ayurveda in India, Kampo in Japan, Hanbang in Korea, and traditional Chinese medicine—all use complex interventions that often involve multiple substances at the same time. They also individualize diagnosis and treatment and maximize the body's inherent healing ability. They advocate treating the "whole" person by addressing their physical, mental, and spiritual attributes rather than focusing on a specific pathogenic process as emphasized in conventional Western medicine (Barnes et al. 2004). Such approaches are particularly appealing when Western medicine is slow, inadequate, or too expensive in addressing Asian patients' concerns.

The growing popularity of Chinese herbals and patent medicines in the United States and the lack of strict federal regulations have led to the possibility of improper labeling and even adulteration of these products with Western drugs or other chemical contaminants. An analysis of 90 representative samples randomly purchased in New York City's Chinatown shows that almost 10 percent of them contained Western pharmaceuticals, undeclared or mislabeled substances, and pharmaceuticals contraindicated in people for whom the product was intended (Miller and Stripp 2007).

Traditional healers may employ a broader perspective than treatment alone when dealing with patients. Some traditional practitioners themselves in the New York Chinatown are not sure of the effectiveness of traditional Chinese medicine in treating TB, but they are also reluctant to refer TB patients to the New York Department of Health's Directly Observed Therapy Program (Ho 2006). Protecting their own reputation is not the only factor in their reluctance to make the referral. They know that some patients have concerns over possible loss of job or deportation, which are more threatening than ineffective treatment. So, even in the case of ineffective treatment, traditional healers may still want to reduce certain patients' contact with modern medicine.

Communication between traditional and Western medicine can be blocked off by both patients and providers. Korean patients would share their biomedical treatment experiences with Hanbang providers, but they do not talk to Western physicians for fear that Western physicians will ridicule them or discourage them from continuing with the traditional treatment. A similar behavior has also been observed in Laotian and Hmong elders (M. Kim et al. 2002). Community-based Western medicine providers are also less likely to refer patients with mental health problems to mainstream programs (Akutsu et al. 2007), which may be more specialized but less culturally competent.

## Underutilization of Mental Health Service

Mental health is probably the area most affected by culture. It is rarely addressed in traditional Chinese medicine. Mental disorder was often considered an indication of one's own sins or one's ancestors'. Being stigmatized brings shame to the whole family. Asian patients tend to feel embarrassed, guilty, and shameful, and they blame themselves. People suffering from emotional or mental problems often would consciously or unconsciously express them in physical terms, particularly through cardiovascular and vestibular complaints. They would seek help from primary care physicians rather than mental health professionals, even though the outcomes are less desirable. Many Asians in primary care settings remain undiagnosed and untreated for mental illnesses. They end up using the emergency rooms and hospitals more, thereby increasing the health care cost (H.J. Chen 2005; Yeung and Schwartz 1986).

## Reduction of Risk Behaviors and Unnecessary Services

On the other hand, plenty of Asian cultural traits and attitudes conducive to health have reduced risk behaviors and unnecessary medical services. Traditional Chinese medicine preaches self-responsibility in prevention and healing. Everyone should live a moderate lifestyle and avoid excessive behavior. When sick, the patient and family have to cooperate with the healer in all aspects of life rather than passively taking pills.

The emphasis on the well-being of the family rather than the individual is instrumental to keeping juvenile delinquency and teenage sex down. This is a major reason for the lower rates in AIDS among Asians (Wortley et al. 2000). The Asian attitude against women smoking, regardless of their SES, has been instrumental to Asian women's much lower smoking rate than that of men (Averbach et al. 2002). Asians are more likely to live with a larger family, which can be a potential source of support to their ill relatives, including schizophrenic patients (Bae and Kung 2000).

## CONVERGING TREND

Despite all of the differences attributed to the Asians' country of origin and care discrepancies in the United States, tendencies toward convergence have emerged in many areas within a few decades of Asians' settlement in the United States. Substantial changes have begun in terms of decline of infectious diseases, increase of Western-style cancer, homogenization of mortality rates and causes, as well as risk behaviors of the younger generation. These tendencies are results from fundamental changes in demography and SES, improvement of living conditions, increased acceptance and availability of Western medicine, as well as Americanization of diet and lifestyle.

### Demographic Changes

A fundamental change is the growth of the U.S.-born Asian population, which is increasingly building a population structure closer to the norm and less twisted by immigration policies. The extraordinary growth rate of the Asian American population—doubling every decade between 1970 and 1990—was very much a rate calculated with a small base. Even with continuous immigration, the overall growth rate has been slowing down to 48 percent between 1990 and 2000, and 27 percent between 2000 and 2005, signaling the shrinking proportion of recent arrivals. Meanwhile, the number and proportion of U.S.-born Asians have been increasing. U.S.-born Asians now comprise 36 percent of the total Asian American population, including 23 percent second generation and 13 percent 3+ generation. (Magazine Publishers of America 2004). These proportions will continue to expand.

Some important converging trends in health are already visible. First of all, certain original differences may not be as big as they appear. The unusually low Asian death rate is actually closer to that of the general U.S. population after accounting for age, the "healthy immigrant effect," higher household income, and particularly the underestimation of Asians on death certificates. Ratios of mortality rates from 1981 to 1991 calculated from death certificates for Chinese, Japanese, and Filipinos to that for whites showed greater variation than corresponding ratios calculated from Medicare records (Lauderdate and Kestenbaum 2002). Mortality rates in Asia vary widely. Life expectancy at birth in 2000 was 62.5 years in India, 67.5 in the Philippines, 69.3 in Vietnam, 71.4 in China, 74.4 in Korea, and 80.7 in Japan. Such large differences were not found among Asian Americans in the Medicare mortality data. Medicare is indeed not just an indicator but also a program of Americanization. Major causes of death have also been becoming similar between Asian and other races. In Massachusetts, the top-five leading causes of death among Asians by the turn of the century were exactly the same five among other races. Even the order of these causes was almost identical across races (Massachusetts Department of Public Health 2000).

## CONVERGING TRENDS

As time goes by, the exposure to the U.S. environment is exerting a leveling effect on Asian immigrants. Studies show that the lower rate of Western-style cancers—such as breast, prostate, and colorectal cancers—can increase within one generation (PK Mills et al. 2005). In a few generations, cancer incidence and mortality rates that varied greatly have shifted toward the average. Starting at lower rates than Caucasians, cancer deaths of Asian males and females increased 277 percent and 324 percent, respectively, between 1980 and 1996, compared to 123 percent and 133 percent for Caucasians during the same period (Xu et al. 2005). Third- and fourth-generation Asian women had a 60 percent higher cancer risk than those born to more recently immigrated parents. Breast cancer rate among Japanese and Filipino women have been creeping up after immigration, same as rates of prostate, colorectal, and other Western-style cancers.

Asians have shown their desire and ability to adopt changes, sometimes even at odds to their genotype. A study of nutrition in Chinese women found milk consumption surprisingly high given its relative absence from traditional diets and the high prevalence of lactose intolerance. Chinese women become more receptive to drinking milk because traditional Chinese culture advocates extra nutrition for child-rearing women. In contrast, cheese remained poorly consumed (Horswill and Yap 1999). But for the same group of people under the same environment, food choice can still be different. Since immigration, Thai Americans have reduced their number of meals, skipped more meals, and delayed breakfast and lunch times. They have replaced Thai snacks such as dessert and tea with sweet and salty items, fruit juice, and soft drinks. They eat out more in American and Chinese restaurants and buy more from supermarkets instead of from Thai stores, which are few and far between. As a whole, changes in Thai food practice parallel those of other Asian groups in the United States (Sukalakamala and Brittin 2006). Koreans who have lived in the United States longer also consume fewer traditional foods. Although dinner remains the most traditional Korean meal, breakfast, lunch, and snacks are increasingly replaced by mainstream foods (EJ Yang et al. 2005, 2007). Chinese American women are engaging in markedly less physical activity than their counterparts in China, thereby losing the protective effects of physical activity on breast cancer risk, following the same course reported for Japanese and Filipino Americans (D. Yang et al. 2003). As a result, prevalence of diabetes among Japanese Americans and Chinese Americans is two to seven times higher than among their counterparts in Japan and China (Joslin Center 2005). Filipina Americans in San Diego County developed higher prevalence of type 2 diabetes and metabolic syndrome than Caucasians, although they are less likely to be obese, to smoke, drink, and take postmenopausal estrogen (Araneta et al. 2002). Despite having a much lower body weight, about 10 percent of Asian Americans have diabetes, exceeding the rate of about 7 percent of Caucasians (Joslin Center 2005).

Using same-language interviews, researchers were able to find a 23 percent rate of psychiatric morbidity among Chinese normal obstetrical patients, which is similar to that in the general population (Yeung and Schwartz 1986). Very slowly, families denying having a disabled child are willing to disclose their secret (Chung 2005). Despite the myth of more self-restraint in sex, Asians adults do contract AIDS (Dhooper 2003), and Asian teenagers do have similarly frequent and unsafe sex as other teenagers. Sexual behaviors of young Asians today resemble more that of their non-Asian cohorts than that of their parents. Unfortunately, Asian high school students have much less conversation about sexual issues with family adults. When negative elements from both Asian and American cultures confluence, younger generations suffer. More Asian high school students felt depressed, had seriously considered suicide, and made a suicide attempt in the past year (Massachusetts Department of Education, 1999).

Although immigrants are in better health than their U.S.-born counter-parts, their health advantages consistently decrease with duration of residence (Frisbie et al. 2001). Asian immigrants who resided in the United States less than five years, between five to nine years, and ten years or more had an odds ratio for activity limitations of 0.45, 0.65, and 0.73, respectively. The longer Asians resided in the United States, the higher their asthma (A. Davis et al. 2006) and breast cancer rates (Sadler et al. 2003). Age-adjusted mortality rate from heart disease among Japanese American men in Hawaii was 40 percent higher than that of their counterparts in Japan (Dhooper 2003). Another study found the ranking of substance abuse among five Asian groups consistent with their ranking of acculturation and SES indicators. Japanese Americans, who are among the earliest Asian immigrants and the most acculturated, have the highest substance abuse rate, while the Vietnamese are the opposite (Price et al. 2002). To some scholars, the continuous deterioration of health advantages associated with immigration during the length of exposure to U.S. society is a negative process of acculturation (Cho and Hummer 2001).

Length of stay and acculturation, however, do not guarantee acceptance and safety in America. Based on data from state government, community surveys, and focus groups, Chung found Asian teenagers particularly vulnerable (Chung 1998, 2005). The myth of model minority has for a long time masked the troubles Asian teenagers are facing. In addition to unsafe sex, sexual harassment, depression, and suicidal tendencies reported earlier, Asian high school students are the group most likely to be threatened or injured with a weapon at school. A Youth Risk

Behavior Survey (Massachusetts Department of Education 1999) in Massachusetts found them more likely to carry a weapon on school property (in the past thirty days: 16% versus 12% Hispanics, 16% blacks, 14% whites, and 15% statewide). One-third of the Asian high school students were involved in at least one physical fight in the past twelve months. Though lower than average, this rate of fighting reflects a loss of the Asian traditional value that emphasizes peace and tolerance. The survey also found that 9 percent of Asian high school students skipped school in the past thirty days because they felt unsafe, compared to 6 percent statewide. This situation is at odds with the Asian emphasis on school attendance, and a major reason for their greater involvement in gangs (17% vs. 10% statewide).

On the other hand, some mainstream American practices have reduced certain risk factors originated in Asia and raised health consciousness and standards. Length of stay in the U.S. is found to be positively correlated with clinical breast examination (TY Wu et al. 2005), smoking cessation, and utilization of mental health services (Barreto and Segal 2005). As cigarette smoking prevalence rates among Asian groups have decreased in California, the incidence of smoking-related cancers is expected to decline. Major infectious diseases such as TB and hepatitis have been loosening their grip in the United States. With mandatory vaccination of California school children against hepatitis B virus infection, the high rates of liver cancer in Asians are expected to decrease within a generation (Kwong et al. 2005; Mills et al. 2005).

Given the fact that each human being is 99.9 percent identical to every other human being, the trend toward convergence under a similar environment should not be surprising. On the other hand, health conditions among Americans will never be the same given the 0.1 percent difference in genes and substantial environmental differences within the United States. How much difference should there be, without being considered as "discrepancies," along "racial" or any other defined aspects? To answer these questions, it is necessary to look into how data are gathered and analyzed, especially how units, samples, and populations are defined. Many figures showing convergence or discrepancy could be results of ill-defined units or mismatch of samples.

## INTERPRETING ASIAN AMERICAN HEALTH IN THE CONTEXT OF "ETHNIC-ENCLAVE COMPLEX"

### Scarcity of Data and Inadequacy of Concepts— The Need for an Enclave Paradigm

Systematic data gathering has lagged behind the rapid growth and changes in the Asian American population. They were not identified as a major racial category until Census 1980 and not covered in major public health studies such as the NHANES surveys. Only 0.01 percent of MED-LINE articles published between 1966 and 2000 mentioned Asian Americans (Ghosh 2003). Lack of ethnic-specific data is reportedly affecting decision making in many areas such as cardiovascular intervention (Mensah et al. 2005; Yancy et al. 2005). The "invisibility" of Asians in policy debates is considered, to a large extent, a result of a paucity of data stemming from the lack of disaggregated data on this heterogeneous group of people (Srinivasan and Guillermo 2000). Of the four major racial categories, Asian Americans were assigned the fewest number of objectives in Healthy People 2000 (MS Chen 1998). Only 0.2 percent of federal health-related grants from 1986 to 2000 mentioned Asian Americans (Ghosh 2003).

Existing data vary greatly in terms of aggregation unit, time frame, quality, variable selection, and definitions. Estimates of health for the whole Asian population mask differences among subgroups (Kuo et al. 1998). Except for a few national surveys and a some reports featuring all members from specific countries such as Filipino (Dela Cruz et al. 2002) and Asian Indians (Jonnalagadda and Diwan 2005), most studies look at a small social unit, a few health conditions, or utilization rates of Asian subgroups. Given the ratio of new to earlier immigrants, the heterogeneity of socioeconomic conditions, the composition of most Asian groups, and their health data can become rather different in a decade.

A major factor that has been drawing attention and resources away from efforts to improve Asian American health is the contradictory assessment of their health conditions. Although smaller, qualitative studies repeatedly present Asians as underserved groups with low income and education, whose access to and quality of care are obstructed by language, cultural, and institutional barriers (e.g., Sullivan and Hatch 1973); larger, quantitative, unsegregated data are more likely to portray Asians as a highly educated, better-off, and healthy population (e.g., Dey et al. 2006; Frisbie et al. 2001). Lumping data from willing and capable Asian respondents at the county level, researchers made sensational statements such as "the life expectance gap between the 3.4 million high-risk urban black males and the 5.6 million Asian female was 20.7 years in 2001" (Murray et al. 2006). Such statements could create misconceptions and unnecessary racial tension because county level data bury the differences in lower-level geographic units. The SES distribution of Asian Americans within each county surrounding the metropolitan center (where most Asians live; see next section) generally vary widely.

The image of a group of healthy and wealthy people who do not need help from society—a "model minority"—was heightened by some sensational reports on the influx of rich Asians taking over a few middle-income neighborhoods on the West Coast. While both images reflected some truth during the 1970s and early 1980s, attempts to generate findings from one end of the socioeconomic spectrum to the whole Asian population have not stopped even after the bipolar model of socioeconomic and health conditions became popular in the 1990s. Although the bipolar model of SES distribution and corresponding discrepancies in Asian health and health care are still in vogue (e.g., MS Chen 1998; Kagawa-Singer and Maxwell 1999; Lubetkin et al. 2003; Wu et al. 2005; Xu et al. 2005), the expansion of the middle-income segment has already exceeded the combined portions of the new immigrant and affluent enclaves in Massachusetts and other metropolitan areas, and the middle-income segment will continue to expand at a faster pace.

The rapidly increasing proportion of Asian Americans settling down in middle-class municipalities is rendering the bipolar model obsolete. No longer living in the poorest neighborhoods next to the metropolitan center, lacking the attention that a few affluent suburbs draw, unfortunately, the situation of most middle-income Asian Americans continues to be speculated from either end of the SES spectrum or polarized.

The data gathering methods were obviously causing sampling bias—Asians willing and able to respond to the surveys tend to be better educated and proficient in English, and Asians subjects in community studies tend to be poorer and sicker than those who could afford to move out. A more fundamental issue is the lack of guidelines to clarify the relationship between the sampling frame (a pool of all people sharing the defined characteristics from which the sample is selected) of "the population-under-study" and "the ultimate population-targeted/implied." Unlike the selection of sample from a defined population, the selection of population-under-study (often used as a proxy or a subpopulation of the population-targeted) has too often been a matter of convenience. This problem is more serious in Asian American studies given the heterogeneity of the population. A statistically significant finding from "a sample of a Chinatown elderly program," for instance, is representative of only the membership of that particular program (the population-under-study), but not representative of "all Chinese elders in such a program in other cities" (a population-implied), let alone "all Asian elders in similar programs in the country" (an even larger population-implied). Given the heterogeneity and rapid changes of the Asian American population, the true means, standard deviations, and ratios fluctuate substantially depending on not just the sample from a population-under-study but also, more importantly, on which population-under-study is chosen to represent the population-targeted. Characteristics of an ethnic group could be quite different if inferred on the basis of findings from members of a certain geographic unit, an insurance plan, a service program, or people sharing a certain medical condition. The remarkable variability in the choice of population-under-study has rendered the already scarce data even more difficult to compare and accumulate.

The aggregate units most often used in the study of Asian American health are ethnic, cultural, or SES groups. Ethnic, cultural, and SES variables, as seen earlier in this chapter, are often but not always associated with health measures, particularly when only a bivariate relationship is considered. Sometimes the term *Asian community* is used to incorporate, consciously or not, both the ethnic/cultural and the SES aspects. The term *community*, however, assumes too many notions that may distort the reality of Asian American life. In its replacement, I propose the framework of "ethnic-enclave-complex" as a more realistic and practical conceptual tool for the desegregation and reaggregation of data.

## Asian American Health in the More Comprehensive Context of "Ethnic Enclave-Complex"

Concepts in the framework "ethnic-enclave-complex" have evolved from actual Asian American experiences (Chung 1986, 1988, 1989, 1992, 1995a, 1995b, 1996, 1998, 2005). Starting in the mid-1960s, Asians have been rapidly settling outside the overcrowded inner-city neighborhoods. For an illustration, let us look at the Greater Boston metropolitan area, where various types of Asian settlements evolved later than those on the West Coast but earlier than others in the country. With a few exceptions, early Asian settlement in Massachusetts was primarily confined to Boston. Within Boston, from 1890 to 1950, Chinatown consistently hosted about 80 percent of the Asian population. This proportion dropped drastically below 20 percent in 1970s because of continuous immigration influx, urban renewal, highway construction, and institutional expansion (J. Brown. 1987). Between 1980 and 1990, the official Asian population size doubled in Boston and tripled in Massachusetts, while Chinatown could hardly squeeze in any more residents. Where have these people gone?

Asian settlement is not random. They generally cluster around metropolitan centers. Census 2000 revealed that over half of all Asians lived in just nine out of the state's 351 cities and towns, the majority of the Cambodians concentrated in just one, Vietnamese in three, and Chinese and Japanese in five. There is also a high degree of multi-Asian co-inhibition, probably due to a security feeling, the need for similar grocery supplies, and health and human services. All of the top ten cities and towns with the largest Chinese, Indian, and Filipino population were also among the same top twenty-five of the 351 municipalities with the largest Asian population in Massachusetts. Almost all of the top ten cities and towns with the largest Japanese, Korean, Vietnamese and other Asians population were among the top thirty. It is becoming more common to find Asian Indians bringing their children to see a Filipino pediatrician, Chinese patients seeing a Vietnamese dentist, and every group eating or taking out at Asian restaurants.

Asian Americans' choice of residence, consumption behavior, health care attitudes, and behaviors are affected by not only their SES but also their culture and connections. More inclusive than the concept of ethnicity, SES, or geography alone, the framework of "ethnic-enclave complex" provides an integrated picture of contemporary Asian American life. While not belonging to "one community," Asian Americans now maintain regular cross-enclave interactions, and occasionally carry out joint actions. The term *enclave* is used instead of *community* because the latter assumes too much homogeneity, cohesiveness, structural and functional sufficiency, and a well-defined boundary. Asian Americans do not share a same background and cohesiveness as assumed in the term *community*. Their common identity, so far, has been mainly "externally imposed" (Espiritu 1992). They often have to go beyond official geographic or administrative boundaries to fulfill their basic needs such as health care and shopping, which are not necessarily ethnic-specific. It is precisely the structural and functional insufficiency that extends ethnic activities beyond the local enclave. An "Asian American enclave-complex" is generally composed of an "ethnic-crossing" and four types of settlements: three types of "ethnic enclaves" ("the new-immigrant enclaves," "enclaves-in-affluent-suburbs," the 1-step-up enclaves", and "non-enclave settlements" (Chung 1995a). Each type of enclave has its own configuration of geography, SES, housing arrangement, consumption pattern, cultural values, and levels and types of ethnic activities (Table 31.1). Enclaves and enclave-clusters can exist without an ethnic-crossing, but then they do not operate as an enclave-complex.

An ethnic-crossing is usually the earliest ethnic settlement located near the metropolitan center, such as the Chinatown in Boston since the late 1800s, the Cambodian settlement in Lowell, and the Vietnamese settlement in Dorchester since the mid-1990s. It assumes a historically and functionally pivotal role of connecting ethnic and non-enclave settlements in the enclave-complex. Though accommodating mainly new immigrants in the beginning, ethnic-crossings also provide ethnic members in the whole metropolitan area with services, food, commodities, and volunteer opportunities. Restricted by their location in busy urban centers, ethnic-crossings eventually cannot absorb the continuous influx of new immigrants. Additional enclaves then spin off and some businesses follow. The term *crossing* is preferred to *center* because later crossings may emerge and ethnic activities do not have to go through the original crossing, hence it is not a center.

New-immigrant-enclaves host recent immigrants who tend to have lower income or educational attainment than other inner-city poor. Though most new immigrants live in the new-immigrant-enclaves, a substantive number of them stay at least briefly with relatives in other enclaves. Indeed, foreign-born Asians, compared to their U.S.-born counterparts, are more likely to live in larger families (21% vs. 13%) (Dey et al. 2006). Depending on their relationship, many recent immigrants would maintain a separate consumption pattern from relatives living under the same roof.

Several years later, new immigrants who landed a secure job or saved up enough money would move to a safer, middle-income town with decent schools and easy access to the ethnic-crossing. These include recent

**Table 31.1** Health Issues in the Asian American Enclave Complex

| | New Immig. Enclave | 1-Step-Up Enclave | Affluent Suburb E. | Non-Enc. Settlemt |
|---|---|---|---|---|
| **Income** | low | middle | high | any level |
| **Household** | singles, incomplete fam. | families, multifamily | family | all forms |
| **Language** | ethnic | English, ethnic | English | English, ethnic |
| **Location** | inner city | near metro-ctr | affluent suburbs | anywhere |
| **Transportation.** | on foot, pub. transp. | on foot, pub. tran, 1 car | 2+ cars | 1+ cars, pub. transp. |
| **Community atmosphere** | visible | incomplete, inconsistent | precarious | nonexistent |
| **Function for residents** | relatively sufficient | incomplete | narrow and specific | none |
| **Role in e.-complex** | business, residential, human services, cultural, political | residential, human services, cultural, political | residential, cultural | residential |
| **Ethnic org. structure** | complete, formal and informal | new, formal, informal | informal, multitown | none |
| **Geo-relationship** | center | easy access to e-cross. | suburb | farther from center |
| **Health envir.** | overcrowding, heavy traffic, air/noise pollution | overcrowding | isolation | isolation |
| **Health access** | local ethnic, E.R., bilingual private practice | local ethnic/ nonethnic, E.R., e-crossing prov. | local nonethnic, e-crossing providers | local nonethnic, E.R.., e-crossing providers |
| **Main health problems** | infectious diseases, asthma, mental prob. | infectious diseases pediatric, chronic dis., mental prob. | chronic diseases | infectious diseases, chronic diseases, mental prob. |

**Table 31.1** *(Continued)*

|  | New Immig. Enclave | 1-Step-Up Enclave | Affluent Suburb E. | Non-Enc. Settlemt |
|---|---|---|---|---|
| **Auxiliary Serv.** | interpretation, health edu. | interpretation, h. edu., transportation | occasional need for transp./ interp. | occasional need for transp./ interp., h.edu |
| **Payment** | public asst., out of pocket | all forms | private insurance | all forms |
| **CAM** | Substantial | Substantial | Sometimes | Sometimes |

college graduates, small-business owners, and blue- and white-collar workers with a stable income. They begin to deal with more non-Asian neighbors, employers, and institutions unfamiliar with Asians. They are forming new 1-step-up enclaves and wading into the American mainstream. The emergence of Asian enclaves in the middle-income sections around metropolitan centers, which host an increasing proportion of the Asian American population, has been the most important trend since the late 1980s (Chung 1995a, 1995b, 1998, 2005). Owners or executives of larger businesses, high-income professionals, and rich immigrants tend to select a few affluent suburbs with the best schools, and may form Asian-enclaves-in-affluent suburb. The ethnic-complex offers a more comprehensive and dynamic perspective than new terms for Asian American settlement such as *ethnoburb* or *Suburban Chinatown*. The ethnoburb has been blessed with an extraordinarily large influx of Asian capital, hosting a large number of Asians with different income levels, increasing the proportion of Asian visibility and posting a larger political potential (Li 1998). Very few Asian settlements could follow the steps of Monterey Park, "the First Suburban Chinatown" (Fong 1994), which has become an international boomtown. Asian populations even in municipalities hosting an ethnic-crossing are generally far from becoming the majority of the host municipality. Their relative political and economic capacity is much weaker.

Further away but still within the metropolitan area are Asian households seeking lower housing cost or shorter distance to work. When Asians in a previously non-enclave environment increase in number and start organizing ethnic activities, a new 1-step-up-enclave or another affluent-suburban-enclave emerges.

Though not closely-knitted together, each type of ethnic enclave plays different roles within a metropolitan area. The need to understand various types of neighborhoods under a metropolitan framework, rather than individual settlements as similar communities separately operating in an unspecific environment, is increasingly acknowledged (Marcuse 1997; Farrell 2008), despite differences in the conceptualization of settlements/neighborhoods/enclaves. Asian enclaves nowadays are distinguishable yet opening up to Asians of all SES and the society-at-large. They are very different from Marcuse's classification of urban settlements (Marcuse 1997). Unlike their predecessors half a century ago, Asian-towns are no longer "classic ghettos" caused by involuntary spatial segregation. Asian enclaves in affluent suburbs are far from "citadels" created by a dominant group to protect or enhance its superior position. Although the 1-step-up-enclaves are "voluntarily developed spatial concentrations," residents are not necessarily members of a group promoting their common welfare, at least not in the beginning of their settlement.

## HEALTH CARE IN ASIAN ENCLAVES

With the conceptual framework "Ethnic-Enclave Complex" setting the stage for sorting out information from various Asian groups, we can begin to segregate and merge health and health care data accordingly.

### Asian Health Care in the Ethnic-Crossing

The typical ethnic-crossing is Chinatown, but it can also be any "Little Tokyo" once spread along the West Coast, a "Little Manila," "Little Saigon," or "Korea-town" sprung up since the 1970s. An ethnic-crossing is where members from the whole metropolitan area find bilingual medical services, traditional healers, herbal supplies, ethnic food, spices, and drinks for their daily living. They will also find social workers to help them apply for public health care, interpretation, and medical escort. They may also find spiritual support, cultural activities, social networking, mental health and counseling services, traveling arrangements, as well as bus service to the casinos. Ethnic-crossings are richer in organizations. In addition to neighborhood groups, Chinatown also hosts organizations for Chinese and Asians across a much larger area, such as Greater Boston and New England. There are charity groups, service agencies, language schools, a merchants' association, a sailors' club, and interest groups for music, arts, calligraphy, martial arts, and sports, as well as a few Chinese and bilingual newspapers.

Mixed with various organizations and commerce are residences in the ethnic-crossing. With the exception of a small number in the gentrified area, the majority of the residents live in old housing stocks, public housing projects, and elderly housing that form the "new-immigrant-enclave within the ethnic-crossing." Chinatown has a long history of being a less healthy place to live (Lui 2002; Craddock 1995). Health hazards reported from living in Chinatown today include residential overcrowding (Myers and Lee 1996), air pollution, secondhand smoke (Brugge et al. 2002b), noise, construction, trash, higher mortality for its workers (King and

Locke 1980), higher children's asthma rates (Lee et al. 2003), higher rates of mental health problems (Sue et al. 1995; Chow et al. 2003), chronic traffic congestion, and higher pedestrian risk (Brugge et al. 2002a).

## New-Immigrant Enclaves

New-immigrant enclaves have increasingly grown outside Chinatown. An increasing number of reports about the poor health conditions, risk factors, and lower utilization gathered their data from these new-immigrant-enclaves. Aside from low SES, language and cultural barriers are main causes for the poorer health conditions and health care. Studies on the Vietnamese enclave in Dorchester, and Cambodians in Lynn and Revere revealed that most Southeast Asians do not consider alcohol and cigarettes as drugs for adults, and few knew where to seek help. Alcohol and other drug use by teenagers had been a major source of conflict between parents and children (Fontanella and Williams 1993a, 1993b).

Less reported is the lack of organizational effort to improve the situation in early new-immigrant enclaves. The high mobility rate of Vietnamese and their distrust of organizations make them particularly difficult to organize. A 1989 Massachusetts state agency study reported that only 5 out of the 453 persons sampled belonged to any organization other than religious ones (Bia 1989). There was a similar experience among Chinese in Allston, Massachusetts, during the 1990s (Chung 1995b). Lacking a longer history and economic power, new-immigrant enclaves are structurally and functionally underdeveloped. It takes these enclaves longer to set up their own ethnic services, as residents could get help from Chinatown. A 1987 Chinatown User survey reported that at least 25 percent of the respondents came from the new-immigrant enclaves (Oriola and Perkins, 1988).

Meanwhile, government and private funding agencies urged individual ethnic groups to form "coalitions" when they apply for grants (Espiritu 1992). Service providers in the new-immigrant enclaves often have to work closely with Chinatown agencies, and their cooperation reinforces the connection between these enclaves. Chinatown agencies in turn hired more non-Chinese Asian workers and even expanded their identity from Chinese to "Asian;" for example, the Asian (previously named Chinese) American Civic Association.

New-immigrant enclaves will grow as long as the scale of current Asian immigration continues. However, the proportion of Asians living in these enclaves will not expand as earlier immigrants will move out and earlier new-immigrant enclaves could turn into ethnic-crossings, like Dorchester for the Vietnamese today.

## Enclaves in Affluent Suburbs

Asians living in other affluent suburbs across the United States generally do not enjoy the high political visibility and economic prominence as those in the ethnoburb, even though many are individually well-off. Many residents in the affluent suburbs maintain close contacts with the rest of the ethnic enclave-complex. A substantial number of them earn their living and provide voluntary service or leadership in the ethnic-crossing. Without help, most of their offspring cannot buy a home in these affluent suburbs in the beginning of their career. Many of them would start their new family in middle-income municipalities nearby to maintain regular family interaction. While mostly being insured and mobile, many affluent suburban Asian residents also host recently arrived relatives who need help in adjusting to American society. Although they live under one roof and may even share meals, newcomers usually want to work hard and become independent. They frequent the ethnic-crossing for English class, ethnic supplies, elderly service, traditional medicine, or Western medicine provided by Asians.

Asian residents may also face certain obstacles that others in affluent suburbs may not. Health providers in the metropolitan center may have more contacts with Asian patients and be more sensitive to their needs. Public health policies there are also more cosmopolitan. In comparison, suburban health providers are less familiar with ethnic problems. The underdiagnosis of TB in Asian Indians by local providers in affluent New Jersey suburbs is one concrete example (Davidow et al. 2003).

## The 1-Step-Up Enclaves

The most important trend at this historical juncture of Asian American settlement in the United States is the rapid and consistent growth of the 1-step-up-enclaves. This rapid growth of Asian enclaves in middle-income municipalities close to the metropolitan center represents a breakthrough in the middle from the bimodal SES distribution of the Asian American population. Because of fluctuations in immigration policies, the SES curve of the Asian population prior to 1990 looked like a U-shaped curve, showing a substantial number with high education/income and a much larger proportion with low education/income, with very few in-between. This "abnormal curve" is representative of neither the American nor any Asian population. Asian Americans' current movement into the middle-income municipalities signals a trend toward the mainstream. These municipalities accommodated an incessant stream of Asians, mostly those who lived for about five or more years in the new-immigrant enclaves now looking for a place to raise their family in an efficient fashion. "Efficiency" here means time, lower transportation cost, and access to ethnic goods and services in the ethnic-crossing. That is why Asians are willing to pool their money and pay a higher price for a house that can host more than one nuclear family. These enclaves also attract the younger generations who want to stay around their parents or who cannot afford moving into the affluent suburbs. This is the place where young professional couples find reliable child care and household chore service at an acceptable price, and where older folks find companions and culturally sensitive elderly services outside of the overcrowded ethnic crossing.

Health issues faced by Asians living outside traditional settlements have raised a few concerns, though their SES and location are not always well defined (Yeung and Schwartz 1986; King and Locke 1987; TY Wu et al. 2006; Haritatos et al. 2007). Mental health researchers reported that "living outside of Chinatown is a source of stress although not severe enough to provoke actual psychiatric morbidity" (Yeung and Schwartz 1986). A study found that Asian Indian women with moderate lower income had the highest level of barriers in obtaining breast cancer screening, higher even than those with the lowest income level. The researchers speculated that since the majority of those in the lowest income group did not have regular mammogram screening, they probably did not encounter the actual barriers experienced in mammogram screening that the middle-income groups did (TY Wu et al. 2006).

The sudden influx of the supposedly self-sufficient Asians had alarmed some local municipalities to the need for better planning. In Quincy, for instance, instead of waiting for Census 1990, two independent needs assessment efforts were conducted in the late 1980s (Parker and Edmonds 1988; Archer and Conroy 1989). On the basis of an Asian population size about twice that counted by Census 1990 and the immigrants' experiences, they estimated the scale and causes of service discrepancy with a sense of urgency. A later "citywide" survey conducted by the city hall, however, placed major Asian needs at a much lower priority. Feeling the pressing needs were inadequately met, advocacy groups and service agencies sponsored another study. Based on a survey responded to by 504 households (to trilingual questionnaires of 140 data-points), 10 focus groups, in-depth interviews, participant observation, and critical analyses of existing figures, Chung presented the first comprehensive assessment of health care and other needs of Asians in the 1-step-up-enclave (Chung 1998). A similar study was later conducted in another 1-step-up-enclave, Malden, focusing specifically on health and disability issues (Chung 2005). By 2000, the Asian population size in these two enclaves alone was already five times larger than that of Chinatown. The following summarizes some major findings on health care issues in these enclaves.

Asians moved into these middle-income municipalities when the heads of their household were within the productive age span. The lack of bilingual services did not deter them in the beginning, and they could also rely on the ethnic-crossing. Within a decade or so, however, their needs for child care and elderly service increased. As local establishments were slow to adjust, about 70 percent of the Asian residents in the cities of Quincy and Malden had to go out of town for medical care.

Unlike their counterparts in new-immigrant enclaves, Asians in 1-step-up-enclaves are less likely to be covered by Medicaid. Many Asians working in small business have no health insurance. Private insurance policies do not cover elderly parents. To deal with sickness, many in these enclaves would skip or delay medical help unless it is for the elderly or children. Some of them would self-treat certain conditions, such as a cold or arthritis, where Western medicine is not particularly effective. Some would obtain drugs from overseas, particularly those who retired but still receive health benefits. Being unfamiliar with the fees and procedures, Asians are reluctant to use the emergency room for primary care purposes unless they are in great pain or are seriously ill.

Insurance barriers and the American health system's unfamiliarity with Asian patients could also cause serious public health problems. For instance, a patient treated for multiple conditions had everything under control until his Mass Health coverage expired. Without insurance, his treatments stopped, his diabetic condition deteriorated, and his dormant tuberculosis (T.B.) came back. He coughed for a long time without seeing a doctor, until he became eligible again for Mass Health. In between, he worked in a restaurant. The Department of Public Health does offer a free T.B. clinic. The public, however, is largely unaware of it. People working in places without paid sick leave would not be eager to receive screening and treatment, as the treatment process takes six to nine months.

Disability rates in Malden, Massachusetts, are higher than what Census 2000 reported. Even as mental disorders are still somatized, signals of mental disorder are on the rise: depression; regular sleep loss; apathy; and worry about money, job, school performance, safety, future, and relatives living elsewhere. In addition, a majority of survey respondents reported unspecific anxiety and unexplained pain. Time constraint due to high expectations, unfamiliarity of environment and procedures, and impatience to accomplish more with less time have all been leading to stress. The long and odd working hours are taking a toll on many Asian families. About half of the respondents worry about negligence, conflicts, or abuse within the family. The harmony and support Asian cultures preach is hard to maintain, particularly during hard times.

Bicultural health care services are growing in the 1-step-up enclaves and contributing to the overall trend of localization of consumption. Still, two decades after the beginning of the Asian influx, health care facilities are far from adequate, as about one-third of the Malden respondents relied on Chinatown alone for medical care.

The ethnic enclave-complex establishes an integrative view of major SES, cultural, geographic, and health information for the understanding of the interactive dynamics of environmental factors Asian Americans are now facing. It provides a theoretically and practically more precise and reliable unit for the desegregation and reaggregation of data. Table 31.1 summarizes the nature of various types of enclaves and respective health issues. (For a detailed set of socioeconomic indicators defining specific features of each type of enclaves, please see Table 31.2. Data from Census 2000 confirm the continuation of the same pattern.)

**Table 31.2** Sample Municipal Settings of Asian Ethnic Enclaves, 1990

| | # Asian | % Asian | Median Household Income | Median Per Capita | Median Price of Single Fam. | Median Monthly Rent* | Renter-Owner Ratio* |
|---|---|---|---|---|---|---|---|
| MA | | 2.4 | $36,952 | $17,224 | $162,800 | $506 | 0.69 |
| Asian | 133,492 | | $34,706 | $12,665 | n.a. | n.a. | 1.50 |
| Boston | | 5.3 | $29,180 | $15,581 | $161,400 | $546 | 2.24 |
| Asian | 30,388 | | $22,504 | $9,406 | n.a. | n.a. | n.a. |
| *Asian Ethnic Crossing* | | | | | | | |
| Chinatown | 3,301 | 88.9 | $12,143 | $7,573 | n.a. | $456 | 22.26 |
| *New Imm. Enclaves* | | | | | | | |
| Allston- | | | | | | | |
| Brighton | 7,604 | 10.8 | $29,384 | $15,773 | $184,000 | $726 | 3.39 |
| Dorchester | 3,725 | 4.4 | $30,000 | $12,500 | $153,000 | $530 | 1.88 |
| Chelsea | 1,435 | 5.0 | $25,144 | $11,559 | $142,000 | $501 | 2.56 |
| *One-Step-Up Enclaves* | | | | | | | |
| Quincy | 5,577 | 6.6 | $35,838 | $17,436 | $161,100 | $599 | 1.05 |
| Malden | 2,815 | 5.2 | $34,344 | $15,820 | $162,920 | $575 | 1.31 |
| Somerville | 2,824 | 3.7 | $32,455 | $15,179 | $165,800 | $591 | 2.23 |
| *Affluent Suburban Enclaves* | | | | | | | |
| Lexington | 1,876 | 6.5 | $67,389 | $30,718 | $282,800 | $902 | 0.22 |
| Newton | 3,760 | 4.5 | $59,719 | $28,840 | $293,400 | $809 | 0.45 |
| Brookline | 4,585 | 8.4 | $45,598 | $29,044 | $377,800 | $629 | 1.32 |

All 1990 census data unless specified. There are several delineations of Chinatown. Figures adopted here come from the Boston Redevelopment Authority (BRA). Dorchester figures are estimated from several BRA Dorchester subdistrict 1990 census summary reports.

* From Edith Hornov, Massachusetts Municipal Profile, 1991–1992, Palo Alto, CA: Information Publications, 1991; and Irene Sege, "Increase in the Diversity as Shown in the Census," *Boston Globe* (July 1, 1991): Metro Section, p.1.

*Source:* "Asian Americans in Enclaves—They Are Not One Community: New Modes of Asian American Settlement," in Asian American Policy Review, #5, 1995. Also in T. Fong and L. Shinagawa, (eds.), *Asian Americans: Experiences and Perspectives,* Upper Saddle River, NJ: Prentice Hall, 2000.

## CONCLUSION

Studies have confirmed some positive and negative impacts of original differences on Asian American health and health care. Biological, cultural, and social factors are all implicated. Although the problems more common in Asia continue to require attention, the needs of earlier immigrants and those who were born in the United States cannot be neglected either. Strong evidence shows that the longer Asians reside in the United States, the more likely their health care behavior, mortality, and morbidity converge with the rest of the country. Although traditional habits persist, Asians' willingness to adjust is also witnessed by their choice of an urban

rather than a rural setting, in which most of them used to live, their acculturation to the American diet, even including those foods at odds with
their habits and genetic responses, and their trust in Western medicine,
including its diagnosis and treatment of chronic diseases and mental disorders. The growing proportion of U.S.-born Asians is also becoming a
major force of Americanization.

Americanization can evolve along different paths depending on one's
SES, culture, geographic location, and many other variables. This chapter offers "the Asian enclave-complex" as a more comprehensive conceptual framework to differentiate and integrate the interaction of major
variables of demography, health condition, health care behavior, and
interventions. Existing data for the enclave-complex is far from detailed
and systematic. However, they reflect the situation in the multifactorial
context, thereby getting closer to the reality than those perceived from
separated perspectives of original differences or societal influences.
Hopefully, the practical and theoretical implications with this approach
will be appreciated soon.

## REFERENCES

Acevedo-Garcia, D., M. Soobader, and L. F. Berkman. 2005. The Differential Effect
of Foreign-Born Status on Low Birth Weight by Race/Ethnicity and Education. *Pediatrics* 115:e20–e30.

Aekplakorn, W., J. Abbott-Klafter, A. Premgamone, B. Dhanamun, C. Chaikittiporn,
V. Chongsuvivatwong, T. Suwanprapisa, W. Chaipornsupaisan, S. Tiptaradol,
and S.S. Lim. 2007. Prevalence and Management of Diabetes and Associated
Risk Factors by Regions of Thailand. Third National Health Examination
Survey 2004. *Diabetes Care* 30:2007–2012.

Aekplakorn, W., P. Bunnag, M. Woodward, P. Sritara, S. Cheepudomwit, S.
Yamwong, T. Yipintsoi, and R. Rajatanavin. 2006. A Risk Score for Predicting
Incident Diabetes in the Thai Population. *Diabetes Care* 29, no. 8:
1872–1877.

Akutsu, P.D., E.D. Castillo, and L.R. Snowden. 2007. Differential Referral Patterns
to Ethnic-Specific and Mainstream Mental Health Programs for Four Asian
American Groups. *American Journal of Orthopsychiatry* 77:95–103.

Alagiakrishnan, K., and A. Chopra. Health and Health Care of Asian Indian
American Elders. http://Stanford.edu/group/ethnoger/asianindian.html

Alegria, M., Z. Cao, T.G. McGuire, V.D. Ojeda, B. Sribney, M. Woo, and D. Takeuchi.
2006. Health Insurance Coverage for Vulnerable Populations: Contrasting
Asian Americans and Latinos in the United States. *Inquiry* 43:231–254.

Andrulis, D.P., L.M. Duchon, and H.M. Reid. 2003. Dynamics of Race, Culture and
Key Indicators of Health in the Nation's 100 Largest Cities and Their Suburbs.
The Social and Health Landscape of Urban and Suburban America Report
Series. SUNY Downstate Medical Center, Brooklyn, New York.

Anjana, M., S. Sandeep, R. Deepa, K.S. Vimaleswaran, S. Farooq, and V.Mohan. 2004. Visceral and Central Abdominal Fat and Anthropometry in Relation to Diabetes in Asian Indians. *Diabetes Care* 27, no. 12:2948–2953.

Araneta, M.G., D.L. Wingard, and E. Barrett-Connor. 2002. Type 2 Diabetes and Metabolic Syndrome in Filipina-American Women. A High-Risk Nonobese Population. *Diabetes Care* 25:494–499.

Araneta, M.G., and E. Barrett-Connor. 2005. Ethnic Differences in Visceral Adipose Tissue and Type 2 Diabetes: Filipino, African-American, and White Women. *Obesity Research* 13, no. 8:1458–1465.

Archer, Bill, and Tom Conroy. "The Asians, Quincy's Newest Immigrants." *Patriot Ledger*, 1989.

Asian and Pacific Islander American Health Forum (APIAHF). Comments on Draft Healthy People 2010 Objectives. http://apiahf.org/hp2010.html.

Averbach, A.R., D. Lam, L.P. Lam, J. Sharfstein, B. Cohen, and H. Koh. 2002. Smoking Behaviors and Attitudes among Male Restaurant Workers in Boston's Chinatown: a Pilot Study. *Tobacco Control* 11, Suppl. 2: ii34–ii37.

Bae, S.W., and W.W. Kung. 2000. Family Intervention for Asian Americans with a Schizophrenic Patient in the Family. *American Journal of Orthopsychiatry* 70, no. 4:532–541.

Baker, S.B., L.H. Nguyen, and J. Dols. 2001. Diabetes-Related Knowledge, Attitudes, and Behaviors in an Asian American Community—Telephone Survey. Poster presented at the One Hundred Twenty-Ninth Meeting of the American Public Health Association, Atlanta, GA, October 23, 2001. http://apha.confex.com/apha/129am/techprogram/paper_27024.htm.

Barnes, P.M., E. Powell-Griner, K. McFann, and R.L. Nahin. 2004. Complementary and Alternative Medicine Use among Adults: United States, 2002. *Advance Data from Vital and Health Statistics* 343, 1–19.

Barnes, P.M., P.F. Adams, and E. Powell-Griner. 2008. Health Characteristics of the Asian Adult Population: United States, 2004–2006. *Advance Data from Vital and Health Statistics* 394, 1–22.

Barreto, R.M., and S.P. Segal. 2005. Use of Mental Health Services by Asian Americans. *Psychiatric Services* 56, no. 6:746–748.

Bates, Lisa M., Dolores Acevedo-Garcia, Margarita Alegría, and Nancy Krieger. 2008. Immigration and Generational Trends in Body Mass Index and Obesity in the United States: Results of the National Latino and Asian American Survey, 2002–2003. *American Journal of Public Health* 98, no. 1:70–77.

Behme, M.T., J. Dupre, S.B. Harris, I.M. Hramiak, and J.L. Mahon. 2003. Insulin Resistance in Latent Autoimmune Diabetes of Adulthood. *Annals New York Academy of Sciences* 1005:374–377.

Bell, M.T. 2004. Immigration: A Megatrends Backgrounder. The Council of State Governments, KY: Lexington.

Bernstein, Nina. 2006. "Recourse Grows Slim for Immigrants Who Fall Ill." *New York Times,* March 3, 2006, Health Section.

Bia, Le Van. 1989. Descriptive Profile and Needs Assessment of Vietnamese People in Massachusetts Department of Mental Health (manuscript).

Biesenbach, G., M.Auinger, M. Clodi, F. Prischl, and R. Kramar. Prevalence of LADA and Frequency of GAD Antibodies in Diabetic Patients with End-Stage Renal Disease and Dialysis Treatment in Austria. *Nephrology Dialysis Transplantation* 20, no. 3:559–565.

Bottazzo, G.F., E. Bosi, C.A.Cull, E. Bonifacio, M. Locatelli, P. Zimmet, I.R. Mackay, and R.R. Holman. 2005. IA-2 Antibody Prevalence and Risk Assessment of Early Insulin Requirement in Subjects Presenting with Type 2 Diabetes (UKPDS 71). *Diabetologia* 48:703–708.

Bourguignon, M. 1988. Chinatown Survey Area Land Use Report. Boston Redevelopment Authority (manuscript).

Boyce, C.A., and V.S. Cain. 2007. Disentangling Health Disparities through National Surveys. *American Journal of Public Health* Vol. 97, no. 1, DOI: 10.2105/AJPH.2006.103960.

Brown, D.W., G.A. Haldeman, J.B. Croft, W.H. Giles, G.A. Mensah. 2005. Racial or Ethnic Differences in Hospitalization for Heart Failure among Elderly Adults: Medicare, 1990 to 2000. *American Heart Journal* 150, no. 3:448–454.

Brown, J. 1987. Profile of Boston's Chinatown Neighborhood, Boston. Boston Redevelopment Authority (manuscript).

Brugge, D., A.C. Lee, M. Woodin, and C. Rioux. 2007. Native and Foreign Born as Predictors of Pediatric Asthma in an Asian Immigrant Population: A Cross Sectional Survey. *Environmental Health* 6:13. http://www.ehjournal.net/content/6/1/13.

Brugge, D., Z. Lai, C. Hill, and W. Rand. 2002. Traffic Injury Data, Policy, and Public Health: Lessons from Boston Chinatown. *Journal of Urban Health* 79, no. 1:87–103.

Brugge, D., W. DeJong, J. Hyde, Q. Lee, C.S. Shih, A. Wong, and A. Tran. 2002. Development of Targeted Message Concepts for Recent Asian Immigrants about Secondhand Smoke. *Journal of Health Communication* 7, no. 1:25–37.

Burgel, Barbara J., Nan Lashuay, Leslie Israel, and Robert Harrison. 2004. Garment Workers in California: Health Outcomes of the Asian Immigrant Women Workers Clinic. *American Association of Occupational Health Nurses Journal* 52, no. 11:465–475.

Car, J., H. Patel, J. Srishanmuganathan, and A. Majeed. 2007. Diabetes Care in Developing Countries. *Canadian Medical Association Journal* 176, no. 2:209–212.

Carlisle, D.M., B.D. Leake, and M.F. Shapiro. 1997. Racial and Ethnic Disparities in the Use of Cardiovascular Procedures: Associations with Type of Health Insurance. *American Journal of Public Health* 87, no. 2:263–267.

Carr, D.B., K.M. Utzschneider, E.J. Boyko, P.J. Asberry, R.L. Hull, K. Kodama, H.S. Callahan, C.C. Matthys, D.L. Leonetti, R.S. Schwartz, S.E. Kahn, and W.Y. Fujimoto. 2005. A Reduced-Fat Diet and Aerobic Exercise in Japanese Americans with Impaired Glucose Tolerance Decreases Intra-Abdominal Fat and Improves Insulin Sensitivity but Not ß-Cell Function. *Diabetes* 54:340–347.

Chen, Huey Jen. 2005. Mental Illness and Principal Physical Diagnoses among Asian American and Pacific Islander Users of Emergency Services. *Issues in Mental Health Nursing* 26, no. 10:1061–1079.

Chen, Jyu-Lin, and Christine Kennedy. 2005. Factors Associated with Obesity in Chinese-American Children. *Pediatric Nursing* 31, no. 2:110–115.

Chen, Moon S., Jr. 1998. Cancer Prevention and Control among Asian and Pacific Islander Americans: Findings and Recommendations. *Cancer* 83, no. S8:1856–1864.

Chen, M.S., Jr., S.M. Shinagawa, D.G. Bal, R.Bastani, E.A. Chow, R.C.S. Ho, L. Jones, S.J. McPhee, R. Senie, V. Taylor, M. Kagawa-Singer, S. Stewart, H.K. Koh, and F.P. Li. 2006. Asian American Network for Cancer Awareness, Research, and Training's Legacy: The First 5 Years. *Cancer* 107, Suppl. 8:2006–2014.

Chen, W., D.B. Petitti, and S. Enger. 2004. Limitations and Potential Uses of Census-Based Data on Ethnicity in a Diverse Community. *Annals of Epidemiology* 14, no. 5:339–345.

Cheung, B.M.Y., N.M.S. Wat, Y.B. Man, S. Tam, G.N. Thomas, G.M. Leung, C.H. Cheng, J. Woo, E.D. Janus, C.P. Lau, T.H. Lam, and K.S.L. Lam. 2007. Development of Diabetes in Chinese with the Metabolic Syndrome—A Six-Year Prospective Study. *Diabetes Care* 30:1430–1436.

Cho, Y., and R.A. Hummer. 2001. Disability Status Differentials across Fifteen Asian and Pacific Islander Groups and the Effects of Nativity and Duration or Residence in U.S. *Social Biology* 48, 3–4:171–195.

Choe, J.H., Koepsell, T.D., Heagerty, P.J., Taylor, V.M. 2005. Colorectal Cancer among Asians and Pacific Islanders in the U.S.: Survival Disadvantage for the Foreign-Born. *Cancer Detection and Prevention* 29, no. 4:361–368.

Chow, J.C.C., K. Jaffee, and L. Snowden. 2003. Racial/Ethnic Disparities in the Use of Mental Health Services in Poverty Areas. *American Journal of Public Health* 93, no. 5:792–797.

Chung, T.L.N. 1983. Chinese Take Very Different Views of Health Services. *Boston Seniority*, July 1983.

———. 1986. Ethnic Difference in Home Care Client Satisfaction. University of Massachusetts Gerontology Institute.

———. 1987. An Analysis of the Political Participation of Chinese Americans. *Ming Pao Monthly*, May 1987 (in Chinese).

———. 1988. Chinese Culture to Keep or Not—Implications from Chinatown Surveys. *Ming Pao Monthly*, July 1988 (in Chinese).

———. 1988. Job Expectation and Opportunities of Asian American Clients. Boston Redevelopment Authority and the South Cove Chinatown Neighborhood Council (manuscript).

Chung, Tom Lun-nap, and the Henderson's Planning Group. 1989. Needs Assessment for the Chinatown Community Center (Parcel C) Project. Boston Redevelopment Authority and the South Cove Chinatown Neighborhood Council (manuscript).

Chung, Tom Lun-nap, Cynthia Ker, Carrie Tang, and Loraine Choi. 1992. Greater Boston Chinese Cultural Association Membership Survey. Greater Boston Chinese Cultural Association (manuscript).

Chung, Tom Lun-nap. 1995a. Asian Americans in Enclaves—They Are Not One Community: New Modes of Asian American Settlement. *Asian American Policy Review,* 5. 78-94. (Also in Fong, T. & L. Shinagawa, (eds.) *Asian Americans: Experiences and Perspectives,* Prentice Hall, 2000. 99-109)

———. 1995b. New Settlement Trends of the Chinese in Greater Boston: Implications for Overseas Chinese Studies. *Bulletin of Ethnology, Academia Sinica,* no. 80. 155-188. (Also in *Overseas Chinese Historical Studies,* Beijing: Oversea Chinese Historical Studies Society, # 2 and # 4, 1998.)

———. 1996. Hate Crimes and the Glass Ceiling—Two Forms of Discrimination against Asian Americans in Massachusetts. MA Asian American Commission & MA Office for Refugees and Immigrants (manuscript).

———. 1998. One Step Closer to the Mainstream? A Comprehensive Assessment of Human Service Needs, Economic and Political Participation of Asian Americans in Quincy, Massachusetts. The Quincy Coalition for the Prevention of Alcohol, Tobacco & Other Drug Problems (manuscript).

———. 2005. Health and Disability Issues of Asian Residents on Malden, Massachusetts. Healthy Malden, Inc., Great Wall Center and Tri-Community Action Program, Inc. (manuscript).

Constantine, M.G., S. Okazaki, and S.O. Utsay. 2004. Self-Concealment, Social Self-Efficacy, Acculturative Stress, and Depression in African, Asian, and Latin American International College Students. *American Journal of Orthopsychiatry* 74, no. 3:230–241.

Corella, D., L. Qi, E.S. Tai, M. Deurenberg-Yap, C.E. Tan, S.K. Chew, and J.M. Ordovas. 2006. Perilipin Gene Variation Determines Higher Susceptibility to Insulin Resistance in Asian Women When Consuming a High-Saturated Fat, Low-Carbohydrate Diet. *Diabetes Care* 29:1313–1319.

Craddock, S. 1995. Sewers and Scapegoats: Spatial Metaphors of Smallpox in Nineteenth-Century San Francisco. *Social Science and Medicine* 41, no. 7:957–968.

Cui, L., J.N. Fang, and M.A. Huang. 2006. Comparison of Distributive Characteristics of Abnormal Blood Lipid between the Han and Korean-Chinese Nationalities in the Urban of Yanbian Area. *Chinese Journal of Clinical Rehabilitation* 10, no. 12:4–6.

Cummins, L.H., A.M. Simmons, and N.W.S. Zane. 2005. Eating Disorders in Asian Populations: A Critique of Current Approaches to the Study of Culture, Ethnicity, and Eating Disorders. *American Journal of Orthopsychiatry* 75, no. 4:553–574.

Dallas, C. 2004. How Scholarly Nursing Literature Addresses Health Disparities for Racial/Ethnic Minority Men. *Association of Black Nursing Faculty Journal* 15, no. 1:10–14.

Davidow, A.L., B.T. Mangura, E.C. Napolitano, and L.B. Reichman. 2003. Rethinking the Socioeconomics and Geography of Tuberculosis among Foreign-Born

Residents of New Jersey, 1994–1999. *American Journal of Public Health* 93, no. 6:1007–1012.

Davis, A.M., R. Kreutzer, M. Lipsett, G. King, and N. Shaikh. 2006. Asthma Prevalence in Hispanic and Asian American Ethnic Subgroups: Results from the California Healthy Kids Survey. *Pediatrics* 118, no. 2:e363–e370.

Davis, J.A. 2005. Differences in the Health Care Needs and Service Utilization of Women in Nursing Homes: Comparison by Race/Ethnicity. *Journal of Women & Aging* 17, no. 3:57–71.

DECODA Study Group. 2003. Age- and Sex-Specific Prevalence of Diabetes and Impaired Glucose Regulation in 11 Asian Cohorts. *Diabetes Care* 26:1770–1780.

Dein, S. 2006. Race, Culture and Ethnicity in Minority Research: A Critical Discussion. *Journal of Cultural Diversity* 13, no. 2:68–75.

Dela Cruz, F.A., M.R. McBride, L.B. Compas, P.R. Calixto, and C.P. Van Derveer. 2002. White paper on the health status of Filipino Americans and recommendations for research. *Nursing Outlook* 50, no. 1:7–15.

Dey, A.N., and J.W. Lucas. 2006. Physical and Mental Health Characteristics of U.S.- and Foreign-Born Adults: United States, 1998–2003. *Advance Data* 369:1–19.

Dhooper, S.S. 2003. Health Care Needs of Foreign-Born Asian Americans: An Overview. *Health and Social Work* 28:63–73.

Dilley, J., A. Ganesan, R. Deepa, M. Deepa, G. Sharada, O.D. Williams, and V. Mohan. 2007. Association of A1C with Cardiovascular Disease and Metabolic Syndrome in Asian Indians with Normal Glucose Tolerance. *Diabetes Care* 30:1527–1532.

Doi, Y., Y. Kiyohara, M. Kubo, T. Ninomiya, Y. Wakugawa, K. Yonemoto, M. Iwase, and M. Iida. 2005. Elevated C-Reactive Protein Is a Predictor of the Development of Diabetes in a General Japanese Population. The Hisayama Study. *Diabetes Care* 28:2497–2500.

Drever, A.I. 2004. Separate Spaces, Separate Outcomes? Neighborhood Impacts on Minority in Germany. *Urban Studies* 41, no. 8:1423–1439.

Eichelberger, L. 2007. SARS and New York's Chinatown: The Politics of Risk and Blame during an Epidemic of Fear. *Social Science and Medicine* 65, no. 6: 1284–1295.

The 8th International Conference on Health Problems Related to the Chinese. 1996. http://www.fcmsdocs.org.

Erosheva, E,E.C. Walton, and D.T. Takeuchi. 2007. Self-Rated Health among Foreign- and U.S.-Born Asian Americans. A Test of Comparability. *Medical Care* 45, no. 1:80–87.

Espiritu, Y.L. 1992. *Asian American Panethnicity, Bridging Institutions & Identities.* Philadelphia, PA: Temple University Press.

Ezenwa, M.O., S. Ameringer, S.E. Ward, and R.C. Serlin. 2006. Racial and Ethnic Disparities in Pain Management in the United States. *Journal of Nursing Scholarship* 38, no. 3:225–233.

Farrell, Chad. 2008. Bifurcation, Fragmentation or Integration? The Racial and Geographical Structure of U.S. Metropolitan Segregation, 1990–2000. *Urban Studies*, 45, 467–499.

Ferketich, A.K., M.E. Wewers, K. Kwong, E. Louie, M.L. Moeschberger, A. Tso, and M. Chen, Jr. 2004. Smoking Cessation Interventions among Chinese Americans: The Role of Families, Physicians, and the Media. *Nicotine and Tobacco Research* 6, no. 2:241–248.

Flynn, Thomas. 1992. Quincy Real Estate Study. University of Massachusetts–Boston, unpublished student paper.

Fong, T. 1994. *The First Suburban Chinatown.* Philadelphia, PA: Temple University Press.

Fontanella, M., and C. Williams. 1993a. Cambodian Community Resident Survey Results. Boston: MA: South Cove Community Health Center.

———. 1993b. Vietnamese Community Resident Survey Results. Boston, MA: South Cove Community Health Center.

Frisbie, W.P., Y. Cho, and R.A Hummer. 2001. Immigration and the Health of Asian and Pacific Islander Adults in the United States. *American Journal of Epidemiology* 153, no. 4:372–380.

Fu, S.S., G.X. Ma, X.M. Tu, P.T. Siu, and J.P. Metlay. 2003. Cigarette Smoking among Chinese Americans and the Influence of Linguistic Acculturation. *Nicotine and Tobacco Research* 5, no. 6:803–811.

Gall, S.B., and T.L. Gall, 1993. *Statistical Record of Asian Americans.* Detroit, MI: Gale Research.

Gary, F.A. 2005. Stigma: Barrier to Mental Health Care among Ethnic Minorities. *Issues in Mental Health Nursing* 26, no. 10:979–999.

Ghosh, C. 2003. Healthy People 2010 and AA/PIs: Defining a Baseline of Information. *American Journal of Public Health* 93, no. 12:2093–2098.

Goel, M.S., E.P. McCarthy, R.S. Phillips, and C.C. Wee. 2004. Obesity among U.S. Immigrant Subgroups by Duration of Residence. *JAMA* 292:2860–2867.

Goetze, R., and M. Johnson. 1991. Chinatown. City of Boston Neighborhood Area Series. Boston Redevelopment Authority, August 1991.

Gorin, S.S., J.E. Heck, B. Cheng, and S.J. Smith. 2006. Delays in Breast Cancer Diagnosis and Treatment by Racial/Ethnic Group. *Archives of Internal Medicine* 166:2244–2252.

GTFHC 1992 (Governor's Task Force on Hate Crimes). 1993. Hate Crimes/Hate Incidents in Massachusetts, Annual Report, 1992.

GTFHC 1993 (Governor's Task Force on Hate Crimes). 1994. Hate Crimes in Massachusetts, Annual Report, 1993.

Haritatos, J., R. Mahalingam, and S.A. James. 2007. John Henryism, Self-Reported Physical Health Indicators, and the Mediating Role of Perceived Stress among High Socio-Economic Status Asian Immigrants. *Social Science & Medicine* 64, no. 6:1192–1203.

He, W., M. Sengupta, V.A. Velkoff, and K.A. DeBarros. 2005. 65+ in the U.S. current Population Reports. Special Studies. http://www.census.gov/prod/2006pubs/p23–209.pdf.

*Herald Monthly.* 1997. Special Issue on Violence among Chinese Youth and Children. June, 1997.

Herrick, C.A., and H.N. Brown. 1998. Underutilization of Mental Health Services by Asian-Americans Residing in the United States. *Issues in Mental Health Nursing* 19, no. 3:225–240.

Hill, L., C.R. Hofstetter, M. Hovell, J. Lee, V. Irvin, and J. Zakarian. 2006. Koreans' Use of Medical Services in Seoul, Korea and California. *Journal of Immigrant & Minority Health* 8, no. 3:273–280.

Ho, M.J. 2004. Health-Seeking Patterns among Chinese Immigrant Patients Enrolled in the Directly Observed Therapy Program in New York City. *International Journal of Tuberculosis and Lung Disease* 8, no. 11:1355–1359.

Ho, M.J. 2004. Sociocultural Aspects of Tuberculosis: A Literature Review and a Case Study of Immigrant Tuberculosis. *Social Science & Medicine* 59, no. 4:753–762.

———. 2006. Perspectives on Tuberculosis among Traditional Chinese Medical Practitioners in New York City's Chinatown. *Culture, Medicine & Psychiatry* 30, no. 1:105–122.

Hong, Betty, and Noushin Bayat. 1999. National Asian American & Pacific Islander Cardiovascular Health Action Plan. Proceedings from the First National AAPI Cardiovascular Health Strategy Workshop, San Francisco, CA, May 8–9, 1999.

Horswill, L.J., and C. Yap. 1999. Consumption of Foods from the WIC Food Packages of Chinese Prenatal Patients on the U.S. West Coast. *Journal of the American Dietetic Association* 99, no. 12:1549–1553.

Horton, J.. 1994. *The Politics of Diversity, Immigrants, Resistance & Change in Monterey Park, California.* Philadelphia, PA: Temple University Press.

Hua, V. 2005. New S. F. Health Campaign Targets Asian community. *San Francisco Chronicle,* October 5, 2005.

Hummer, Robert, Maureen Benjamin, and Richard Rogers. 2004. Racial and Ethnic Disparities in Health and Mortality among the U.S. Elderly Population. In *Critical Perspectives on Racial and Ethnic Differences in Health in Late Life*, ed. N. Anderson, R. Bulatao, and B. Cohen, Ch. 3, 53-94 Washington, DC: National Academies Press.

Hung, R.. 2004. Asian-American Civic and Political Participation in Boston Enclaves: The Role of Resources and Community Organizing. Paper presented at WOW3, Workshop in Political Theory and Policy Analysis, Indiana University, Bloomington, Indiana, June 2–5, 2004.

Hwang, W.C. 2006. The Psychotherapy Adaptation and Modification Framework: Application to Asian Americans. *American Psychologist* 61, no. 7:702–715.

Im, E.O.. 2003. Symptoms Experienced during Menopausal Transition: Korean Women in South Korea and the United States. *Journal of Transcultural Nursing* 14, no. 4:321–328.

Im, E.O., and W. Chee. 2005. A Descriptive Internet Survey on Menopausal Symptoms: Five Ethnic Groups of Asian American University Faculty and Staff. *Journal of Transcultural Nursing* 16, no. 2:126–135.

Impact Quincy. Minutes of the September 16, 1992 Asian Focus Group Meeting. Quincy Coalition for the Prevention of Alcohol, Tobacco & Other Drug Problems. Quincy, MA, 1992.

Impact Quincy. Public Health Problem # 1: Alcohol. Quincy Coalition for the Prevention of Alcohol, Tobacco & Other Drug Problems. Quincy, MA, 1995.

Ishii, M., G. Hasegawa, M. Fukui, H. Obayashi, M. Ohta, M. Ogata, K. Yoshioka, Y. Kitagawa, K. Nakano, T. Yoshikawa, and N. Nakamura. 2005. Clinical and Genetic Characteristics of Diabetic Patients with High-Titer (>10,000 U/ml) of Antibodies to Glutamic Acid Decarboxylase. *Immunology Letters* 99, no. 2:180–185.

Iso, H., C. Date, K. Wakai, M. Fukui, A. T., and the JACC Study Group. 2006. The Relationship between Green Tea and Total Caffeine Intake and Risk for Self-Reported Type 2 Diabetes among Japanese Adults. *Annals of Internal Medicine* 144, no. 8:554–562.

Jasso, G., D.S. Massey, M.R. Rosenzweig, and J.P. Smith. 2004. Immigrant Health: Selectivity and Acculturation. In *Critical Perspectives on Racial and Ethnic Differences in Health in Late Life*, ed. Norman Anderson, R. Bulatao, and B. Cohen, Ch. 7, 227-268. Washington, DC: National Academies Press.

Jayne, R.L., and S.H. Rankin. 2001. Application of Leventhal's Self-Regulation Model to Chinese Immigrants with Type 2 Diabetes. *Journal of Nursing Scholarship* 33, no. 1:53–59.

Jonnalagadda, S., and S. Diwan. 2005. Health Behaviors, Chronic Disease Prevalence and Self-Rated Health of Older Asian Indian Immigrants in the U.S. *Journal of Immigrant Health* 7, no. 2:75–83.

Joslin Center. 2005. http://aadi.joslin.harvard.edu/introduction/why-asian.asp (accessed on December 16, 2005).

Kagawa-Singer M., and A.E. Maxwell. 1999. Breast Cancer Screening in API American Women. In *Preventing and Controlling Cancer in North America: A Cross-Cultural Perspective*, ed. D. Weiner, 147–163. Westport, CT: Praeger.

Kandula, N.R., D.S. Lauderdale, and D.W. Baker. 2007. Differences in Self-Reported Health among Asians, Latinos, and Non-Hispanic Whites: The Role of Language and Nativity. *Annals of Epidemiology* 17, no. 3:191–198.

Kang, E.S., S.Y. Park, H.J. Kim, C.W. Ahn, M. Nam, B.S. Cha, S.K. Lim, K.R. Kim, and H.C. Lee. 2005. The Influence of Adiponectin Gene Polymorphism on the Rosiglitazone Response in Patients with Type 2 Diabetes. *Diabetes Care* 28:1139–1144.

Karter, A. J.. 2003. Race and Ethnicity: Vital Constructs for Diabetes Research. *Diabetes Care* 26, no. 7:2189–2193.

Kearney, L.K., M. Draper, and A. Baron. 2005. Counseling Utilization by Ethnic Minority College Students. *Cultural Diversity and Ethnic Minority Psychology* 11, no. 3:272–285.

Khang, Y.H., J.W. Lynch, and G.A. Kaplan. 2005. Impact of Economic Crisis on Cause-Specific Mortality in South Korea. *International Journal of Epidemiology* 34, no. 6:1291–1301.

Kiang, P., and C. Sagara, eds. 1992. *Recognizing Poverty in Boston's Asian American Community.* Boston, MA: The Boston Foundation.

Killoran, M., and A. Moyer. 2006. Surgical Treatment Preferences in Chinese-American Women with Early-Stage Breast Cancer. *Psycho-Oncology* 15, no. 11:969–984.

Kim, M., H.R. Han, K.B. Kim, and D.N. Duong. 2002. The Use of Traditional and Western Medicine among Korean American Elderly. *Journal of Community Health* 27, no. 2:109–120.

Kim, S.M., J.S. Lee, J. Lee, J.K. Na, J.H. Han, D.K. Yoon, S.H. Baik, D.S. Choi, and K.M. Choi. 2006. Prevalence of Diabetes and Impaired Fasting Glucose in Korea. Korean National Health and Nutrition Survey 2001. *Diabetes Care* 29:226–231.

King, H., and F.B. Locke. 1980. Chinese in the United States: A Century of Occupational Transition. *International Migration Review* 14, no. 1:15–42.

———. 1987. Health Effects of Migration: U.S. Chinese in and outside the Chinatown. *International Migration Review* 21, no. 3, Special Issue: Migration and Health: 555–576.

King, R.C.. 2000. Racialization, Recognition, and Rights: Lumping and Splitting Multiracial Asian Americans in the 2000 Census. *Journal of Asian American Studies* 3.2:191–217.

Kozuki, Y., and M.G. Kennedy. 2004. Cultural Incommensurability in Psychodynamic Psychotherapy in Western and Japanese Traditions. *Journal of Nursing Scholarship* 36, no. 1:30–38.

Kronenberg, F., L.F. Cushman, C.M. Wade, D.Kalmuss, and M.T. Chao. 2006. Race/Ethnicity and Women's Use of Complementary and Alternative Medicine in the United States: Results of a National Survey. *American Journal of Public Health* 96, no. 7:1236–1242.

Kuo, J., and K. Porter. 1998. Health Status of Asian Americans: United States, 1992–94. *Advance Data* 298:1–16.

Kwong, S.L., M.S. Chen., K.P. Snipes, D.G. Bal, and W.E. Wright. 2005. Asian Subgroups and Cancer Incidence and Mortality Rates in California. *Cancer* 104, Suppl. 12:2975–2981.

Landin-Olsson, M.. 2002. Latent Autoimmune Diabetes in Adults. *Annals of the New York Academy of Sciences* 958:112–116.

Lauderdale, D.S., and P.J. Rathouz. 2000. Body Mass Index in a U.S. National Sample of Asian Americans: Effects of Nativity, Years since Immigration and Socioeconomic Status. *International Journal of Obesity* 24, no. 9:1188–1194.

Lauderdale, D.S., V. Kuohung, S.L. Chang, and M.H. Chin. 2003. Identifying Older Chinese Immigrants at High Risk for Osteoporosis. *Journal of General Internal Medicine* 18, no. 7:508–515.

Lauderdale, D.S., and . Kestenbaum. 2002. Mortality Rates of Elderly Asian American Populations Based on Medicare and Social Security Data. *Demography* 39, no. 3:529–540.

Law, S., M. Hutton, and D. Chan. 2003. Clinical, Social, and Service Use Characteristics of Fuzhounese Undocumented Immigrant Patients. *Psychiatric Services* 54, no. 7:1034–1037.

Le, V.B. 1989. Descriptive Profile & Needs Assessment of Vietnamese People in Massachusetts. Department of Mental Health.

Lee, J., E.C. Pomeroy, S.K. Yoo, and K.T. Rheinboldt. 2005. Attitudes toward Rape: A Comparison between Asian and Caucasian College Students. *Violence against Women* 11, no. 2:177–196.

Lee, S.C., G.T.C. Ko, J.K.Y. Li, C.C. Chow, V.T.F. Yeung, J.H. Critchley, C.S. Cockram, and J.C.C. Chan. 2001. Factors Predicting the Age When Type 2 Diabetes is Diagnosed in Hong Kong Chinese Subjects. *Diabetes Care* 24, no. 4:646–649.

Lee, T., D. Brugge, C. Francis, and O. Fisher. 2003. Asthma Prevalence among Inner-City Asian American Schoolchildren. *Public Health Reports* 118, no. 3:215–220.

Lee, Z.S.K., J.C.N. Chan, V.T.F. Yeung, C.C. Chow, M.S.W. Lau, G.T.C. Ko, J.K.Y. Li, C.S. Cockram, and J.A.J.H. Critchley. 1999. Plasma Insulin, Growth Hormone, Cortisol, and Central Obesity among Young Chinese Type 2 Diabetic Patients. *Diabetes Care* 22, no. 9:1450–1457.

Leong, P., S. Tumanyan, B. Blicher, A. Yeung, and K. Joshipura. 2007. Periodontal Disease among Adult, New-Immigrant, Chinese Americans in Boston with and without Diabetes—A Brief Communication. *American Association of Public Health Dentistry* 67, no. 3: 171–173.

Leung, T.Y., and C.M. Leung. 2002. Insight into the Psychosocial Aspects of Huntington's Disease in Chinese Society. *International Journal of Psychiatry in Medicine* 32, no. 3:305–310.

Lew, R., and S.P. Tanjasiri. 2003. Slowing the Epidemic of Tobacco Use among Asian Americans and Pacific Islanders. *American Journal of Public Health* 93, no. 5:764–768.

Li, W. ed. 2006. *From Urban Enclave to Ethnic Suburbs: New Asian Communities in Pacific Rim Countries.* Honolulu: University of Hawaii Press.

Li, W. 1998. Ethnoburb versus Chinatown: Two Types of Urban Ethnic Communities in Los Angeles. Paris, December 8–11, 1997. Article 70, put online on December 10, 1998. Modified on May 15, 2007. http://www.cybergeo.eu/index1018.html (accessed on May 6, 2008).

Li, W.W., A.L. Stewart, N.A. Stotts, and E.S. Froelicher. 2005. Cultural Factors and Medication Compliance in Chinese Immigrants Who Are Taking Antihypertensive Medications: Instrument Development. *Journal of Nursing Measurement* 13, no. 3:231–252.

Li, Z.B., T.H. Lam, S.Y. Ho, W.M. Chan, K.S. Ho, M.P. Li, G.M. Leung, and R. Field-ing. 2006. Age- versus Time-Comparative Self-Rated Health in Hong Kong Chinese Older Adults. *International Journal of Geriatric Psychiatry* 21, no. 8:729–739.

Liao, D., P.J. Asberry, J.B. Shofer, H. Callahan, C. Mathys, E.J. Boyko, D. Leonetti, S.E. Kahn, M. Austin, L. Newell, R.S. Schwartz, and W.Y. Fujimoto. 2002. Improvement of BMI, Body Composition, and Body Fat Distribution with Lifestyle Modification in Japanese Americans with Impaired Glucose Toler-ance. *Diabetes Care* 25, no. 9:1504–1510.

Light, I., 1972. *Ethnic Enterprise in America; Business and Welfare among Chinese, Japanese, and Blacks.* Berkeley: University of California Press.

Lin, J.S., A. Finlay, A. Tu, and F.M. Gany. 2005. Understanding Immigrant Chinese Americans' Participation in Cancer Screening and Clinical Trials. *Journal of Community Health* 30, no. 6:451–466.

Liu, H.M. 1998. The Resilience of Ethnic Culture: Chinese Herbalists in the American Medical Profession. *Journal of Asian American Studies* 1.2:173–191.

Lorenzo, M.K., A.K. Frost, and H.Z. Reinherz. 2000. Social and Emotional Func-tioning of Older Asian American Adolescents. *Child and Adolescent Social Work Journal* 17, no. 4:289–304.

Lubetkin, E.I., H.Jia, and M.R. Gold. 2003. Use of the SF-36 in Low-Income Chinese American Primary Care Patients. *Medical Care* 41, no. 4:447–457.

Lui, M.T.Y. 2002. Race and Disease in Urban Geography. *Reviews in American History* 30, no. 3:453–462.

Lyon, Jonathan. 1991. Domestic Violence, Southeast Asian Refugees, and the Public Health: A Qualitative Study. Master's thesis, Tufts University.

Ma, G.X. 1999. Between Two Worlds: The Use of Traditional and Western Health Services by Chinese Immigrants. *Journal of Community Health* 24, no. 6:421–437.

Ma, G.X., S.E. Shive, C.Y. Fang, Z.D. Feng, L. Pararneswaran, A. Pham. 2007. Knowledge, Attitudes, and Behaviors of Hepatitis B Screening and Vaccina-tion and Liver Cancer Risks among Vietnamese Americans. *Journal of Health Care for the Poor and Underserved* 18, no. 1:62–73.

Mackenzie, E.R., L. Taylor, B.S. Bloom, D.J. Hufford, and J.C. Johnson. 2003. Eth-nic Minority Use of Complementary and Alternative Medicine (CAM): A National Probability Survey of CAM Utilizers. *Alternative Therapies in Health & Medicine* 9, no. 4:50–56.

Magazine Publishers of America. Asian-American Market Profile. 2004. www.magazine.org/content/files/market_profile_asian.pdf.

Maker, A.H., P.V. Shah, and Z. Agha. 2005. Child Physical Abuse: Prevalence, Characteristics, Predictors, and Beliefs about Parent-Child Violence in South Asian, Middle Eastern, East Asian, and Latina Women in the United States. *Journal of Interpersonal Violence* 20, no. 11:1406–1428.

Makimoto, K. 1998. Drinking Patterns and Drinking Problems among Asian-Americans and Pacific Islanders. *Alcohol Health & Research World* 22, no. 4:270-275.

Marcuse, P. 1997. The Ghetto of Exclusion and the Fortified Enclave: New Patterns in the U.S. *American Behavioral Scientist* 41:311–326.

Massachusetts Department of Education. 1999. Triennial School Survey (TSS).

Massachusetts Department of Education. 1999. Youth Risk Behavior Survey (YRBS).

Massachusetts Department of Elder Affairs. 2005. Status of the Elderly.

Massachusetts Department of Mental Health, Executive Office of Human Services. 1989. Refugee Mental Health Needs Assessment: A Key Informant Study. Massachusetts.

Massachusetts Department of Public Health. 1994–1998. Behavior Risk Factor Surveillance Survey (BRFSS).

Massachusetts Department of Public Health. 1998. A Profile of Health among Massachusetts Adults.

Massachusetts Department of Public Health.1995–1999. Behavior Risk Factor Surveillance Survey (BRFSS).

Massachusetts Department of Public Health. 1998–2000. A Profile of Massachusetts Adults with Disabilities.

Massachusetts Department of Public Health. 2000. Massachusetts Death.

Massachusetts Department of Public Health. 2004. Massachusetts Health Status Indicators by Race and Hispanic Ethnicity (MHSI).

Massachusetts Executive Office of Public Safety, Criminal History Systems Board, Crime Reporting Unit (MAEOPS). 1991. Hate Crime in Massachusetts, Preliminary Annual Report, January–December, 1990.

Massachusetts Executive Office of Public Safety, Criminal History Systems Board, Department of Public Safety, Crime Reporting Unit (MAEOPS). 1992. Hate Crime/Hate Incidents in Massachusetts, 1991 Annual Report.

Massachusetts Office of Refugees and Immigrants. 1989. Refugees and Immigrants in Massachusetts: A Demographic Report.

Massachusetts Office of Refugees and Immigrants. 1990. Demographic Update. Vol.1, No.1.

Matejkova-Behanova, M.. 2001. Latent Autoimmune Diabetes in Adults (LADA) and Autoimmune Thyroiditis (Minireview). *Endocrine Regulations* 35:167–172.

Maxwell, A.E., R. Bastani, and U.S. Warda. 2000. Demographic Predictors of Cancer Screening among Filipino and Korean Immigrants in the United States. *American Journal of Preventive Medicine* 18, no. 1:62–68.

McBean, A.M., S.L. Li, D.T. Gilbertson, and A.J. Collins. 2004. Differences in Diabetes Prevalence, Incidence, and Mortality among the Elderly of Four Racial/Ethnic Groups: Whites, Blacks, Hispanics, and Asians. *Diabetes Care* 27, no. 10:2317–2324.

McDevitt, H.O. 2005. Characteristics of Autoimmunity in Type 1 Diabetes and Type 1.5 Overlap with Type 2 Diabetes. *Diabetes* 54:S4–S10.

McNeely, M.J., and E.J. Boyko. 2004. Type 2 Diabetes Prevalence in Asian Americans: Results of a National Health Survey. *Diabetes Care* 27, no. 1:66–69.

————. 2005. Diabetes-Related Comorbidities in Asian Americans: Results of a National Health Survey. *Journal of Diabetes and Its Complications* 19, no. 2:101–106.

Mensah, G.A., A.H. Mokdad, E.S. Ford, K.J. Greenlund, and J.B. Croft. 2005. State of Disparities in Cardiovascular Health in the United States. *Circulation* 111, no. 10:1233–1241.

Miller B.A., L.N. Kolonel, L. Bernstein, J.L. Young, Jr., G.M. Swanson, D. West, C.R. Key, J.M. Liff, C.S. Glover, G.A. Alexander, et al. (eds). Racial/Ethnic Patterns of Cancer in the United States 1988–1992, National Cancer Institute. NIH Pub. No. 96-4104. Bethesda, MD, 1996.

Miller, G.M., and R. Stripp. 2007. A Study of Western Pharmaceuticals Contained within Samples of Chinese Herbal/Patent Medicines Collected from New York City's Chinatown. *Legal Medicine* 9, no. 5:258–264.

Mills, P.K., R.C. Yang, and D. Riordan. 2005. Cancer Incidence in the Hmong in California, 1988–2000. *Cancer* 104, no. 12 (Suppl.): 2969–2974.

*Ming Pao Daily.* 2005. The Chinese Community is Shocked by the Rapid Increase of AIDS., July 27, 2005.

*Ming Pao Daily.* 2005. The High Mortality Rate of Colon Cancer is Preventable. July 27, 2005.

MISER (Massachusetts Institute for Social and Economic Research). 1992. Revised Projected Total Population and Age Distribution for 1995 and 2000, Massachusetts Cities and Towns, March 13, 1992.

MISER (Massachusetts Institute for Social and Economic Research). 1997. Preliminary 1995 Population Estimates, Components of Change, Massachusetts Cities and Towns, April 8.

MISER (Massachusetts Institute for Social and Economic Research). 1992. Poverty Status of Persons in 1989: Massachusetts Cities, Towns, and Selected Other Areas, 1990 Census of Population and Housing, Summary Tape File 3, April 16.

Misra, A., J.S. Wasir, and R.M. Pandey. 2005. An Evaluation of Candidate Definitions of the Metabolic Syndrome in Adult Asian Indians. *Diabetes Care* 28, no. 2:398–403.

Montonen, J., R. Järvinen, P. Knekt, M. Heliövaara, and A. Reunanen. 2007. Consumption of Sweetened Beverages and Intakes of Fructose and Glucose Predict Type 2 Diabetes Occurrence. *Journal of Nutrition* 137:1447–1454.

Moon, A., J.E. Lubben, and V. Villa. 1998. Awareness and Utilization of Community Long-Term Care Services by Elderly Korean and Non-Hispanic White Americans. *Gerontologist* 38, no. 3:309–316.

Morenoff, J., and Lynch, J. 2004. What Makes a Place Healthy? Neighborhood Influences on Racial/Ethnic Disparities in Health over the Life Course. In *Critical Perspectives on Racial and Ethnic Differences in Health in Late Life,* ed. N. Anderson, R. Bulatao, and B. Cohen, Ch. 11. 406–449. Washington, DC: National Academies Press.

Mui, A.C., S.Y. Kang, L.M. Chen, and M.D. Domanski. 2003. Reliability of the Geriatric Depression Scale for Use among Elderly Asian Immigrants in the USA. *International Psychogeriatrics* 15, no. 3:253–271.

Murray, C.J.L., S.C. Kulkarni, C. Michaud, N. Tomijima, M.T. Bulzacchelli, T.J. Iandiorio, and M. Ezzati. 2006. Eight Americas: Investigating Mortality Disparities across Races, Counties, and Race-Counties in the United States. *PLoS Medicine* vol.3, no. 9, e260:1513–1524.

Myers, D., and S.W. Lee. 1996. Immigration Cohorts and Residential Overcrowding in Southern California. *Demography* 33, no. 1:51–65.

Myers, H., and W.C. Hwang. 2004. Cumulative Psychosocial Risks and Resilience: A Conceptual Perspective on Ethnic Health Disparities in late Life. In *Critical Perspectives on Racial and Ethnic Differences in Health in Late Life,* ed. N. Anderson, R. Bulatao and B. Cohen, Ch. 13. 492-539. Washington, DC: National Academies Press.

Naik, R.G., and J.P. Palmer. 2003. Latent Autoimmune Diabetes in Adults (LADA). *Reviews in Endocrine and Metabolic Disorders* 4, no. 3:233–241.

National Diabetes Education Program, Southeast Asian Subcommittee of the Asian American/Pacific Islander Work Group. 1992. Silent Trauma: Diabetes, Health Status, and the Refugee Southeast Asians in the United States.

National Asian Women's Health Organization. 2002. Making a Difference: Highlights from a National Symposia Series on Asian Americans and Diabetes.

National Institute of Diabetes and Digestive and Kidney Diseases Press Office (NIDDK), Millions of Asian Americans and Pacific Islanders at Increased Risk for Type 2 Diabetes. 2004. National Institutes of Health News released September 29, 2004.

Newman, J.M., and R. Linke. 1982. Chinese Immigrant Food Habits: A Study of the Nature and Direction of Change. *Royal Society of Health Journal* 102, no. 6:268–271.

Ng, M.C.Y., S.C. Lee, G.T.C. Ko, J.K.Y. Li, W.Y. So, Y. Hashim, A.H. Barnett, I.R. Mackay, J.A.J.H. Critchley, C.S. Cockram, and J.C.N. Chan. 2001. Familial Early-Onset Type 2 Diabetes in Chinese Patients: Obesity and Genetics Have More Significant Roles Than Autoimmunity. *Diabetes Care* 24, no. 4:663–671.

Ngo-Metzger, Q., E.P. McCarthy, R.B. Burns, R.B. Davis, F.P. Li, and R.S. Phillips. 2003. Older Asian Americans and Pacific Islanders Dying of Cancer Use Hospice Less Frequently Than Older White Patients. *American Journal of Medicine* 115, no. 1:47–53.

Ngo-Metzger, Q., S.H. Kaplan, D.H. Sorkin, B.R. Clarridge, and R.S. Phillips. 2004. Surveying Minorities with Limited-English Proficiency: Does Data Collection Method Affect Data Quality among Asian Americans? *Medical Care* 42, no. 9:893–900.

Odo, C., and A. Hawelu. 2001. Eo na Mahu o Hawai'i: The Extraordinary Health Needs of Hawaii's Mahu. *Pacific Health Dialog* 8, no. 2:327–334.

Office of Disease Prevention & Health Promotion, Department of Health and Human Services. 1988. Disease Prevention/Health Promotion, the Facts.

Oh, J.Y., Y.S. Hong, Y.A. Sung, and Elizabeth Barrett-Connor. 2004. Prevalence and Factor Analysis of Metabolic Syndrome in an Urban Korean Population. *Diabetes Care* 27:2027–2032.

Okazaki, S. 2000. Treatment Delay among Asian-American Patients with Severe Mental Illness. *American Journal of Orthopsychiatry* 70, no. 1:58–64.

O'Malley, Robert. 1994. Fields Corner, Dorchester. *Sampan*, August 5, 1994.

Oppenheimer, G.M. 2001. Paradigm Lost: Race, Ethnicity, and the Search for a New Population Taxonomy. *American Journal of Public Health* 91, no. 7:1049–1055.

Oriola, D., and G. Perkins. 1988. *Chinatown User Survey*. Boston: Boston Redevelopment Authority.

Palmer, J.P. 2002. Beta Cell Rest and Recovery—Does It Bring Patients with Latent Autoimmune Diabetes in Adults to Euglycemia? *Annals of the New York Academy of Sciences* 958:89–98.

Palmer, J.P., and I.B. Hirsch. 2003. What's in a Name. Latent Autoimmune Diabetes of Adults, Type 1.5, Adult-Onset, and Type 1 Diabetes. *Diabetes Care* 26:536–538.

Pan, W.H., K.M. Flegal, H.Y. Chang, W.T. Yeh, C.J. Yeh, and W.C. Lee. 2004. Body Mass Index and Obesity-Related Metabolic Disorders in Taiwanese and U.S. Whites and Blacks: Implications for Definitions of Overweight and Obesity for Asians. *American Journal of Clinical Nutrition* 79, no. 1:31–39.

Pan, X.R., G.W. Li, Y.H. Hu, J.X. Wang, W.Y. Yang, Z.X. An, Z.X. Hu, J. Lin, J.Z. Xiao, H. Bi. Cao, P.A. Liu, X.G. Jiang, Y.Y. Jiang, J.P. Wang, H.Z., H. Zhang, P.H. Bennett, and B.V. Howard. 1997. Effects of Diet and Exercise in Preventing NIDDM in People with Impaired Glucose Tolerance: The Da Qing IGT and Diabetes Study. *Diabetes Care* 20:537–544.

Park, H.S., S.Y. Lee, S.M. Kim, J.H. Han, and D.J. Kim. 2006. Prevalence of the Metabolic Syndrome among Korean Adults According to the Criteria of the International Diabetes Federation. *Diabetes Care* 29:933–934.

Parker, V., and S. Edmonds. 1988. *Quincy Gateway City Newcomer Needs Assessment*. Boston: Edmonds & Parker Housing & Community Services.

Pelczarski, Y., and S.P. Kemp. 2006. Patterns of Child Maltreatment Referrals among Asian and Pacific Islander Families. *Child Welfare* 85, no. 1:5–31.

Pinnelas, D., R. De La Torre, J. Pugh, C. Strand, and S.F. Horowitz. 1992. Total Serum Cholesterol Levels in Asians Living in New York City: Results of a Self-Referred Cholesterol Screening. *New York State Journal of Medicine* 92, no. 6:245–249.

Ponce, N.A., S. Huh, and R. Bastani. 2005. Do HMO Market Level Factors Lead to Racial/Ethnic Disparities in Colorectal Cancer Screening? A Comparison between High-Risk Asian and Pacific Islander Americans and High-Risk Whites. *Medical Care* 43, no. 11:1101–1108.

Price, R.K., N.K. Risk, M.M. Wong, and R.S. Klingle. 2002. Substance Use and Abuse by Asian Americans and Pacific Islanders: Preliminary Results from Four National Epidemiologic Studies. *Public Health Reports* 117, Suppl. 1:S39–S50.

Qiu, Y., and H. Ni. 2003. Utilization of Dental Care Services by Asians and Native Hawaiian or Other Pacific Islanders: United States, 1997-2000. *Advance Data* 336: 1–11.

Quincy Department of Planning and Community Development. 1994. Neighborhood Associations Conduct Needs Assessment. City of Quincy Community Development Digest, Spring 1994.

Quincy Housing Authority. Quincy Housing Authority 1995 Annual Report. Quincy, MA 1995.

Quincy Mayor's Special Hearing Panel on Alcohol Abuse. Recommendations for Community Action, Final Report. Quincy, MA, April 16, 1996.

Ramachandran, A., C. Snehalatha, K. Satyavani, S. Sivasankari, and V. Vijay. 2003. Type 2 Diabetes in Asian-Indian Urban Children. *Diabetes Care* 26:1022–1025.

Ramachandran, A., S. Ramachandran, C. Snehalatha, C. Augustine, N. Murugesan, V. Viswanathan, A. Kapur, and R. Williams. 2007. Increasing Expenditure on Health Care Incurred by Diabetic Subjects in a Developing Country. A Study from India. *Diabetes Care* 30:252–256.

Rissanen, J., H. Wang, R. Miettinen, P. Karkkainen, P. Kekalainen, L. Mykkanen, J. Kuusisto, P. Karhapaa, L. Niskanen, M. Uusitupa, and M. Laakso. 2000. Variants in the Hepatocyte Nuclear Factor 1-alpha and 4-alpha Genes in Finnish and Chinese Subjects with Late-Onset Type 2 Diabetes. *Diabetes Care* 23, no. 10:1533–1538.

Robbins, J.M., and D.A. Webb. 2006. Hospital Admission Rates for a Racially Diverse Low-Income Cohort of Patients with Diabetes: The Urban Diabetes Study. *American Journal of Public Health* 96, no. 7:1260–1264.

Rosenthal, D.A., D. Wong, K.M. Blalock, and D.A. Delambo. 2004. Effects of Counselor Race on Racial Stereotypes of Rehabilitation Counseling Clients. *Disability & Rehabilitation* 26, no. 20:1214–1220.

Ryu, H., W.B. Young, and C. Park. 2001. Korean American Health Insurance and Health Services Utilization. *Research in Nursing & Health* 24, no. 6:494–505.

Ryu, H., W.B. Young, and H. Kwak. 2002. Differences in Health Insurance and Health Service Utilization among Asian Americans: Method for Using the NHIS to Identify Unique Patterns between Ethnic Groups. *International Journal of Health Planning & Management* 17, no. 1:55–68.

Sadler, G.R., L. Ryujin, T. Nguyen, G. Oh, G. Paik, and B. Kustin. 2003. Heterogeneity within the Asian American Community. *International Journal for Equity in Health* 2, no. 12: 1–9

Sanjeevi, C.B., G. Gambelunghe, A. Falorni, A. Shtauvere-Brameus, and A. Kanungo. 2002. Genetics of Latent Autoimmune Diabetes in Adults. *Annals of the New York Academy of Sciences* 958:107–111.

Sayeed, M. Abu, H. Mahtab, P.A. Khanam, Z.A. Latif, S.M. K. Ali, A. Banu, B. Ahren, and A.K.A. Khan. 2003. Diabetes and Impaired Fasting Glycemia in a Rural Population of Bangladesh. *Diabetes Care* 26:1034–1039.

Sharma, S., S.P. Murphy, L.R. Wilkens, L. Shen, J.H. Hankin, B. Henderson, and L.N. Kolonel. 2003. Adherence to the Food Guide Pyramid Recommendations among Japanese Americans, Native Hawaiians, and Whites: Results from the Multiethnic Cohort Study. *Journal of the American Dietetic Association* 103, no. 9:1195–1198.

Shelley, D., M. Fahs, R. Scheinmann, S. Swain, J. Qu, and D. Burton. 2004. Acculturation and Tobacco Use among Chinese Americans. *American Journal of Public Health* 94, no. 2:300–307.

Shin, H., H. Song, J. Kim, and J.C. Probst. 2005. Insurance, Acculturation, and Health Service Utilization among Korean-Americans. *Journal of Immigrant Health* 7, no. 2:65–74.

Shin, H.S., H.R. Han, and M.T. Kim. 2007. Predictors of Psychological Well-Being amongst Korean Immigrants to the United States: A Structured Interview Survey. *International Journal of Nursing Studies* 44, no. 3:415–426.

Sincavage, J.R. 2005. Fatal Occupational Injuries among Asian Workers. *Monthly Labor Review* 128, no. 10:49–55.

Smith, A.. Moving to Malden. *Sampan,* July 15, 2005. p. 6.

So, A.Y.C.. 1984. Ethnic Doctors in Los Angeles's Chinatown. *Journal of Ethnic Studies* 11, no. 4:75–82.

Sorgi, M. 1993. Doing Business in the Asian Community. *Quincy Business News,* September 1993.

Soriguer-Escofet, F., I. Esteva, G. Rojo-Martinez, S.R. de Adana, M. M. Merelo, M. Aguilar, F. Tinahones, J.M. García-Almeida, J.M. Gómez-Zumaquero, A. L. Cuesta-Muñoz, J. Ortego, J.M., and Diabetes Group of the Andalusian Society of Endocrinology and Nutrition. 2002. Prevalence of Latent Autoimmune Diabetes of Adults (LADA) in Southern Spain. *Diabetes Research and Clinical Practice* 56, no. 3:213–220.

South Cove Community Health Center. 2004. Production Report, Malden Only, January 1, 2004–December 31, 2004, unpublished report.

Srinivasan, S., and T. Guillermo. 2000. Toward Improved Health: Disaggregating Asian American and Native Hawaiian/Pacific Islander Data. *American Journal of Public Health* 90, no. 11:1731–1734.

Stevens, G.D., L. Shi, and L.A. Cooper. 2003. Patient-Provider Racial and Ethnic Concordance and Parent Reports of the Primary Care Experiences of Children. *Annals of Family Medicine* 1, no. 2:105–112.

Sue, S., D.W. Sue, L. Sue, and D.T. Takeuchi. 1995. Psychopathology among Asian Americans: A Model Minority? *Cultural Diversity and Mental Health* 1, no. 1:39–51.

Sukalakamala, S., and H.C. Brittin. 2006. Food Practices, Changes, Preferences, and Acculturation of Thais in the United States. *Journal of the American Dietetic Association* 106, no. 1:103–108.

Sullivan, C., and K. Hatch. 1973. *The Chinese in Boston, 1970,* (6th printing), Boston: Action for Boston Community Development (ABCD).

Sun, A., E. Wong-Kim, S. Stearman, and E.A. Chow. 2005. Quality of Life in Chinese Patients with Breast Cancer. *Cancer* 104, Suppl. 12:2952–2954.

Tan, C.E., S. Ma, D. Wai, S.K. Chew, and E.S. Tai. 2004. Can We Apply the National Cholesterol Education Program Adult Treatment Panel Definition of the Metabolic Syndrome to Asians? *Diabetes Care* 27:1182–1186.

Tan, H.H., and S.C. Lim. 2001. Latent Autoimmune Diabetes in Adults (LADA): A Case Series. *Singapore Medical Journal* 42, no. 11:513–516.

Tanjasiri, S.P., S.P. Wallace, and K. Shibata. 1995. Picture Imperfect: Hidden Problems among Asian Pacific Islander Elderly. *Gerontologist* 35, no. 6:753–760.

Tashiro, C.J. 2006. Identity and Health in the Narratives of Older Mixed Ancestry Asian Americans. *Journal of Cultural Diversity* 13, no. 1:41–49.

Taylor-Piliae, R.E., and E.S. Froelicher. 2007. Methods to Optimize Recruitment and Retention to an Exercise Study in Chinese Immigrants. *Nursing Research* 56, no. 2:132–136.

Tong, P.C., A.P. Kong, W.Y. So, X. Yang, C.S. Ho, R.C. Ma, R. Ozaki, C.C. Chow, C.W. Lam, J.C.N. Chan, and C.S. Cockram. 2007. The Usefulness of the International Diabetes Federation and the National Cholesterol Education Program's Adult Treatment Panel III Definitions of the Metabolic Syndrome in Predicting Coronary Heart Disease in Subjects with Type 2 Diabetes. *Diabetes Care* 30:1206–1211.

Tong, P.C., K.F. Lee, W.Y. So, M.H. Ng, W.B. Chan, M.K. Lo, N.N. Chan, and J.C. Chan. 2004. White Blood Cell Count Is Associated With Macro- and Microvascular Complications in Chinese Patients with Type 2 Diabetes. *Diabetes Care* 27:216–222.

Torsch, V.L., and G.X. Ma. 2000. Cross-Cultural Comparison of Health Perceptions, Concerns, and Coping Strategies among Asian and Pacific Islander American Elders. *Qualitative Health Research* 10, no. 4:471–489.

Tri-City Community Action Program, Inc. (TRI-CAP). 2004. 2003–2005 Community Action Plan, November 2002 Revision.

Tsai, J.L., Y. Chentsova-Dutton, L. Freire-Bebeau, and D.E. Przymus. 2002. Emotional Expression and Physiology in European Americans and Hmong Americans. *Emotion* 2, no. 4:380–397.

Tu, S.P., S.L. Jackson, Y. Yasui, M. Deschamps, T.G. Hislop, and V.M. Taylor. 2005. Cancer Preventive Screening: A Cross-Border Comparison of United States and Canadian Chinese Women. *Preventive Medicine* 41, no. 1:36–46.

Tuomi, T., A. Carlsson, H. Li, B. Isomaa, A. Miettinen, A. Nilsson, M. Nissen, B.O. Ehrnstrom, B. Forsen, B. Snickars, K. Lahti, C. Forsblom, C. Saloranta, M.R. Taskinen, and L.C. Groop. 1999. Clinical and Genetic Characteristics of Type 2 Diabetes with and without GAD Antibodies. *Diabetes* 48, no. 1:150–157.

U.S. Census Bureau. 2002. The Asian Population: 2000, Census 2000 Brief. 2/2002.

Urakami, T., S. Kubota, Y. Nitadori, K. Harada, M. Owada, and T. Kitagawa. 2005. Annual Incidence and Clinical Characteristics of Type 2 Diabetes in Children as Detected by Urine Glucose Screening in the Tokyo Metropolitan Area. *Diabetes Care* 28:1876–1881.

U.S. Census Bureau News. Nation's Population 1/3 Minority, released on May 10, 2006.

U.S. Bureau of the Census. Detailed Population Characteristics, Massachusetts, 1980, PC90-1-D23, Table 219.

————. Social & Economic Characteristics, Massachusetts, 1990, CP-2-23, Table 50.

Ver Ploeg, M., and E. Perrin, eds. 2004. *Eliminating Health Disparities: Measurement and Data Needs*. Washington DC: National Academies of Sciences.

Wang, J.J., H. Gang, J. Lappalainen, M.E. Miettinen, Q. Qiao, and J. Tuomilehto. 2005. Changes in Features of the Metabolic Syndrome and Incident Impaired Glucose Regulation or Type 2 Diabetes in a Chinese Population. *Diabetes Care* 28:448–450.

Wang, J.J., Q. Qing, M.E. Miettinen, J. Lappalainen, G. Hu, and J. Tuomilehto. 2004. The Metabolic Syndrome Defined by Factor Analysis and Incident Type 2 Diabetes in a Chinese Population with High Postprandial Glucose. *Diabetes Care* 27:2429–2437.

Wang, Y., M.C.Y. Ng, S.C. Lee, W.Y. So, P.C.Y. Tong, C.S. Cockram, J.A.J.H. Critchley, and J.C.N. Chan. 2003. Phenotypic Heterogeneity and Associations of Two Aldose Reductase Gene Polymorphisms with Nephropathy and Retinopathy in Type 2 Diabetes. *Diabetes Care* 26:2410–2415.

Wanger Associates. 1994. The Greater Boston Asian American Community. Research prepared for the Malden Hospital. Newton, MA.

Watanabe, R.M., M.H. Black, A.H. Xiang, H. Allayee, J.M. Lawrence, and T.A. Buchanan. 2007. Genetics of Gestational Diabetes Mellitus and Type 2 Diabetes. *Diabetes Care* 30:S134–S140.

Wei, J.T., and M. Loo. Prostate Biopsies in Chinese American Men. Chinese American Health Issues. http://www.camsociety.org.

Wei, J.N., F.C. Sung, C.Y. Li, C.H. Chang, R.S. Lin, C.C. Lin, C.C. Chiang, and L.M. Chuang. 2003. Low Birth Weight and High Birth Weight Infants Are Both at an Increased Risk to Have Type 2 Diabetes among Schoolchildren in Taiwan. *Diabetes Care* 26:343–348.

Weinick, R.M., and N.A. Krauss. 2000. Racial/Ethnic Differences in Children's Access to Care. *American Journal of Public Health* 90, no. 11:1771–1774.

Weiss, L. 1994. Timing Is Everything. *Atlantic Monthly*, January 1994.

Winker, M.A. 2004. Measuring Race and Ethnicity: Why and How? *JAMA* 292, no. 13:1612–1614.

Woo, P.P.S., J.J. Kim, and G.M. Leung. 2007. What is the Most Cost-Effective Population-Based Cancer Screening Program for Chinese Women? *Journal of Clinical Oncology* 25, no. 6:617–624.

Wortley, P.M., R.P. Metler, D.J. Hu, and P.L. Fleming. 2000. AIDS among Asians and Pacific Islanders in the United States. *American Journal of Preventive Medicine* 18, no. 3:208–214.

Wu, T.Y., J. Bancroft, and B. Guthrie. 2005. An Integrative Review on Breast Cancer Screening Practice and Correlates among Chinese, Korean, Filipino, and Asian Indian American Women. *Health Care for Women International* 26, no. 3:225–246.

Wu, T.Y., B. West, Y.W. Chen, and C. Hergert. 2006. Health Beliefs and Practices Related to Breast Cancer Screening in Filipino, Chinese and Asian-Indian Women. *Cancer Detection & Prevention* 30, no. 1:58–66.

Xu, Y., M.C. Ross, R. Ryan, and B. Wang. 2005. Cancer Risk Factors among South-east Asian American Residents of the U.S. Central Gulf Coast. *Public Health Nursing* 22, no. 2:119–129.

Yancy, C.W., E.J. Benjamin, R.P. Fabunmi, and R.O. Bonow. 2005. Discovering the Full Spectrum of Cardiovascular Disease: Minority Health Summit 2003: Executive Summary. *Circulation* 111, no. 10:1339–1349.

Yang, D., L. Bernstein, and A.H. Wu. 2003. Physical Activity and Breast Cancer Risk among Asian-American Women in Los Angeles: A Case-Control Study. *Cancer* 97, no. 10:2565–2575.

Yang, E.J., H.K. Chung, W.Y. Kim, L. Bianchi, and W.O. Song. 2007. Chronic Diseases and Dietary Changes in Relation to Korean Americans' Length of Residence in the United States. *Journal of the American Dietetic Association* 107, no. 6:942–950.

Yang, E.J., J.M. Kerver, and W.O. Song. 2005. Dietary Patterns of Korean Americans Described by Factor Analysis. *Journal of the American College of Nutrition* 24, no. 2:115–121.

Yang, L., Z.G. Zhou, G. Huang, L.L. Ouyang, X. Li, X. Yan. 2005. Six-Year Follow-up of Pancreatic Beta Cell Function in Adults with Latent Autoimmune Diabetes. *World Journal of Gastroenterology* 11, no. 19:2900–2905.

Yang, X., B. Hsu-Hage, H. Zhang, L. Yu, L. Dong, J. Li, P. Shao, and C. Zhang. 2002. Gestational Diabetes Mellitus in Women of Single Gravidity in Tianjin City, China. *Diabetes Care* 25:847–851.

Yau, Y.. 1997. A Portrait of the Director of the Chinese Detoxification Center. *Sing Tao Weekly*, June 22, 1997.

Yee, A., and T.L.N. Chung. 1991. "Under-Utilization" of Physician Service and the Chinese Health Culture. University of Massachusetts Gerontology Institute.

Yeh, G.Y., D.M. Eisenberg, T.J. Kaptchuk, and R.S. Phillips. 2003. Systematic Review of Herbs and Dietary Supplements for Glycemic Control in Diabetes. *Diabetes Care* 26:1277–1294.

Yeung, W.H., and M.A. Schwartz. 1986. Emotional Disturbance in Chinese Obstetrical Patients: A Pilot Study. *General Hospital Psychiatry* 8, no. 4:258–262.

Ying, Y.W., and M. Han. 2007. The Longitudinal Effect of Intergenerational Gap in Acculturation on Conflict and Mental Health in Southeast Asian American Adolescents. *American Journal of Orthopsychiatry* 77, no. 1:61–66.

Yu, E.S.H., E.H. Chen, K.K. Kim, and S. Abdulrahim. 2002. Smoking among Chinese Americans: Behavior, Knowledge, and Beliefs. *American Journal of Public Health* 92, no. 6:1007–1012.

Yu, E.S.H., K.K. Kim, E.H. Chen, and R.A. Brintnall. 2001. Breast and Cervical Cancer Screening among Chinese American Women. *Cancer Practice* 9, no. 2:81–91.

Yu, E.S.H., K.K. Kim, E.H. Chen, R.A. Brintnall, and W.T. Liu. 2001. Colorectal Cancer Screening among Chinese Americans: A Community-Based Study of Knowledge and Practice. *Journal of Psychosocial Oncology* 19, no. 3–4:97–112.

Yu, E.S.H., E. H. Chen, K.K. Kim, and S. Abdulrahim. 2002. Smoking among Chinese Americans: Behavior, Knowledge, and Beliefs. *American Journal of Public Health* 92, no. 6:1007–1012.

Yu, M.Y., O.S. Hong, and A.D. Seetoo. 2003. Uncovering Factors Contributing to Under-Utilization of Breast Cancer Screening by Chinese and Korean Women Living in the United States. *Ethnicity & Disease* 13, no. 2:213–219.

Yu, M.Y., T.Y. Wu, and D.W. Mood. 2005. Cultural Affiliation and Mammography Screening of Chinese Women in an Urban County of Michigan. *Journal of Transcultural Nursing* 16, no. 2:107–116.

Yu, S.M., Z.J. Huang, and G.K. Singh. 2004. Health Status and Health Services Utilization among U.S. Chinese, Asian Indian, Filipino, and Other Asian/Pacific Islander Children. *Pediatrics* 113, no. 1 :101–107.

# Chapter 32

# Impact of Trauma and War

## Douglas Nam Le

Since the 1970s trauma has been a topic of increasing interest and relevance to the field of mental health (Herman 1997). In recent years public-health researchers as well as trauma survivors have linked the experience of trauma to its biological sequelae and to its role as a social determinant of health (Hollifield 2002; Weisberg 2002; Chen 2007; Boscarino 2008; Kinzie 2008). This chapter elucidates the impact of trauma, war, and violence on health primarily from the experiences of Cambodian and Vietnamese communities in the United States. Southeast Asian refugee communities have survived extreme loss, human atrocity, and structural violence in Asia and the United States; yet the history of these communities has also demonstrated an extraordinary capacity for resiliency, survival, and strength. From an initial discussion of historical and theoretical perspectives on trauma, there follows a summary and analysis of the consequences of trauma in relation to mental health, physical health, and somatization; and resultant barriers to utilizing accessible and quality health care for Southeast Asians in the United States. The conclusion highlights strategies for addressing historical trauma, promoting the health of Asian American trauma survivors, and for supporting community development with this population.

## SOUTHEAST ASIAN COMMUNITIES IN THE UNITED STATES

During the 1960s and 1970s the nations of the Southeast Asian peninsula experienced devastating warfare. This included the United States invasion of Vietnam and subsequent civil war—also known as the "Vietnam Conflict," or in Vietnam the "American War"—and the United States' covert bombing and military operations in Cambodia and Laos.

What resulted from these wars were years of civil unrest in Vietnam, Cambodia, and Laos, including the rise of the Khmer Rouge regime and the "Killing Fields" between 1975 and 1979. Many of the generation who lived through these wars also experienced a complex history of political unrest and armed conflict prior to this period, which included colonization under France, occupation by Japan during World War II, and movements for national liberation from the 1950s onward. Beginning in 1975, millions of Southeast Asians fled their war-torn states as refugees, and many resettled and built new lives in the United States.

For the numerous waves of refugees from Southeast Asia to the United States, the first point of arrival was often a refugee camp in Thailand, the Philippines, Hong Kong, or Malaysia. Families would experience various lengths of stays at refugee camps, up to fifteen years, as they were processed for resettlement or repatriated depending on their ability to make a case for refugee status. Upon arrival in the United States, measures of refugee policy were taken to disperse the relatively small population of Southeast Asian refugees and prevent the formation of ethnic enclaves. This was seen as a step to reduce the economic burden of resettlement on receiving communities, and to facilitate their social and economic integration. Despite the efforts of the U.S. government to disperse resettled refugees geographically, they often migrated to reconnect with social networks and extended families across state lines.

According to the 2000 U.S. census, there are more than 1.8 million Southeast Asians of Cambodian, Hmong, Laotian, and Vietnamese descent living in the United States. Sociodemographic indicators show Southeast Asian communities experience sociopolitical barriers that can limit their capacity to access mainstream institutions. Among all Asian and Pacific Islander (API) communities in the United States, Southeast Asian households are among the most frequent to speak a language other than English at home (91–95%), and Vietnamese households have the highest rates of being linguistically isolated (45%) compared to all other API ethnic households. Data from the 2000 U.S. census also indicate that Southeast Asians represent four of the top five ethnic groups with high rates of limited English proficiency— 61 percent among Vietnamese, 58 percent among Hmong, 53 percent among Cambodians, and 52 percent among Laotians (APIAHF 2005).

Similar to other Asian American communities in the United States, Southeast Asians represent the full spectra of socioeconomic strata, educational attainment, and work sectors. Many Southeast Asian Americans are in professional occupations, and still more have become small business owners to support their families in the United States and in Asia. Nevertheless, it is important to recognize where Southeast Asian communities still face challenges regarding socioeconomic status and education, which remain vital indicators for security and prosperity in the United States. Many Southeast Asians who settled in the United States as refugees initially lacked fluency in English, transferable labor skills, and other forms of social capital to rebuild their lives. The U.S. Refugee Act of 1980 provided for federal programs to assist refugees through the Office of Refugee Resettlement. In the form of resettlement and social service programs, the U.S. government provided English instruction, employment skills training, and orientation on American values and behaviors in U.S.-operated refugee camps through Asia, as well as through mutual aid associations (MAAs) and other community based-organizations in receiving U.S. communities. Aid to Families with Dependent Children (AFDC), which had been a program designed in the 1930s during the construction of the American welfare state, was one of the primary sources of support allocated to resettled refugees through cash assistance. Although these welfare programs were intended to ease the instrumental and cognitive demands of resettlement, they only provided for basic subsistence. Changes in federal welfare policy during the mid-1990s ended entitlements that facilitated access to public benefits for those with refugee status.

Poverty and low levels of educational attainment in these communities are both the direct and indirect results of their histories of armed conflict, flight, and resettlement. Among API groups in the United States, per capita income is the lowest among Southeast Asians, notably $6,631 for Hmong and $10,215 for Cambodians. These two groups also have the highest rates of poverty, with 73 percent of Hmong households and 54 percent of Cambodian households living at or below 200 percent of the poverty line in 2000. These numbers are particularly startling when compared to the poverty rate found in the general U.S. population (22%) and among all Asian Americans (28%). Southeast Asians also possess the lowest levels of educational attainment when compared to other API groups (Barnes 2008). According to the 2000 U.S. census between 38 percent and 59 percent of Southeast Asian Americans had attained less than a high school degree, compared to 20 percent within the general U.S. population and 19 percent among Asian Americans (APIAHF 2005). Systems of education in Southeast Asian countries vary, and historically, access to formal education in Southeast Asian nations have been vulnerable to the tides of political movements and armed conflict in these nations. Many Southeast Asians who have since arrived to the United States as refugees or immigrants have been resettled in disparate communities with limited connections with other Southeast Asians or in centers of urban poverty and violence. These experiences are among the numerous ecological factors, characterized through key demographic and socioeconomic indicators, that have impacted the health status and overall development of many Southeast Asian communities.

## TRAUMA EXPERIENCE

Trauma is an emotional or psychological injury usually resulting from an extremely stressful or life-threatening situation, and it is often attributed to post-traumatic stress disorder (PTSD). PTSD was first categorized as an anxiety disorder in the *Diagnostic and Statistical Manual of Mental Disorder* (DSM-III) of the American Psychological Association in 1980. The classification of PTSD as a clinically diagnosable psychological condition gave recognition to trauma within the field of mental health. This was a groundbreaking moment for the various social and political movements that had advocated for the institutional acceptance of trauma, which has had a fractured and often silenced history in Europe and the United States. Since then, the application of the term *trauma* and the discourse surrounding it has encompassed the most public acts of aggression and political oppression, as well as the most intimate expressions of violence.

Although a single event can have a traumatic effect on its witness, it is more often the "constellation of lived experiences" of an individual, or shared within a community that structures the impact of trauma on the health, social environments, and self-efficacy of trauma survivors (Erikson 1995). Pervasive forms of violence such as racism or homophobia, and disenfranchisement related to living in poverty are examples of the milieu in which trauma can operate. For all survivors, this web of life events begins with the individual's environment, which exposed her or him to the trauma; the traumatic episode itself; and finally, the challenging work of processing the trauma and rebuilding a life. Foster identifies four migration stages through which immigrants and refugees experience traumatic events that have a potential to effect mental health and overall well-being 1) premigration trauma; 2) traumatic events experienced during flight and migration; 3) stressors related to accessing systems of asylum, assessment, and resettlement; and 4) distress resulting from instrumental demands in the country of resettlement due to unemployment, lack of work or educational opportunities, and discrimination (Foster 2001).

Within this scheme of analysis there exist many examples of traumatic events and other stressors unique to the Southeast Asian American experience. Military combatants in these wars as well as civilian survivors of military operations experienced innumerable trauma events, including loss of family, displacement, physical injury and rape, exposure to Agent Orange and similar chemical defoliants, and being close to death. During the Khmer Rouge regime in Cambodia, educated and professional classes were targeted for execution, and society as a whole was reorganized into state-run work and training camps. Survivors of the Khmer Rouge "Killing Fields" experienced forced labor, murder of and forced separation from family, torture, untreated medical illness, and starvation. At the end of the wars, those who fled as boat people from Vietnam or across mountain and jungle regions from Laos and Cambodia faced starvation, risk of death, acts of violence and exploitation (i.e. rape and robbery), and attack by military forces en route. Former Vietnamese soldiers who were allies of the U.S. government were sent to reeducation camps where they underwent prolonged torture, interrogation, and deprivation for periods extending from six months to almost ten years. Refugee camps operated throughout the region to contain and process the mass displacements of peoples from Cambodia, Laos, and Vietnam were another site of trauma experience. Many camp residents lived in congested quarters, and only bare necessities of food and medical care were provided at most sites. There were also limited opportunities for work or education in the camps. Though now safe at these camps, families often experienced extreme liminality in engaging with government bureaucracies, recounting traumatic experiences to gain refugee status, and awaiting resettlement. Upon resettlement in the United States or elsewhere, Southeast Asians would experience myriad new stressors as they struggled to rebuild their lives.

Numerous tools have been developed to accurately and sensitively assess trauma, depression, and related psychological disturbances in Southeast Asian refugee populations. Mollica and colleagues were the first to develop and validate successfully the Hopkins Symptom Checklist as a facile tool in assessing major depression and anxiety among Laotian, Cambodian, and Vietnamese refugees (Mollica 1987). They later developed the Harvard Trauma Questionnaire to be the first valid and reliable cross-cultural assessment tool relating trauma experiences and symptoms to PTSD criteria for Southeast Asian populations (Mollica et al. 1992). Clinicians have also studied the validity of the Harvard Trauma Questionnaire and Hopkins Symptom Checklist for patient screening and assessment (Fawzi 1997). The Comprehensive Trauma Inventory-104 is a more recently developed assessment tool that has been proven to be reliable and valid for Southeast Asian trauma survivors; it assesses a broader range of traumatic war-related events in a broader range of refugees than currently available instruments (Hollifield et al. 2006). Such assessment tools document the level of exposure to and frequency of traumatic experiences such as physical injury, torture, starvation, armed combat, and unnatural death of a friend or family member. They also assess patients' reporting of trauma-related symptoms from feelings of social isolation, depression and hopelessness to symptoms of flashbacks and hyperarousal. There is divergent evidence regarding the efficacy of clinical treatment for PTSD and its associated conditions such as major depression for Southeast Asians. Several studies highlight the positive health outcomes from talk therapy or group therapy when developed in a culturally relevant manner (Hwang 2006), whereas others document limitations in western modalities for treatment (Boehnlein 2004; Watters 2001).

To understand the impact of trauma, it is critical for public health practitioners to understand how for trauma survivors this continuum of life events strongly influences all aspects of health and health care seeking behaviors. These include health communication, disease prevention, health care access, community outreach, health outcomes, and program planning. A critical analysis of the histories of migration to and settlement in the United States is also needed to explain the impact of trauma on health for Asian Americans. For Asian American communities that have experienced war and violence, public health models need to integrate trauma as a contributing factor to the maintenance of overall health and well-being.

## EFFECTS OF TRAUMA ON COMMUNITY HEALTH

Upon arrival in the receiving country, migrants face the stressors of acculturation, overt discrimination, and hindered social relations. However, the experience of migration involves many situations that are imbued with uncertainty, disorientation, and stress from the moment that a refugee leaves his or her homeland. Numerous stressors, including the traumas of war, persecution, and dislocation, become sites where a refugee can experience severe trauma, and these events will often challenge the psychological health and emotional homeostasis of migrants. Migrants leave their home countries for various economic, social, and political reasons; often the migration is a choice, but there are times when it is forced. Individuals who are forced to migrate as a result of political, social, or economic oppression and violence—refugees and asylum seekers—experience the trauma of migration most acutely. There are countless points in a refugee's experience that leave him or her vulnerable to victimization, and there are few sites of healing or opportunities to cope with this stress.

### Mental Health and Emotional Well-being

Because of past experience of significant trauma such as famine, armed conflict, or loss of relatives, first-generation Southeast Asian refugees differ in their high risk for PTSD, major depression, and various anxiety disorders. Refugees who are fleeing political violence and warfare know that they can never return. Refugees also know that they may not even survive the journey abroad. Once they arrive in their nations of asylum, many refugees must face the difficulties of adaptation following the experience of traumatic separation. This experience of loss produces a perplexing dichotomy of emotions. Immigrants and refugees know that their situations in the United States are not particularly enviable, but those who have been left behind are even worse off. Most individuals are able to cope with these feelings over time as they begin to adapt to their new communities of resettlement; however, for many, past events continue to have an impact on their present health.

The majority of the literature on the mental health of Southeast Asian communities in the United States reflects the work conducted in the first decade of resettlement. Many of these studies were conducted in clinical settings, often emphasizing the assessment of psychological distress and contributing factors related to recent trauma or acculturative stressors. Although the literature on Southeast Asian communities does indicate a reduction in depression and other forms of psychological distress up to ten years after resettlement (Tran et al. 2007; Steel et al. 2002), numerous studies also support that more than three decades after refugee resettlement pervasive emotional and behavioral disturbances persist among community members, including PTSD, major depression, anxiety disorder, and schizophrenia (Marshall 2005). These conditions are primarily seen in members of the first generation, who are now approaching advanced age, have developed comorbid chronic diseases such as diabetes, and who often face compounded barriers to accessing health and mental health services such as limited English proficiency and social isolation (Sorkin 2008). Those who lost loved ones or have migrated to the United States alone face heightened barriers and isolation because they often lack supportive networks.

The contributing risk factors related to poor mental health for Southeast Asians are complex and interrelated. Past war-related trauma, stressors related to migration and resettlement, and day-to-day stressors such as family conflict and financial stress have all been identified as risk factors for PTSD and major depression among Southeast Asian refugees (Blair 2000). Ben-Sira identifies three types of demands that qualify the stressors that refugees and immigrants experience in the process of adaptation: instrumental demands, cognitive demands, and affective demands. Instrumental demands are the points of stress that are caused within the political or economic circumstances of an immigrant's situation. English proficiency, a reliance on public benefits that determines a family's options for work, and the availability of transferable work skills are such demands that can be additional burden to adjustment. Undocumented status within a country can be another instrumental demand. Cognitive demands that refugees and immigrants face include adaptation to a new culture and environment, and difficulties that arise from language-discordant communication. Within the cognitive demands that refugees experience are overt discrimination and rejection at the hands of their receiving nation and its people. Finally, affective demands can be understood to be the experience of object-person relations, including intergenerational conflict, social isolation, and social relations. For migrants who make the journey with family members or friends, close object-person relations often serve as support in light of severe instrumental and cognitive demands. However, the intensity of affective demands can further challenge the psychological well-being of migrants as they try to reconstruct their social worlds (Ben-Sira 1997).

National studies of mental health status among Asian Americans have found that nativity is associated with risk for all psychiatric disorders, and that foreign-born Asian Americans exhibit less risk for psychiatric disorders. Overtime risk for psychiatric disorder increases with years of residence in the United States (Breslau 2006). Chung and Kagawa-Singer conducted the first-ever study of psychological distress among Southeast

Asians in a nonclinical population. They found that premigration trauma events and experiences at refugee camps were significant predictors for psychological distress even five years or more after resettlement. Psychological distress also varied across Southeast Asian ethnic groups in the study, where Cambodians experienced the highest levels of stress when compared to Laotians and Vietnamese. For Cambodians the primary concern related to stress were premigration issues; however, Vietnamese and Laotians reported both premigration and postmigration issues, such as acculturation, as sources of stress (Chung and Kagawa-Singer 1993). In a study comparing self-reported health status and chronic medical conditions between Vietnamese and white non-Hispanic Californians over 55, the Vietnamese were significantly more likely to report mental problems, but less likely to have their medical providers discuss mental health with them (Sorkin 2008).

The impact of trauma in Southeast Asian communities also varies across generations. The first generation of Southeast Asian refugees and immigrants represents those who survived the war and its numerous consequences. They had lost or left behind family, and had sacrificed to flee and resettle abroad. Members of the second generation often have little to no experience with the war, and only know as much of the history as their parents are able to share. In addition to growing up and developing their unique identity in the United States, they can be expected to support the family financially, respond to instrumental needs (e.g., assistance with interpretation and navigating public systems), and fulfill certain filial obligations and similar cultural expectations. Schapiro et al. conducted a study of three generations within a recent Vietnamese immigrant community investigating psychological distress, experiences with resettlement, acculturation, biculturalism, and premigratory stressors. They found that young adult Vietnamese in the sample fared the best on numerous indicators, as they were the most acculturated, most bicultural, and least depressed. The second generation also had the healthiest self-reported status, was more often employed, and had the highest income. Despite this, young adults reported the most dissatisfaction with life in the United States and had most family conflict. This demonstrates that although a higher level of acculturation can serve as a protective factor against psychological stress, acculturation and social capital can also become stressors in a bicultural context. The most compelling finding from this study was the conclusion that current adjustment factors played a significantly more important role in determining mental health outcomes than war-related traumas and other premigratory stressors (Schapiro et al. 1999).

A final cognitive demand on Asian American immigrants and refugees that remains under-researched is the effect of discrimination and social violence on health and mental health. Discrimination can be experienced along a bias continuum including, but not limited to, race, perceived appearance, language proficiency and accent, religion, age, and gender identity. In a national study of Asian Americans, Gee et al. found that self-reported discrimination was associated with greater odds of having any DSM-IV categorized disorder, depression, or anxiety disorder in the previous year even when controlling for significant sociodemographic characteristics, health status, chronic physical conditions, poverty, and acculturative stress, among other factors, for Asian Americans across the United States (Gee et al. 2007).

## Physical Health and Chronic Disease

Past trauma and the subsequent development of PTSD have a documented impact on the physical health well-being of Southeast Asians. A report analyzing health characteristics among Asian Americans from the National Health Interview Surveys between 2004 and 2006 found Vietnamese Americans to have the highest rate (19%) of reporting fair or poor health; and Vietnamese women (28%) were more than twice as likely as Vietnamese men (11%) to be in fair or poor health (Barnes 2008). Cambodian and Vietnamese youth have been found to have low self-reported health status when compared to their peers of both immigrant and nonimmigrant heritage (Algrem 2007). There are numerous prevalent health conditions that disproportionately affect Southeast Asians of both genders—including hypertension and stroke, diabetes, hepatitis B, liver disease, and lung cancer—and Southeast Asian women, including breast and cervical cancer. There are numerous behavioral and environmental risk factors for Southeast Asians that explain the high morbidity of these conditions, such as diet and exercise, smoking and alcohol consumption, family history, and utilization of early preventative screening for cancers. However, there is also an inextricable and compounding relationship between persistent psychological conditions and physical health. In one study of PTSD conducted in a primary care setting, 46 percent of Southeast Asian refugee patients had a reported history of trauma but no PTSD, and 37 percent met DSM-IV criteria for PTSD. Southeast Asians with PTSD have been reported to have a significantly greater number of current and lifetime medical conditions than patients with other anxiety disorders excluding PTSD. Diagnosis of PTSD was identified to be a stronger predictor of a number of reported medical conditions than trauma history, physical injury, lifestyle factors, or comorbid depression (Weisberg et al. 2002). The comorbidity of psychological distress, such as major depression, and chronic illness, such as diabetes, can compound the effects of both physical and psychological conditions, increase health utilization through ambulatory care visits or prescription use, and significantly increase health care expenses per patient with a comorbid condition (Egede 2002).

Diabetes is an emerging health crisis for Vietnamese and Cambodian communities in the United States that are particularly affected by trauma.

Although there is still a critical lack of reliable data on diabetes and its associated risk factors for these communities, numerous studies utilizing community-based samples have documented unique disparities in the burden of diabetes for Vietnamese and Cambodian Americans. These studies document the rate of diabetes to be between 5.3 percent and 6.1 percent for Vietnamese Americans, and 5.1 percent for Cambodian Americans (CDC 2004; Barnes 2008). Diet, exercise, obesity, and family history are prevalent risk factors for diabetes among Vietnamese and Cambodians, as found in other communities who share this disparity. However, Southeast Asians also experience unique historical and systemic factors that place them at elevated risk for developing diabetes. Not surprisingly, rates for diabetes have been found to be as high as 13 percent for Cambodians and 14 percent for Vietnamese in studies representative of trauma survivors (Kinzie 2008). This finding is significant, considering that one study found that in the adult first-generation Cambodian refugee population of Long Beach, California, 62 percent experience post-traumatic stress disorder (PTSD), and as many as 51 percent have major depression (Grant et al. 2006). Famine and malnutrition have also been linked to the development of diabetes later in life (National Diabetes Education Program 2006). For some Southeast Asian refugees, malnutrition was a recurring experience. The exodus from Vietnam or Cambodia, whether by land or sea, involved several days to several weeks of travel, and food was often scarce. Survivors who experienced the Khmer Rouge work camps or the "reeducation camps" for former U.S. allies in Vietnam after the war endured long periods of time when food was withheld or simply not available. Chemical defoliants were used throughout Southeast Asia during the war, and towns and villages were often razed as a military tactic. As a result, exposure to dioxins present in Agent Orange and other chemical defoliants used during the war have also been linked to birth defects in civilian populations (Ngo 2006), and elevated risk for diabetes and cardiovascular disease among Southeast Asian refugees and U.S. veterans of the Vietnam War (Carpenter 2008).

## Somatization

Somatization is a unique presentation of trauma and its effects in the bodies of trauma survivors. It is a psychiatric diagnosis applied to patients who chronically and persistently report physical symptoms not directly related to any medical condition; it is comorbid with mood and anxiety disorders. Common symptoms are sexual disinterest, headache, chronic pain or weakness, and gastrointestinal problems. Although somatization is not exclusive to Southeast Asians and other survivors of trauma, persistent mental and physical illness and barriers in cultural knowledge and communication between Southeast Asian patients and their health care providers create a unique perspective on somatization in the context of the impact of trauma on health. An international study of psychological disorders in the primary care setting by the World Health Organization documented that between 45 and 95 percent of patients with depression also reported somatic symptoms. Presentation of somatic symptoms was more common at clinical sites where patients lacked an ongoing relationship with their medical provider (Simon et al. 1999).

The process of somatization is one way by which survivors of trauma cope with past events and recent stressors in order to build resiliency. In the Southeast Asian community there is an array of response mechanisms to trauma that serve as both protective factors against poor health outcomes, as well as those that impact the health of the individual and the family negatively. Experiencing traumatic life events and witnessing community or family violence can lead to major depression (Fox 1999), PTSD, and other forms of psychological distress (Ho 2008). Survivors and witnesses of violence have also been shown to commit violence as an adaptive response to victimization, torture, and trauma. For Southeast Asian communities, this has translated into elevated risks for suicide, intimate partner violence, child abuse within the home, and gang violence. Serious violence committed by Southeast Asian young people has been correlated to experiences of traumatic and stressful life events. Ngo and Le report that high levels of acculturation, intergenerational and intercultural conflict, as well as self-reported individualism placed Southeast Asian youth at increased risk for serious violence, whereas social support served as a protective factor (Ngo and Le 2007). Limited studies related to excessive alcohol consumption, substance use and abuse, and disordered gambling have been documented in relatively low rates among Southeast Asians, compared to the common perception of these behaviors in the community. In a community-based sample of Cambodians in Long Beach, California, Marshall identified the rate of lifetime disordered gambling at 13 percent, significantly lower than what has been reported in the literature (Marshall 2009). A comparable study of alcohol consumption and binge drinking in the same community of Cambodians reports that approximately one-quarter of respondents had consumed any alcohol in the past 30 days, and 2 percent reported binge drinking. U.S.-born Southeast Asians were approximately three times more likely than their foreign-born counterparts to have used an illicit substance in the past month (Wong et al. 2007).

The history of migration for Southeast Asian refugees, including exposure to traumatic events such as torture, armed conflict, or internment, has a great effect on the prevalence of mental and physical conditions, as well as health outcomes. With particular regard to postmigration and acculturative stressors, manifestations of mood or anxiety disorders and psychosomatic symptoms are heightened. Situations of emotional instability produce strained social relations and the occurrence of interpersonal violence, substance abuse, and other socially detrimental behaviors in many cases. Related to PTSD, emotional numbness may also develop, manifest in feelings of detachment and an inability to feel emotions such as intimacy, tenderness, and sexuality. Suicidal ideation and action are also results of precarious emotional states in some cases. Acculturative stress can therefore produce numerous psychological, physical, and psychosomatic conditions among Southeast Asians; however, these outcomes are not a given for all. The manifestation of these conditions and their outcomes depend on a variety of group and individual characteristics, and the context of the migration and resettlement.

## TRAUMA AND ACCESS TO HEALTH CARE

### Utilization of Health Care Services

To provide linguistically accessible and culturally competent health care services to Southeast Asian communities in the United States, health care systems must include staff and medical providers who speak Southeast Asian languages and who understand those cultures and histories. Rates of service utilization, subjective satisfaction, and perceived helpfulness were found to vary by generation, whereby second- and third-generation Asian Americans reported higher on these indicators. Southeast Asians continue to be underrepresented in the health care workforce. The 2000 U.S. census counts 249 physicians per 100,000 of the American population, and 257 physicians per 100,000 white Americans. However, these rates among Southeast Asians remain low, with only 24 Hmong, 28 Laotian, and 40 Cambodian physicians per 100,000 people in each ethnic subgroup. This disparity exists in the nursing profession as well, where there are an estimated 794 nurses per 100,000 Americans and 872 white nurses per 100,000 white Americans, and rates among Hmong (49), Cambodian (144), Laotian (169), and Vietnamese (288) remain low per 100,000 in their respective communities (APIAHF 2005).

One study of utilization of mental health services by Asian Americans found that 8.6 percent of the sample had availed of any type of mental health services, and 34.1 percent of Asian Americans who had a probable diagnosis of a psychological condition sought services (Abe-Kim et al. 2007). Some barriers to adequate utilization of health care services by Southeast Asians have been identified to be cultural. One example of a cultural belief that may hinder patients from seeking health care is the belief within Southeast Asian cultures that suffering is inevitable and disease is related to fate (Uba 1992). For Southeast Asians who experience extreme loss and similar traumatic experiences premigration, these experiences can reaffirm this belief. A lack of familiarity and subsequent distrust of medical systems in the United States can also lead to apprehension in accessing health care services. Similarly, medical providers' lack of understanding of Southeast Asian patients' cultural beliefs regarding health and disease prevention, which includes the utilization of cultural and alternative medicines, prevent the integration of medical professionals' best practices and patients' self-determination in the provision of care (Uba 1992). A study by Ngo-Metzger et al. identifies important qualities of health care from the perspectives of limited English proficient Southeast Asian patients. They perceive their medical providers' knowledge, interest, and acceptance of cultural and alternative medicine as characteristics of high quality care. Professional and gender-concordant interpreters, as opposed to children or family members, were also endorsed as important characteristics of quality care (2003).

Other studies have documented that cultural barriers play a lesser role in underuse of health care services by Southeast Asians. These studies also found that structural barriers such as high cost and language present significantly more critical challenges in a community member's ability to access health care services (Wong et al. 2006). However, cultural and structural barriers do not apply to all segments of the community in their health seeking behaviors. Marshall et al. correlate traditionally identified barriers to health care access to relatively high rates of health care utilization in their study of a Cambodian refugee community in California. Limited English proficiency, unemployment, low levels of formal education, and disabled or retired status were contributing factors to 70 percent of their sample seeing a medical provider and 46 percent a mental health provider. Additionally, women and respondents receiving government assistance were more likely to seek services than men and those not receiving any public benefits (Marshall et al. 2006). These findings are not completely surprising as community members endorsing those social and demographic characteristics are likely to rely on social and medical services provided in their communities.

## Language Access and Literacy as Barriers to Care

Knowledge of available services in local communities, as related to patients' levels of acculturation, English proficiency, and supportive networks, also plays a key factor in patients' ability to access health care in Southeast Asian communities. The bonds within families and coethnic networks are one tool that refugees use to navigate the process of acculturation once they arrived in the United States. The social capital resulting from close interpersonal contacts became the most available source of information regarding instrumental demands, such as finding a language-concordant physician or enrolling in health insurance. The children of these households often became the navigator of public systems and interpreters in the health care setting for parents and elders who have less cultural knowledge of U.S. systems or have limited English proficiency.

There is a growing body of literature that underscores the importance of language communication and literacy in medically underserved communities, such as Southeast Asians, in the United States. In light of the complex medical and mental health needs of Southeast Asian communities, these instrumental barriers to adequate health care are magnified. Southeast Asian patients with limited English proficiency (LEP) and who rely on interpreters have been found to be more likely to have questions about their health care and not to ask them when compared to those patients who did not have to use an interpreter. Similarly, LEP Southeast Asian patients who rated their experience with interpreters highly were more likely to rate the health care they received highly as well (Green et al. 2005). In regions of the country where there are significant Southeast Asian populations—such as Long Beach and San Jose, California, Lowell, Massachusetts, or Houston, Texas—there are often community-based health care services or hospital-based providers and language access programs that meet the linguistic and cultural needs of this community. However, in other regions with smaller or emerging communities these resources are often scarce.

In health care settings where language assistance is required but not available, the quality of that care can be greatly compromised. Studies have found that Asian Americans, and especially those with limited English proficiency, are likely to report lower self-reported overall health status when compared to non-Hispanic whites and Latinos in national samples. This trend persists even when controlled for socioeconomic status (Kandula 2007). Anh et al. document frequent use of cultural and alternative medicine (CAM) in the primary care setting among two-thirds of Vietnamese and Chinese Americans with limited English proficiency in one national study. However, only 7.6 percent of these patients reported discussing their use of CAM with their physician (Anh et al. 2006). This study shows one of the many barriers that language discordance creates between patient and medical provider, thus impacting the quality of care. Anh also reports that for patients in the study discussions with their physicians about patients' use of CAM were associated with better ratings of quality care. Southeast Asian patients with language-discordant providers also report receiving less health education, poorer interpersonal care, and lower quality care overall when compared to those with language-concordant providers. Although the use of interpreters did mitigate differences in health education received by patients in both groups, it did not affect the quality of care reported by patients with language-discordant providers (Ngo-Metzger et al. 2007).

Literacy and educational attainment of patients can also be a confounding barrier to accessible and culturally competent health care. When compared to the general U.S. population and other Asian American subgroups, Southeast Asians consistently have lower levels of lifetime formal education in certain segments of the community. A proportion of monolingual

Southeast Asian immigrants and refugees are also illiterate in their own language because of lack of access to formal education. One study has identified literacy as a contributing factor to Vietnamese women's modified use and appropriate adherence to medication prescribed by Western physicians (O'Callaghan and Quine 2007). Southeast Asian elders who lack English proficiency and formal education face challenges communicating with their medical providers about cancer or may present misconceptions and negative attitudes about cancer prevention. As a result, literacy and language discordance become barriers to effective utilization of preventative cancer screening in an at-risk group (Nguyen et al. 2008).

## TRAUMA-INFORMED CARE

From experience of Southeast Asian communities in the United States, resiliency necessitates holistic support to cope with psychological distress, to integrate past traumatic events, and to manage current health concerns. Survival and community development require maintaining economic subsistence, traditional culture, and social networks. An understanding of the pervasive impact of trauma on health for Southeast Asian communities in the United States is critical to create resources to support survivors and to promote the overall development and well-being of these communities. These are practical strategies already in use in communities across the country, and they have proven to be effective in mitigating the impact of trauma on emotional well-being and physical health, as well as in reducing barriers to accessing health care for Southeast Asian Americans. This relevant model is not exclusive to Southeast Asian communities, and it can be replicated with other Asian American and immigrant communities who have survived traumatic events, including natural disasters, armed conflict, or family violence. There is also resonance with communities who experience numerous pervasive forms of violence and trauma such as discrimination, government surveillance and deportation, and persistent poverty.

### Cultural Competence toward Resiliency

It is important to recognize resiliency in the Southeast Asian community and protective factors against psychological distress or ill health (Hsu et al. 2004). The majority of first- or 1.5-generations refugee and immigrant Southeast Asians in the United States have lived through myriad traumatic events as a direct result of the wars in Southeast Asia or through a consequence of these conflicts, such as internment under the Khmer Rouge or participating in the refugee exodus. In light of these challenges, narratives of the Southeast Asian American experience are often characterized by experiences of survival, loss, isolation, and despair. And yet resiliency and processes of recovery at the individual and family levels serve as critical forces to rebuild Southeast Asian communities in the United States. In the clinical setting a patient may present resiliency through cultural bereavement as opposed to PTSD if the patient has experienced a process of recovery. In this situation empathy from a provider and affirmation of patients' histories are critical to providing culturally appropriate care (Davis 2000). In the development of interventions to promote health and manage chronic conditions such as diabetes, Southeast Asian patients will identify American lifestyles, mistrust of the U.S. medical system, and a lack of understanding among providers of patients' cultural and spiritual beliefs as deterrents to optimal health. Conversely, patients endorse healthy traditions and beliefs relevant to their culture as access points through which both to communicate health promotion messages and encourage empowering care management behaviors (Devlin et al. 2000). In this perspective the preservation of cultural views and identities becomes a tool for health maintenance and promotion.

## Empowering Family and Social Networks

For Southeast Asian communities, traumatic events experienced both premigration and postmigration have a significant impact on the well-being of families and social networks. In their study of PTSD and refugee children, Heptinstall et al. reported a significant correlation between the number of traumatic events premigration and children's PTSD scores. Postmigration stressors such as insecure asylum status or financial difficulties within the family were significantly associated with higher depression scores among children (Heptinstall et al. 2004). Another study of Southeast Asian youth and their parents resettled in the United States found that parent refugee status facilitated youth involvement in serious violence, and it was also significantly related to family/partner violence by youth (Spencer 2006).

After resettlement, conflicts within families between parents and children along the lines of communication, school performance, personal behavior, and antisocial behavior bear weight on parents' self-reported health status, though there are differences in how these dynamics play out in Vietnamese and Cambodian families (Boehnlein et al. 1995). Intergenerational and intercultural conflict has also been documented to have significant impacts on major depression and other psychological distress among both Southeast Asian young people and their parents (Ngo 2006). In the management and treatment of these conditions, it is critical to engage multiple generations of family members in interventions that address mental distress and other disorders (Ying 2007). It is often the case that in Southeast Asian families in which heads of the household and elders have limited English proficiency, low levels of literacy and other forms of social capital, young people and adult children play a critical role in managing household affairs, interpreting medical care, and navigating public systems. Although this increases families' ability to adapt and meet their instrumental needs, this cultural brokering by young people can lead to family conflict and additional stressors related to the reversal of traditional family roles (Trickett 2007).

Though the family and the larger community are the setting for these factors that contribute to negative behaviors, barriers to quality health care, and poor health outcomes, it is also through families and social networks that social capital and communal resources are leveraged within the Southeast Asian community. This phenomenon is rooted in practical, self-reliant strategies for survival developed in communities after resettlement. There is also a cultural resonance for this. Frye conducted a review of health promotion literature and folklore pertaining to Southeast Asians to identify key, effective cultural themes. Kinship solidarity and the preservation of equilibrium emerged as critical values for health promotion in this population (Frye 1995). In the context of health care these themes serve as effective mechanisms for delivering health maintenance and promotion messages. They also serve as adaptive values that promote the resiliency of Southeast Asian communities in response to the myriad instrumental, cognitive, and social demands in the United States.

## Integration of Services and Care Models

Although prevalent mental distress among Southeast Asian Americans is rooted in traumatic experiences premigration, there is clear evidence that the instrumental and acculturative demands of raising bicultural families, finding work, and navigating government benefits also act as stressors. Integrative, community-based interventions mitigate the impact of these demands on clients and complement cognitive-behavioral therapy and other modalities of treatment. There are numerous examples of the successful integration of care models in the literature. Miller recommends that providers move beyond psychotherapy and other clinic-based mental health services to integrate community interventions and supportive services in the treatment of pervasiveness of mental illness in Southeast Asian communities. This method addresses the reluctance of many refugees to utilize conventional psychological or psychiatric services (Miller 1999).

A study of the use of cultural and alternative medicines among a sample of Cambodian community members diagnosed with PTSD, major depression, or alcohol use disorder found that community members utilized both Western sources of care for treatment of mental health as well as CAM. The study demonstrated that few patients used CAM exclusively and that CAM is not a barrier to accessing Western modalities of care for mental health (Berthold 2007). Among patients with type 1 and 2 diabetes, depressive symptoms were associated with greater diabetes symptom reporting, poorer physical functioning, and less adherence to exercise regimens and diet. There was a significant association between depressive symptoms and HbA1c levels in type 1, but not type 2 diabetic patients. Because of their association with clinical aspects of diabetes care such as diabetes symptom reporting and adherence to diabetes self-care, depressive symptoms are important to recognize in treating patients with diabetes (Ciechanowski et al. 2003). Silove et al. undertook a study of Vietnamese patients' satisfaction with mainstream mental health services compared to a refugee-centered setting. Patients reported greater satisfaction with treatment provided at the refugee-centered clinic, which results the authors interpreted to be related to better navigation of services and improved communication between the provider and the patients and families (Silove et al. 1999). A health care system that is responsive to the community's unique needs and attributes must be integrative in its approach to serving Southeast Asians.

## CONCLUSION

More than thirty years after the massive displacement of people from Southeast Asia as a result of war and political turmoil, Vietnamese, Laotian, Hmong, and Cambodian families and communities across the United States continue to grow and change. Many Southeast Asian Americans have attained success and prosperity as an outcome of their strength and their capacity to survive despite very difficult odds. Adaptation to the systems, culture, and language of the United States has served as a protective factor from poor health for many community members. Most importantly, the reconstitution of social networks and value systems, and processes of mutual aid and support have also made possible the development of these communities. Nevertheless, historical traumas and acculturative stressors have exposed these communities to serious mental health disorders and chronic illnesses. Today this impact is most felt among elders in the community who were the first generation of refugees and who now are confronted with multifaceted health and social needs. In Southeast Asian communities where concentrated poverty, violence, and social disenfranchisement still persist, the need for outreach, tailored health care services, community organizing, and broader community development become ever more critical. Because of the insidious effect of trauma in the Southeast Asian American experience, it is not possible to heal and to promote health without engaging the well-being of the community holistically.

## REFERENCES

Abe-Kim J, Takeuchi DT, Hong S, Zane N, Sue S, and Spencer MS. 2007. Use of mental health-related services among immigrant and US-born Asian Americans: Results from the National Latino and Asian American study. *American Journal of Public Health* 97 (1): 91–98.

Almgren G, Magarati M, and Mogford L. 2009. Examining the influences of gender, race, ethnicity, and social capital on the subjective health of adolescents. *Journal of Adolescence* 32 (1): 109–133.

Anh A, Ngo-Metzger Q, Legedza AT, Massagli MP, Clarridge BR, and Phillips RS. 2006. Complementary and alternative medical therapy use among Chinese and Vietnamese Americans: prevalence, associated factors, and effects of patient-clinician communication. *American Journal of Public Health* 96 (4): 647–653.

Asian and Pacific Islander American Health Forum. 2005. Diverse communities, diverse experiences: the status of Asian Americans and Pacific Islander in the U.S. http://www.apiahf.org/resources (accessed July 20, 2008).

Barnes P, Adams PF, and Powell-Griner E. 2008. Health characteristics of the Asian adult population: United States, 2004–2006. *Advanced Data* (394): 1–22.

Ben-Sira, Z. 1997. *Immigration, stress, and readjustment.* Westport, CT: Praeger Publishers.

Berthold S, Wong EC, Schell TL, Marshall GN, Elliott MN, and Takeuchi DT. 2007. U.S. Cambodian refugees' use of complementary and alternative medicine for mental health problems. *Psychiatric Services* 58 (9): 1212–1218.

Blair, R. 2000. Risk factors associated with PTSD and major depression among Cambodian refugees in Utah. *Health and Social Work* 25 (1): 23–30.

Boehnlein J, Kinzie JD, Sekiya U, Riley C, Pou K, and Rosborough B. 2004. A ten-year treatment outcome study of traumatized Cambodian refugees. *Journal of Nervous and Mental Disease* 192 (10): 658–663.

Boehnlein J, Tran HD, Riley C, Vu KC, Tan S, and Leung PK. 1995. A comparative study of family functioning among Vietnamese and Cambodian refugees. *Journal of Nervous and Mental Disease* 183 (12): 768–773.

Boscarino J. 2008. Psychobiologic predictors of disease mortality after psychological trauma: implications for research and clinical surveillance. *Journal of Nervous and Mental Disease* 196 (2): 100–107.

Breslau J, and Chang DF. 2006. Psychiatric disorders among foreign-born and US-born Asian-Americans in a US national survey. Social Psychiatry and Psychiatric Epidemiology 41(2): 943–950.

Carpenter DO. 2008. Environmental contaminants as risk factors for developing diabetes. *Reviews on Environmental Health* 23 (1):59–74.

Centers for Disease Control and Prevention. 2004. Health Status of Cambodian and Vietnamese Selected Communities, United States, 2001–2004. *Morbidity and Morality Weekly Report* 53 (33): 760–764.

Chen A, Keith VM, Leong KJ, Airriess C, Li W, Chung KY, and Lee CC. 2007. Hurricane Katrina: prior trauma, poverty and health among Vietnamese-American survivors. *International Nursing Review* 54 (4): 324–331.

Chung R, and Kagawa-Singer M. 1993. Predictors of psychological distress among Southeast Asian refugees. *Social Science and Medicine* 36 (5): 631–639.

Ciechanowski P, Katon WJ, Russo JE, and Hirsch IB. 2003. The relationship of depressive symptoms to symptom reporting, self-care and glucose control in diabetes. *General Hospital Psychiatry* 25 (4): 246–252.

D'Amico E, Schell TL, Marshall GN, and Hambarsoomians K. 2007. Problem drinking among Cambodian refugees in the United States: How big of a problem is it? *Journal of Studies on Alcohol and Drugs* 68 (1): 11–17.

Davis R. 2000. Refugee experiences and Southeast Asian women's mental health. *Western Journal of Nursing Research* 22 (2): 144–163.

Devlin H, Roberts M, Okaya A, and Xiong YM. 2006. Our lives were healthier before: focus groups with African American, American Indian, Hispanic/Latino, and Hmong people with diabetes. *Health Promotion Practice* 7 (1): 47–55.

Egede L, Zhang D, and Simpson K. 2002. Comorbid depression is associated with increased health care use and expenditures in individuals with diabetes. *Diabetes Care* 25 (3): 464–470.

Erikson K. 1995. Notes on Trauma and Community. In *Trauma: Explorations in Memory*, ed. C. Caruth. Baltimore, MD: Johns Hopkins University Press.

Fawzi M, Pham T, Lin L, Nguyen TV, Ngo D, Murphy E, and Mollica RF. 1997. The validity of posttraumatic stress disorder among Vietnamese refugees. *Journal of Trauma and Stress* 10 (1): 101–108.

Foster R. 2001. When immigration is trauma: Guidelines for the individual and family clinician. *American Journal of Orthopsychiatry* 71 (2): 153–170.

Fox P, Cowell JM, and Montgomery AC. 1999. Southeast Asian refugee children: violence experience and depression. *International Journal of Psychiatric Nursing Research* 5 (2): 589–600.

Frye B. 1995. Use of cultural themes in promoting health among Southeast Asian refugees. *American Journal of Health Promotion* 9 (4): 269–280.

Gee G, Spencer M, Chen J, Yip T, and Takeuchi DT. 2007. The association between self-reported racial discrimination and 12-month DSM-IV mental disorders among Asian Americans nationwide. *Social Science and Medicine* 64 (10): 1984–1996.

Grant N, Marshall S, Berthold M, Schell TL, Elliott MN, Chun CA, and Hambarsoomians K. 2006. Rates and correlates of seeking mental health services among Cambodian refugees. *American Journal of Public Health* 96 (10): 1829–1835.

Green A, Ngo-Metzger Q, Legedza AT, Massagli MP, Phillips RS, and Iezzoni LI. 2005. Interpreter services, language concordance, and health care quality: Experiences of Asian Americans with limited English proficiency. *Journal of General Internal Medicine* 20 (11): 1050–1056.

Heptinstall E, Sethna V, and Taylor E. 2004. PTSD and depression in refugee children — Associations with pre-migration trauma and post-migration stress. *European Child & Adolescent Psychiatry* 13 (6): 373–380.

Herman, Joan. 1997. *Trauma and recovery.* New York, NY: Basic Books.

Ho J. 2008. Community violence exposure of Southeast Asian American adolescents. *Journal of Interpersonal Violence* 23 (1): 136–146.

Hollifield M, Warner TD, Lian N, Krakow B, Jenkins J, Kesler J, Stevenson J, and Westermeyer J. 2002. Measuring trauma and health status: A critical review. *Journal of the American Medical Association* 288 (5): 611–621.

Hollifield M, Warner TD, Jenkins J, Sinclair-Lian N, Krakow B, Eckert V, Karadaghi P, and Westermeyer J. 2006. Assessing war trauma in refugees: Properties of the Comprehensive Trauma Inventory-104. *Journal of Traumatic Stress* 19 (4): 527–540.

Hsu E, Davies CA, and Hansen DJ. 2004. Understanding mental health needs of Southeast Asian refugees: historical, cultural, and contextual challenges. *Clinical Psychology Review* 24 (2): 193–213.

Hwang C. 2006. The psychotherapy adaptation and modification framework: Application to Asian Americans. *American Psychologist* 61 (7): 702–715.

Kandula N, Lauderdale DS, and Baker DW. 2007. Differences in self-reported health among Asians, Latinos, and non-Hispanic whites: The role of language and nativity. *Annals of Epidemiology* 17 (3): 191–198.

Kinzie J, Riley C, McFarland B, Hayes M, Boehnlein J, Leung P, and Adams G. 2008. High prevalence rates of diabetes and hypertension among refugee psychiatric patients. *Journal of Nervous and Mental Disease* 196 (2): 108–112.

Marshall G, Berthold SM, Schell TL, Elliott MN, Chun CA, and Hambarsoomians K. 2006. Rates and correlates of seeking mental health services among Cambodian refugees. *American Journal of Public Health* 96 (10): 1829–1835.

Marshall G, Elliot MN, and Schell TL. 2009. Prevalence and correlates of lifetime disordered gambling in Cambodian refugees residing in Long Beach, CA. *Journal of Immigrant and Minority Health* 11 (1): 35–40.

Miller K. 1999. Rethinking a familiar model: Psychotherapy and the mental health of refugees. *Journal of Contemporary Psychotherapy* 29 (3): 183–306.

Mollica R, Caspi-Yavin Y, Bollini P, Truong T, Tor S, and Lavelle J. 1992. The Harvard Trauma Questionnaire: Validating a cross-cultural instrument for measuring torture, trauma, and posttraumatic stress disorder in Indochinese refugees. *Journal of Nervous and Mental Disease* 180 (2): 111–116.

Mollica R, Wyshak G, de Marneffe D, Khuon F, and Lavelle J. 1987. Indochinese versions of the Hopkins Symptom Checklist-25: A screening instrument for the psychiatric care of refugees. *American Journal of Psychiatry* 144 (4): 497–500.

National Diabetes Education Program, US DHHS. 2006. Silent Trauma: Diabetes, Health Status, and the Refugee. http://www.ndep.nih.gov/diabetes/pubs/SilentTrauma.pdf (accessed July 20, 2008).

Ngo A, Taylor R, Roberts CL, Nguyen TV. 2006. Association between Agent Orange and birth defects: systematic review and meta-analysis. *International Journal of Epidemiology* 35 (5): 1220–1230.

Ngo-Metzger Q, Masagli MP, Clarridge BR, Manocchia M, Davis RB, Iezzoni LI, and Phillips RS. 2003. Linguistic and cultural barriers to care. *Journal of General Internal Medicine* 18 (1): 44–52.

Ngo-Metzger Q, Sorkin DH, Phillips RS, Greenfield S, Massagli MP, Clarridge B, and Kaplan SH. 2007. Providing high-quality care for limited English proficient patients: The importance of language concordance and interpreter use. *Journal of General Internal Medicine* 22 (2 Suppl): 324–330.

Nguyen G, Barg FK, Armstrong K, Holmes JH, and Hornik RC. 2008. Cancer and communication in the health care setting: Experiences of older Vietnamese immigrants, a qualitative study. *Journal of General Internal Medicine* 23 (1): 45–50.

O'Callaghan C, and Quine S. 2007. How older Vietnamese Australian women manage their medicines. *Journal of Cross-Cultural Gerontology* 22 (4): 405–419.

Shapiro J, Douglas K, de la Rocha O, Radecki S, Vu C, and Dinh T. 1999. Generational differences in psychosocial adaptation and predictors of psychological distress in a population of recent Vietnamese immigrants. *Journal of Community Health* 24 (2): 95–113.

Silove D, Manicavasagar V, Beltran R, Le G, Nguyen H, Phan T, and Blaszczynski A. 1997. Satisfaction of Vietnamese patients and their families with refugee and mainstream mental health services. *Psychiatric Services* 48 (8): 1064–1069.

Simon G, VonKorff M, Piccinelli M, Fullerton C, and Ormel J. 1999. An international study of the relation between somatic symptoms and depression. *New England Journal of Medicine* 341 (18): 1329–1335.

Sorkin D, Tan A, Hays RD, Mangione CM, and Ngo-Metzger Q. 2008. Self-reported health status of Vietnamese and non-Hispanic white older adults in California. *Journal of the American Geriatrics Society* 56 (8): 1543–1548.

Spencer J, and Le TN. 2006. Parent refugee status, immigration stressors, and Southeast Asian youth violence. *Journal of Immigrant and Minority Health* 8 (4): 359–368.

Steel Z, Silove D, Phan T, and Bauman A. 2002. Long-term effect of psychological trauma on the mental health of Vietnamese refugees resettled in Australia: A population-based study. *Lancet* 360 (9339): 1056–1062.

Tran T, Manalo V, and Nguyen VTD. 2007. Nonlinear relationship between length of residence and depression in a community-based sample of Vietnamese Americans. *International Journal of Social Psychiatry* 53 (1): 85–94.

Trickett E, and Jones CJ. 2007. Adolescent culture brokering and family functioning: A study of families from Vietnam. *Cultural Diversity with Ethnic Minorities in Psychology* 13 (2): 143–150.

Uba L. 1992. Cultural barriers to health care for Southeast Asian refugees. *Public Health Reports* 107 (5): 544–548.

Watters C. 2001. Emerging paradigms in the mental health care of refugees. *Social Science and Medicine* 52 (11): 1709–1718.

Weisberg R, Bruce SE, Machan JT, Kessler RC, Culpepper L, and Keller MB. 2002. Nonpsychiatric illness among primary care patients with trauma histories and posttraumatic stress disorder. *Psychiatric Services* 53 (7): 848–854.

Wong E, Marshall GN, Schell TL, Elliott MN, Hambarsoomians K, and Chun CA. 2006. Barriers to mental health care utilization for U.S. Cambodian refugees. *Journal of Counseling and Clinical Psychology* 74 (6): 1116–1120.

Wong F, Huang ZJ, Thompson EE, De Leon JM, Shah MS, Park RJ, and Do TD. 2007. Substance use among a sample of foreign- and U.S.-born Southeast Asians in an urban setting. *Journal of Ethnicity and Substance Abuse* 6 (1): 45–66.

Ying Y, and Han MY. 2007. The longitudinal effect of intergenerational gap in acculturation on conflict and mental health in Southeast Asian American adolescents. *American Journal of Orthopsychiatry* 77 (1): 61–66.

# Chapter 33

# Voices of the Community
## Socioeconomic Factors Influencing Access to Health Care for API Communities in New York City

### Sapna Pandya

*Nitin is a 35-year-old immigrant from India on a H1B visa. He has a fluency in English that some third- and fourth-generation Americans do not have. He has a graduate school degree—something that over three-fourths of the U.S. population lacks—and a job—something that a good 5 percent of Americans do not have (Bureau of Labor Statistics 2008). Nitin knows he is lucky to have all these privileges. However, what Nitin does not have is health insurance. Now, on a daily basis, this was not something that concerned Nitin much. He was healthy, worked out, kept himself fit. But one day, he checked his blood pressure and it was terribly elevated. He was not quite sure what it meant, but that morning while showering, he was suddenly attacked by a spell of dizziness. Nitin could not stand up without holding the shower wall, and when he glanced at himself in the mirror, he saw something he had not noticed ever before: his left eye seemed to droop a little. After a visit to the ER, Nitin discovered that he was at serious risk for a stroke and needed to continue making visits to the specialists there. This visit to the ER may jeopardize his hopes of getting a green card, but without which his own life could be in jeopardy. However, the hospital also charged him a bill of $10,000, just for this initial assessment. How is Nitin to make these choices? Between paying his rent and paying his hospital bill? Between saving his immigration process and saving his life?*

## REMODELING THE MINORITY

Underlying the various barriers to health care access for Asian and Pacific Islander (API) communities in the United States is a widespread systemic issue that, though seemingly obvious, unfortunately often gets overlooked or complicated—the problem of socioeconomic class. That is to say, in addition to linguistic, cultural, immigration-related, and other discriminatory factors, API communities face *financial* hurdles both on the road to getting health care and while receiving services—indeed, financial hurdles lie at the very heart of these other concerns. Several, and long-standing, research studies have suggested that "people with higher socioeconomic status have better health and longer lives than those with lower socioeconomic status" (Robert and House 2000).

Though to date, few studies have been published that look specifically at the relationship between socioeconomic status and health outcomes specifically among API communities in the United States, ample data exist that demonstrate the economic burden of health care and health care coverage in the country. This data will be used as a starting point in a discussion on how lack of financial resources exacerbates health care disparities for API communities, with an eye to New York City in particular.

Behind the "model minority myth" that has been chasing API communities lies the sad reality of the poverty that many community members in New York City face. This reality is made clear by disaggregating demographic data collected through census and other means according to geography, ethnicity, and visibility. For example, according to the 2006 American Community Survey, although fewer than 10 percent of the families at or below poverty in New York State are reportedly Asian alone or in combination with other races, 20 percent of families below poverty in New York County are Asian. Further, poverty rates for individuals 65 years and older in New York County are just shy of 50 percent—that is half of Asian elders living in poverty in New York County. Compare this to 20 percent for the total population in the same area. Published data can also be skewed because APIs with lower incomes, API small-business owners, limited-English proficient APIs, and undocumented and uninsured APIs are usually left out of census collection.

It is also important to consider the ways in which API poverty gets hidden by generally reported statistics. Although it is true that Asians in New York City reported a higher median household income compared with the general population in the 2006 American Community Survey, Asian per capita income was almost 15 percent below the city average. If we only consider the household income, we may blind ourselves to the fact that API households have on average a higher number of householders—each wage-earner is earning far less than non-APIs, and there are more people among whom earned income has to be shared.

## AN UNHEALTHY REALITY

As urban scholar John Powell of Ohio State notes, "Studies that fail to account for the intersection of poverty and race and its impact on the entire metropolitan area simply repackage and recycle old and disappointing attempts at urban reform" (Powell http://www.citymayors.com/society/us_blackmen.html). Indeed, it is important to consider the ways in which living with limited means can directly impact health access and subsequently health status for API immigrants. For example, with regard to housing, several studies have suggested that low-wage API workers and elderly APIs often live "in congested and substandard housing, which pose risks to their health (Zhan 2003, 285). For the two-thirds of API children that are brought up in poverty in New York City, the effects of a poor childhood may be felt later in life, as "exposure to poor economic and social conditions during childhood can affect not only the health of people during childhood, but their later health in adulthood as well, even if their adult social and economic conditions are favorable."

Research suggests that "communities with lower socioeconomic levels may offer less healthy housing, work places, and recreational options, with greater potential exposure to toxins such as lead paint, asbestos, and pest infestation" (Evans and Kantrowitz 2002). Studies even state that living in communities with lower socioeconomic levels is "associated with a greater likelihood of smoking, higher blood pressure and cholesterol levels ... even after controlling for individual socioeconomic status" (Reijneveld 1998) and that "obesity among low-income Asian Americans is rising at alarming rates statewide" (Chen http://www.news.ucdavis.edu/sources/poverty_health.lasso).

Besides these most direct ways that poor housing conditions brought on by poverty can be linked to poor health outcomes, it is also important to think about how the costs of housing is related to financial flexibility to pay for health care; this issue will be discussed more in depth later in this chapter. In New York City, the median monthly gross rent was $920 in 2005 (Lee 2006). For an API couple in which only one partner is working (which is common among many API immigrant families), earning $1166 is considered living at the poverty level. This would mean that for an API family living in poverty, over three-fourths of their monthly income would be spent on rent alone. Not much is left after rent is paid for health insurance premiums, or even to pay the sliding-fee at municipal hospitals. This is likely one of the main reasons why API immigrants have one of the highest uninsured rates in the country, in particular for women, who are more likely not to be wage-earners. In California, 28 percent of API women and 37 percent of noncitizen API women are uninsured as compared to 21 percent of the larger Californian population (Zhan 2003, 150). This data is even more striking when disaggregated by gender, as 40 percent of Korean women (Zhan 2003, 150) and South Asian women

(APICHA 2005) are uninsured, or even by occupation, when we consider that 80 percent of South Asian taxi workers in New York City are uninsured (Interview 2005).

The noted social entrepreneur Paul Farmer states that "in the wealthy countries of the Northern hemisphere, the relatively poor often travel far and wait long for health care inferior to that available to the wealthy" (Farmer 2005). This is true of poor API immigrants, many of whom travel far and wait long for care that is especially inferior because it is in a language that they don't speak, being dispensed by providers that are not sensitive to their cultural needs. In Los Angeles, one of the largest homes to low-income API populations, over 40 percent of API immigrants speak English "less than very well" or, in other words, are considered Limited English Proficient (LEP). This number has been disaggregated in several metropolitan areas as well, such as New York City, where 70 percent of Chinese immigrants and 60 percent of Bangladeshi immigrants are considered LEP; the majority of these populations comprise low-wage workers. Because Medicaid does not comprehensively cover the cost of providing language services, many poor API immigrants are not offered phone interpreters or in-person interpreters, despite hospital directives and governmental policies (such as the recent NYC Mayoral Executive Order 120 in summer 2008) that urge municipal agencies to provide these services to their LEP patients. As a result of this gap, individuals avoid going to a medical provider, and when they do go, they face large hurdles in understanding the provider's instructions and giving consent for procedures.

## NOT A FAIR CHOICE

Though often overlooked, of notable importance is the way in which poverty impacts one's perception of their rights to health care. API immigrants from lower socioeconomic status (SES) often do not avail of services that they could be eligible for despite progressive rules and policies that are actually in place to assist these communities. Oftentimes this is due to the tricky balancing act that API immigrants have to negotiate; choosing between housing and health, as mentioned earlier, or tending to one's health or one's immigration process, for example. To prepare a full visa packet, an immigrant can expect to pay an average of $2000 to $3000, though oftentimes this cost runs up to $12,000 depending on the complexity of the case, where they are filing, and so on (How Much 2007).

We must also consider the fact that though an individual may need to, and also desire to seek out regular medical care or obtain health insurance, structural barriers prevent him or her from doing so. Take, for instance, the example of New York City, where API immigrants are overrepresented in certain industries—the restaurant industry, child care services, taxi and limousine services, construction work, and food delivery—all of which require long shifts with little scope for flexible hours, which means less flexible time to access primary care medical facilities. Because individuals working in these industries cannot access primary care because of their working hours, they put off seeing a medical professional until the problem is too severe to bear, and they are at the stage that they need emergency attention. This problem is exacerbated by the fact that though the vast majority of API immigrants are working, many are not given any semblance of health benefits by their employer, even in the case of workman's compensation in case of emergency. A recent report among South Asians in New York City demonstrated that nine out of ten domestic workers were not provided health coverage (Human Rights Watch 2006).

Though data show that immigrants do in fact use emergency rooms less than native-born Americans, hospital studies have demonstrated that immigrants do use the emergency room more often than they use primary care facilities. However, these studies often fail to point out that this is not a fair choice because working twelve-hour shifts, seven days a week (such as many taxi workers do, for example) does not leave much time to check out that perhaps-threatening headache you have been having. As a lot of data have evidenced, "people who cannot afford to pay for health often go without it" (Zhan 2003, 306).

Though there are ample examples of how immigrants make contributions to the United States, many immigrants have internalized the sentiment that they somehow do not deserve public benefits in this country, and, as such, they are reluctant to avail of services when needed. The Internal Revenue Service (IRS) counted contributions totaling over $400 billion from documented immigrants last year, and according to the Social Security Administration's actual figures, more than two-thirds of what they call "other-than-legal" (a.k.a. "undocumented") immigrants are paying payroll taxes. In other words, API immigrants, whether documented or undocumented, *are* contributing to public benefits such as Medicaid, Medicare, Family Health Plus, food stamps, and the like, even if they do not realize this, and even if they are not participating and making use of these programs themselves. This includes everybody, from the low-wage worker to the corporate executive, though, of course, we know that the cost of not using public benefits to the low-wage worker is much greater. For the undocumented low-wage API immigrant, this means that though they are dutifully filing taxes, sometimes paying back taxes to make up for years they were not aware they had to pay (e.g., if they are seeking asylum), they still cannot use Medicaid dollars to finance their health care, and they will not get Social Security benefits when they reach retirement age.

Such injustices contribute to the feeling many poor API immigrants have that they do not deserve to take advantage of health benefits, and they also contribute to the lack of complete knowledge among API immigrants about their eligibility. Though API elderly have a relatively high usage rate of the Medicaid program, many API immigrants do not know about the program, their eligibility for it, and "nor do they have the financial support to pay for basic health care costs" (Zhan 2003, 298). This problem is of course exacerbated when individuals also face language barriers, as discussed earlier, as well as by the fact that Medicaid and Medicare, and indeed the entire American health care system, are very new concepts to recent immigrants, in particular those from low-income backgrounds.

Because of the lack of awareness regarding health access barriers for API immigrants, too little attention, and thereby little funding, goes toward these communities. In fact, in the document Healthy People 2000, a federal tool to help outline health objectives in the country, only eight objectives targeted API communities as compared to six times this number targeting black communities, and three times this number targeting Latino populations (Zhan 2003, 300). This type of gross invisibility is exacerbated by the model minority myth referenced in this chapter's opening paragraphs. Public health researchers have stated that "the observed disparities in health are driven largely by a complex set of causal processes rather than by selection or by artifactual mechanisms" (Goldman 2001). It is therefore crucial that we consider the complex, underlying ways in which socioeconomic class impacts the health of our API communities in the United States.

## REFERENCES

Asian Pacific Islander Coalition against HIV/AIDS (APICHA), Inc. (2005). "South Asian Immigrant Women's HIV/AIDS Related Issues: An Exploratory Study of New York City."

Bureau of Labor Statistics, Department of Labor, April 2008.

Moon S. Chen Jr., professor of public health sciences and co-leader of the Cancer Prevention and Control Program at UC Davis Cancer Center. http://www.news.ucdavis.edu/sources/poverty_health.lasso.

G. Evans and Elyse Kantrowitz. "Socioeconomic Status and Health: The Potential Role of Environmental Risk Exposure." Annual Review of Public Health 23 (2002): 303–331.

P. Farmer. Pathologies of Power: Health, Human Rights, and the New War on the Poor. Berkeley and Los Angeles: University of California Press, 2005; 143.

N. Goldman. "Social Inequalities in Health Disentangling the Underlying Mechanisms." Ann N Y Acad Sci 954 (2001): 118–139.

"How Much Does an Immigration Attorney Cost?" January 2007, http://www.costhelper.com/cost/finance/immigration-attorney.html.

Interview with New York Taxi Workers Association, 2005.

Moon Wha Lee, compiler. Selected Findings of the 2005 New York City Housing and Vacancy Survey. New York: New York City Department of Housing Preservation and Development, 2006.

John A. Powell, former director of Ohio State's New Institute for the Study of Race and Ethnicity in the Americas. http://www.citymayors.com/society/us_blackmen.html.

S.A. Reijneveld. "The Impact of Individual and Area Characteristics on Urban Socioeconomic Differences in Health and Smoking." *International Journal of Epidemiology* 27 (1998): 33–40.

S.A. Robert and J.S. House. "Socioeconomic Inequalities in Health: An Enduring Sociological Problem." In *Handbook of Medical Sociology*, eds. C.E. Bird, P. Conrad, and A.M. Fremont. Upper Saddle River, NJ: Prentice Hall, Inc., 2000; 79–97.

"Swept under the Rug: Abuses against Domestic Workers around the World," Human Rights Watch, 2006. www.hrw.org/reports/2006/wrd0706/wrd0706web.pdf.

Lin Zhan. *Asian Americans: Vulnerable Populations, Model Interventions, and Clarifying Agendas*. Boston: Jones and Bartlett Publishers, Inc., 2003.

# PART VII

---

# Lifestyles and Health

# Chapter 34

# Socioeconomic and Cultural Barriers to Preventive Health

## Kenny Kwong

The purpose of this chapter is to explore socioeconomic and cultural barriers to preventive health among Asian Americans and understand their specific needs and experiences when they seek preventive health care. The Systems Model of Clinical Preventive Care (Walsh and McPhee 1992) and their related concepts will be presented as useful tools in understanding the patients' view on and behavior in preventive health care activities and in highlighting factors that may influence patients in engaging in preventive health behavior. This chapter explores the cultural views of health and illness among Asian Americans, assesses their beliefs and attitude toward preventive health screening, and identifies socioeconomic and health care systemic barriers that affect their access to preventive health services. Several case examples, based on real people who participated in a study by this author, will be included to illustrate the concepts and principles to improve access and overcome barriers to preventive health among Asian Americans. Recommendations to enhance and improve access to preventive health will also be presented.

The task of improving Asian Americans' access to preventive care is easier said than done. The first and foremost challenge of all is to define what their needs are, because there have not been many studies done on this group. The Asian American population was not identified as a separate minority population group before the 2000 census (Chen 2005). There is a significant information gap in ethnic-specific disease incidence and statistics within the Asian American populations. Very little information is available on the incidences and treatment of various illnesses among specific subgroups of Asian American populations. If there is any health literature on Asian Americans at all, they are focused on documenting the existence and extent of health disparities rather than on explaining why these disparities exist. Even fewer studies have examined psychosocial and cultural variables that may affect access to preventive health screening and treatment of specific subgroups within the Asian American populations. The relatively low incidence of certain types of diseases causes health care experts, government officials, and the Asian American community to overlook the importance of health promotion and preventive health services for these populations. It also creates a false impression that Asian Americans as a group are not at risk for certain diseases, and that they are capable of taking care of their own needs and therefore do not need preventive health services.

The poor and medically underserved populations often encounter numerous barriers to preventive health care. These barriers include poverty, substandard and overcrowded housing, crime, lack of resources such as transportation and child care, as well as lack of knowledge and skills in negotiating the health care system (Langer 1999). Many studies have reported that socioeconomic status (SES), as measured by education and income, is a major factor affecting quality of health and health disparity (Cutler et al. 2006; Adams et al. 2003; Adler and Newman 2002). Several studies consistently reported that low education, low income, and lack of health insurance are associated with lower participation in cancer screenings among Asian Americans (Islam et al. 2006; Juon et al. 2004; Lee et al. 2006). Low SES is also associated with higher risk of cancer incidence, morbidity, mortality, as well as poor cancer survival (Ward et al. 2004; Bradley et al. 2002; Kagawa-Singer 1995). Poor Asian Americans are often overwhelmed by various situations such as poor physical health, poor living conditions, and unemployment. They may not consider preventive health care a priority and engage in preventive health screening practices unless they can seek and receive services from health care organizations that are responsive to their specific needs and coping patterns (Hopps et al. 1995). Moreover, cultural beliefs, attitudes, and life experiences may also affect their reaction to body discomforts, health maintenance, daily activities, food preference, and various treatment and health practices (Ashing et al. 2003; Engstrom 2006). The lack of English proficiency also forces many of them to stay in closely-knit communities and avoid needed health care services. All these barriers make it difficult for them to access preventive health services and to seek prompt treatment for diseases. It is therefore important for health care providers and public health professionals to understand barriers to preventive health and health education among Asian Americans, especially those with low socioeconomic status, and improve their access to services by designing culturally sensitive and consumer friendly programs that meet the needs of this population.

## CONCEPTUAL FRAMEWORK

The Health Belief Model and the Systems Model of Clinical Preventive Care (Walsh and McPhee 1992) and their related concepts provide a useful framework for studying the patient's perspective and health-related behavior, which in turn helps develop health education and health promotion strategies that are effective to the target population.

The Health Belief Model (HBM) was originally developed by Rosenstock (1974) and Becker, Drachman, and Kirschy (1974) to study why people failed to accept disease prevention activities and early detection screening tests. Key dimensions of this model include *perceived susceptibility, perceived severity* of illness, and *perceived barriers to* and *benefits of* carrying out recommended health-related behavior or preventive health activities. In order for an individual to take action and avoid a disease, he would need to believe that he is personally *susceptible* to the disease even in the absence of symptoms, that occurrence of the disease would have at least some degree of *severity* on certain aspects of his life, that taking an action would be *beneficial* to him by reducing his susceptibility to the disease or by reducing its severity, and that taking action itself would not be impeded by *barriers* such as cost, transportation, convenience, embarrassment, or other negative factors. The combined factors help predict whether an individual would engage in health-related behavior or not. However, Rosenstock (1974) noted that the combination of these factors may not result in actual behavior unless some *instigating events* or *cues* occurred to trigger the behavior. In the case of preventive health screening, instigating events may be internal, such as experience of symptoms or perception of bodily changes, or they may be external, such as the impact of environmental events or media communication (Strecher and Rosenstock, 1997). Rosenstock (1974) also added other variables such as diverse demographic, socio-psychological, and structural variables to the HBM because these may affect an individual's perception of susceptibility, severity, benefits, and barriers, and therefore indirectly influence health-related behavior.

Rosenstock and colleagues (1988) later modified the HBM by incorporating *self-efficacy* as an important variable. They argued that in order to effect behavior change, the individual needs to feel that he or she is competent to carry out that change. Self-efficacy, derived from social learning theory, is defined as "the conviction that one can successfully execute the behavior required to produce the outcomes" (Bandura 1977, p. 79). The concept of self-efficacy in explaining the initiation and maintenance of behavioral change has been supported by a substantial body of literature (Wood 2008; Bandura 2004; Strecher and Rosenstock 1997). Rosenstock (1990) later modified the concept of self-efficacy and used the *value expectancy* concept to predict health-related behavior. For the individual to practice preventive health behavior, he needs to have "the desire to avoid illness or to get well (value)" (p. 40) and believe that a specific health behavior is available for him to prevent illness (expectancy).

The PRECEDE-PROCEED Planning Framework proposed by Green and Kreuter (2005) complements the HBM by identifying the skills, resources, or social support needed by an individual to perform preventive health behavior and to plan and evaluate health intervention. The Planning Framework consists of a multiple-phase process with the basic notion that health behaviors are complex, multidimensional, and are influenced by a variety of factors (Gielen et al. 2008), namely *predisposing, enabling,* and *reinforcing* factors. Because health and health risks are determined by multiple factors, efforts to effect behavioral, social, and environmental change must also be multidimensional (Green and Kreuter, 2005). This framework emphasizes the important role of social and environmental factors in determining health behaviors and health outcomes.

Building on the HBM and the Planning Framework, Walsh and McPhee (1992) developed the Systems Model of Clinical Preventive Care (the Model) that can be applied to study a variety of preventive care activities and situations (Naleway et al. 2006; Lane et al. 2000). The Model contains components of psychosocial, behavioral, communication, and health education theories. This Model is unique in its focus on both patient and physician factors in influencing patient preventive care activities. The physician's performance of preventive care activities and physician referral are also influenced by *predisposing, enabling,* and *reinforcing* factors. Both patient and physician factors are independently influenced by other factors such as health care delivery system factors, preventive activity factors, and situational factors. Table 34.1 outlines all these patient and physician factors, contextual, and system factors as described in the Model. All these factors interact with each other in influencing the likelihood of whether any preventive activity is performed or not.

In summary, the Health Belief Model, the Systems Model of Clinical Preventive Care, and their related concepts are useful tools in identifying factors that may influence patients in engaging in preventive health activities. They are also helpful in revealing the relationships among and between these factors and various health outcomes. Based on the Systems Model, a review of literature will focus on the following areas: (1) cultural influences in preventive health; (2) beliefs and attitudes toward preventive health; (3) socioeconomic barriers; and (4) health care delivery systems barriers to preventive health.

**Table 34.1** Factors Influencing Patients in Engaging in Preventive Health Activities

- **Patient predisposing factors**
  Patient beliefs, attitudes, expectations, motivation, self-efficacy, and health internal locus of control.

- **Patient enabling factors**
  Education, health knowledge, skills, income, and physiologic factors.

- **Patient reinforcing factors**
  Social support and inherent reinforcement value of the preventive activity.

- **Physician predisposing factors**
  Physician beliefs, attitudes, prior clinical experiences, and personal health practices.

- **Physician enabling factors**
  Training, knowledge of screening recommendations, and the availability of educational tools and materials.

- **Physician reinforcing factors**
  Patient satisfaction with the physician's preventive care orientation, communication with other physicians, and peer support and approval.

- **Health care delivery system factors**
  Access to care, availability of technology and personnel, organizational priorities, reimbursement, and coordination with community resources

- **Preventive activity factors**
  Preventive activity and costs, risks, effectiveness, and efficacy of the activity.

- **Situational factors**
  Triggers to health behavior, which include internal cues such as symptoms and external cues such as physician encouragement or reminders.

## CULTURE AND PREVENTIVE HEALTH

Culture is "the sum of beliefs, practices, habits, likes, dislikes, norms, customs, rituals" (Spector 2000, p. 78). Culture is revealed through the unique shared values, beliefs, and practices that are directly or indirectly associated with health-related behavior (Pasick et al. 1996). Health behavior and practice is the outcome of knowledge, attitudes, and beliefs embedded in the context of life circumstances and experiences (Pasick 1997). Each cultural group is different and unique in defining health and well-being, perceiving the causes of disease, misfortune, and death (Spector 2000); and identifying appropriate preventive health activities and effective treatment strategies to ensure the survival and well-being of its members (Kagawa-Singer 1996). It is important for health care professionals to be familiar with the cultural beliefs and practices of Asian Americans and understand how patients and their families interpret the causes of certain diseases and the recommended regimen for disease prevention, screening, and treatment. As Kagawa-Singer (1996) stated, patients will only incorporate recommended medical regimens when these recommendations fit into their belief systems and are relevant to their lives at a specific point in time. They also need to believe that the changes are worth the effort to try and that they have the resources to do so.

Cross-cultural studies have also shown that culture affects how symptoms are expressed and manifested; when help and services are being sought; when individuals are in physical, emotional, or psychological pain; what healing or treatment procedures are considered acceptable to the individual; as well as the meaning ascribed to the return to health or a feeling of well-being (Pedersen et al. 2008; Engstrom 2006; DHHS 2001). Individuals from a specific cultural background may have a very different set of values, beliefs, and understanding of health screening procedures and treatment process that differ from that of their health care providers. In Case Example 1, a patient revealed her experience of cancer screening services in the United States as compared to that in China. She concluded that her experience with the medical system in China was very different, and in her mind somewhat "superior" to that of the United States.

### Case Example 1—Two Countries, Two Systems

Patients who came from China had health care experience from two different health care systems, one in their country of origin, and one in the U.S. Because both systems have different sets of screening guidelines, diagnosis, treatment process, and treatment outcomes, it may create confusion for them, especially when they have to seek follow up care in the U.S. for a pre-existing condition that was once treated in China. A Chinese patient talked about her diagnosis and treatment of "hyperplasia of mammary glands," a condition which was considered as "pre-cancerous" in China which required treatment. She compared her cancer screening experience in the U.S. with that in China.

I believe that I am at risk for breast cancer and that's why I have been participating in cancer screening at the health center for the last 3 years. I am very concerned about my health. I was diagnosed of "mammary gland fibroma" (breast fibroid) in China when I was 20 years old. One time when I took a bath and touched my breast, I felt something. The lump was like a ball rolling inside my breast. I went to see a doctor and found out I had mammary gland fibroma. This was believed to be a precursor of breast cancer. But it was not cancer yet because the lump in my breast moved . . . I had surgery and was hospitalized for 10 days. Then, the doctors suggested that I had regular check up thereafter . . .

When I was in the hospital, they did a biopsy to test if my breast lumps were benign or malignant. After the test, the doctor told me that the result was negative. However, there were six other patients who had the same abnormality in their breasts. Four had fibroma. I was lucky because mine was just benign. They even let me look at the size of both breast fibroids, one was bigger and the other was smaller . . .

In China, the Chinese government had no specific cancer screening guidelines nor assumed any responsibilities of offering testing . . . Whether you get preventive health care depends on whether your "employment unit" offers gynecological check up or not. My "unit" provided screening services on breast and cervix . . . In the U.S., there is no diagnosis called "hyperplasia of mammary glands" (HMG). The diagnosis for breast abnormality in this country is just whether there is cancer or not. In China, there is more follow up once a patient is diagnosed of HMG . . . They would tell you whether you had HMG and asked you to take medication to control hyperplasia. . . . I believed those diagnosed with breast cancer or with breast problems might also have had HMG. That's why in China, after taking the x-ray, they would tell you if you had HMG or not. If you did, they asked you to take medications to eliminate hyperplasia in the breasts . . .

The doctors in China asked me to take herbal pills. Some patients took them but I did not. I didn't think "hyperplasia of mammary glands" was a big problem. I don't like taking herbal pills. A few of my co-workers also have HMG. In China, they tell you whether your HMG is "prolific" or not. Patients can actually see the extent of HMG level from x-ray films. The doctor can show you which part of your breast has HMG. If you have a serious case of HMG, you need to take medications. My coworker took the pills and her HMG decreased drastically . . . On the contrary, Western-based medical system has no specific treatment or medications for HMG . . . These herbal pills can be picked up in the hospital in China, but in the U.S., those medications are not available. In China, both Chinese medicines and Western medicines are available in the hospital . . . In the U.S., after taking an x-ray, we were only told if we had cancer or not, or if we had other abnormality in our breasts. There was no "transitional" stage, such as before cancer developed . . . Here in the U.S., they did not tell me the exact problem of my breast . . . In China, doctors tell you whether you have HMG. They said that women with HMG have higher risks of developing into breast cancer. They then prescribe medicine to you."

In cross-cultural medical practice, there are often negative or unintended consequences for treatment when the physician provides medical intervention without understanding the patient's perception of illness, treatment, and well-being. Dyche and Zayas (1995) recommend that physicians discuss medical issues with the patient sensitively and collaboratively by being persistent in asking what the patient thinks is wrong and how serious it is, how the illness affects the patient's life, and what the patient thinks can help. In addition, the concept of social support for patients with serious diseases appears to differ in different cultures. Who provides social support, what kind of social support is considered appropriate and desired, and perceived adequacy of social support are different in different cultures (Wellisch et al. 1999). For example, in oncology practice of Western medicine, emotional support in the form of expression of feeling is often assumed to be important in helping patients cope with cancer (Kagawa-Singer 1996). However, in many other cultures, material support and "doing for" the patient is considered more appropriate because the culture stresses emotional support without words (Uba 1994). In such cultures, talking about dysphoric emotions may create greater distress. It can be detrimental to the patient because it will not change the situation. Therefore, when providing social support to patients, it is important to know what is culturally appropriate and acceptable and what is not in order for intervention to be effective (Kagawa-Singer 1996).

Cultural factors can enhance or impede participation in health education and screening activities. Several studies found that cultural factors are more likely to be barriers to preventive health screening and early detection activities among culturally diverse groups (Liang et al. 2004; Spector 2000; Kagawa-Singer 1995). However, other studies indicate that many immigrants from Asian cultures endorse *prevention* as an essential and important concept, and use some forms of health measures—such as herbal remedies, acupuncture, and other traditional medical treatments—to strengthen the body, resist disease, and improve health and physical well-being (Ahn et al. 2006; Spector 2000; Ma 1999). In Asian culture, prevention includes health promotion as well as balance and harmony in health behaviors, lifestyle, and daily diet. Based on holistic views of health, many traditional Asians practice preventive health through exercising regularly, maintaining a balanced and healthy diet, and using herbs and soups to promote health and prevent disease. In fact, these practices are consistent with what Western medicine is currently advocating in health promotion and disease prevention.

There are many factors influencing the extent to which members of a specific culture participate in disease prevention and screening. These factors include the patients' birthplace and the level of acculturation or assimilation to the new host society (Hedeen et al. 1999); their cultural attitude toward bodily functions and the power of indigenous healers (McBride et al. 1998); their level of trust in Western health care (Ma 2000); their general and specific health beliefs; their practices concerning health, diet, and access to screening; and their expectation concerning the quality of patient-provider interaction and communication in the health care setting (Liang et al. 2004; Olsen and Stromborg 1993). Underutilization of preventive health screening services among ethnic minorities is often attributed to factors such as language difficulties, lack of cancer information in the patient's language, and fear of cancer (Hoeman et al. 1996; Lee 1998).

A thorough understanding of the cultural characteristics of the target population and of how those characteristics affect health behavior is important to ensure the success of intervention. In designing culturally appropriate health promotion activities, Pasick et al. (1996) recommended "cultural tailoring," the development of interventions, strategies, messages, and health materials to conform to specific cultural characteristics, rather than "cultural targeting," the identification of a population subgroup for the purpose of ensuring exposure of that subgroup to the intervention. Pasick et al. argued that "cultural tailoring" allows health care providers and health educators to move from beneath the surface of race and ethnicity to those factors that directly influence behavior and health.

## Asian American Beliefs and Attitudes toward Preventive Health

Cultural values, beliefs, attitudes, and personal experiences affect a person's reaction to illness, health maintenance, changes in life, and various health promotion and treatment practices (Spector 2000). In the United States, health care practice is guided by a scientific, evidence-based, biomedical approach. It is questionable whether this approach to preventive health screening and treatment is optimal when working with Asian Americans who are seeking health care according to their specific cultural beliefs and personal practice. Health care professionals need to be sensitive to their own cultural background and perspective and how these affect their practice (Panos and Panos 2000). Otherwise, they may misunderstand their patients, miss valuable diagnostic cues, and encounter higher rates of patient noncompliance with preventive health screening guidelines. Therefore, understanding the notion of preventive care and the meaning of diseases in the Asian American culture and the specific health beliefs and practices of the Asian American populations is essential to providing quality health screening services and treatment.

An important first step in improving access to quality health care is to recognize that the American health care system is itself a cultural system that reflects American values, which may be very different from the values in Asian culture (Kagawa-Singer 1996). The basic tenet of the American health care system, which is founded on Judeo-Christian values, states that life is sacred and should be preserved at all costs, that individual, autonomous decision-making ability should be emphasized and supported, and that nobody should suffer (Silberfarb 1982). In contrast, a health care principle held by many traditional Asians is that individual life is not sacred, that the welfare of the group and the community is more important than that of the individual, that decisions are made by group consensus, and that suffering in life is inevitable (Kagawa-Singer 1996).

To speak of "Asian American culture" as a singular, distinct, and coherent entity is misleading (Uba 2002). Although Buddhism, Confucianism, and Taoism underlie many Asian traditional cultural values and belief systems, there are also major differences among Asian cultures (Uba 1994). For example, Filipinos are most often Catholic, whereas Koreans are likely Protestants. A large number of Southeast Asians are Buddhists. Different Asian American groups may not reconcile the same Asian cultural traditions because they have come from different countries. They also hold traditional values to varying degrees because of differences in generation status, gender, economic class, and geographical locations

(Uba 2002). Asian American cultural values are discussed here to provide some understanding of the differences between Asian American values and Euro-American values and the implications of these differences for the health behavior of Asian Americans.

Asian culture has a long history and tradition distinct from that of Western culture. Health care values held by most Asians who hold traditional values emphasize harmony in relationships, respect, self-control, yin-yang balance, interdependency, collectivism, and precedence of group interests and family needs over individual interests (Spector 2000; Ino and Glicken 1999; Uba 1994) as opposed to Western values that encourage direct expression, independence, and individual autonomy (Ma 1999). These values and beliefs impact the lives of Asians in a manner different from Western philosophies or religions (Uba 1994; Ino and Glicken 1999; Chen 1996).

The basic tenet of Buddhism is that all life is suffering, and that suffering originates from undue desires (Carter 1994; Ino Glicken 1999). This belief is contrary to the basic philosophy of the Western health care system that nobody should suffer. Buddhism also believes that all living beings are doomed to ride the "wheel of life" through endless cycles of birth, growth, maturity, aging, illness, and death unless they seek the enlightenment of Buddhism (Carter 1994). Buddhism stresses seeking enlightenment through being diligent and selfless and avoiding undue desires (Kagawa-Singer 1996). Therefore, emotional restraint and coping with life's suffering for the quality of one's next life have special implications in Asian culture (Ino and Glicken 1999).

Confucianism teaches the importance of family, filial piety, respect for the elders, and the virtue of the individual as illuminated by observing the basic relationships of society as well as maintaining social harmony at all levels of society (Spector 2000; Ino and Glicken 1999). Collectivist values in Confucianism emphasize that common good or the pursuits and needs of the community takes precedence over the pursuits and needs of the individual. Collectivist values, as contrary to individualist values in the West, affect health beliefs and health behavior of Asian Americans in many ways (Pasick et al. 1996). First, collectivists see the entire family as the most credible source of health information. Therefore, one models one's health behavior after family members as opposed to the individualistic perspective that sees health care providers and unrelated others as having greater credibility (Pasick et al. 1996). Most health care services in the United States are provided to encourage the individual to be self-sufficient and autonomous in his decision making even when he is sick. However, Asian Americans tend to believe in group identity, interdependency, and consensus modes of decision making (Jenkins and Kagawa-Singer 1994). Therefore, efforts in promoting more individualistic values by health care providers may create discomfort for Asian Americans, because oftentimes problems are shared and discussed among family members (Sue and Sue 2007). Rather, peer support and encouragement as well as family involvement should be utilized more to promote access to preventive care.

Based on psychological theories of individual decision making, the Preventive Behavior Model (Murdaugh and Verran 1987) combines the concept of *health value orientation* with the concept of *health internal locus of control* in predicting preventive health behavior. *Health value orientation* is the importance paid to health by the individual and the standard on which health choices are made. *Health internal locus of control* is the belief that health is determined by one's action and by one's rational choice. The design and the implementation of the majority of preventive health screenings in the United States are based on these concepts of enhancing the patient's ability to control disease by engaging in preventive screening activities. However, the Western belief that health is determined by one's effort is contrary to the Taoist value of the East that asserts that health is a state of spiritual and physical harmony with nature (Spector 2000). Taoism teaches harmony between human beings and nature, and it is concerned with the metaphysical and mystical process of "Tao" or the Way (Ino and Glicken 1999). The person follows the principle of "wu-wei" or nonaction, which means that he should always act in accordance with nature and not against it. Taoism promotes the belief that nature has the ultimate authority over the course of one's life and existence (Ino and Glicken 1999) and that one is not in complete control of nature or one's destiny.

The holistic concept is an important concept in traditional Asian culture that affects the prevention and treatment of diseases. Based on the holistic concept, the human body is regarded as an internal organism (Spector 2000, p. 197). Pathologies and diseases are always considered in conjunction with other organs and tissues of the entire body. Special attention is paid to the integration of the human body as an internal organism with the external environment. The onset, development, and change of disease conditions are considered in conjunction with the social and environmental changes (p. 198). Traditional Asians believe that diseases are only "preventable" or "controllable" by maintaining balanced energy levels and eating properly (Hoeman et al. 1996). These values and perceptions are reflected in their strong adherence to a holistic approach with traditional beliefs in yin-yang balance, hot-cold principle, harmony with nature, medicinal foods, self-diagnosis, and alternative treatment practices. Case Example 2 is an account of an old Chinese man who embarked on a journey to China looking for inspiration, enlightenment, and alternative treatment methods for his health condition. He eventually found his own path of integrated healing approaches that worked miraculously to "cure" the ailments from which he suffered.

**Case Example 2—A Pathfinder's Account on a "Miracle Cure"**

Many patients experience nothing but frustration, anxiety, fear, and confusion when seeking health care services. They often could not find a satisfactory treatment for their condition. So they decided to create their own path by looking into alternative treatment options. The following is an account of an old Chinese patient who for years looked for inspiration, enlightenment, and alternative treatment methods for his prostate problems.

"I had prostate problems for a long time and I tried many medications. Then I went to China and tried to find out from Chinese traditional medicine what I could do with my prostate problems . . . I visited well-known practitioners of Chinese traditional medicine . . . I was then introduced to a Buddhist monk in the mountains of ChengDu. This old monk taught me a special exercise called "prostate exercise" to strengthen my prostate. Western doctors may think that this is absurd . . . But I have taken western medications for a long time and it can only help my problem in a limited way . . . Exercising can prevent cancer. In China, there was a saying that "*qi gong* can prevent cancer" . . . Exercising can strengthen our immune system and the cancer cells won't attack our body . . . The Chinese doctor told me to practice *qi gong* and "exercise" my prostate. He said these methods were effective in treating my prostate problem . . .

It was quite simple. Every time we practice *qi gong*, we can exercise our bladder as well. Hold it tight and then relax. They called it "bladder exercise." After each bowel movement or urination, you "exercise your bladder" by contracting your abdomen muscles and then relaxing it. The movement looks like the gesture of men having orgasm during sexual intercourse. They said it was good for your prostate. If one does not care about having a large prostate, this person must be sexually active because he has lots of exercise in his prostate . . . Since I learned about this "prostate exercise," I practice it almost every day. I can now do it everywhere even when I am outside. I can even show it to you.

When I returned from China, I saw my urologist for a check-up. Two years in a row, my doctor was surprised to find that my prostate has shrunk to its original size. He said I looked much younger, more like a 30-year-old man. I told the doctor that I wanted to cut down my medication and asked whether it would be okay or not. The doctor said it was up to me . . . The doctor said he could not feel my prostate when he did a digital rectal examination. I told him what I did when I was in China. I also told the doctor about the "theory" of exercising the prostate."

This patient also went on to learn other types of exercise that benefited his health, such as *kung fu* and *judo*. He also learned about food groups that were known to be rich in antioxidants and had been persistent in exercising and eating a healthy diet. As a result, not only did his symptoms of prostate enlargement and arthritis disappear, he was also healthier in general.

For many immigrant Asians, Western diagnostic procedures are not used for screening purposes but for a health problem only; therefore they do not understand why so many diagnostic tests are necessary (Spector 2000). A patient who has no experience with preventive care may not comprehend the concept of screening for a disease that he or she probably does not have. Therefore, despite the fact that they take some health measures, they may not necessarily accept the Western approach to disease prevention. For instance, cancer has a very negative connotation in the Asian American community (Sun et al. 2005; Jenkins and Kagawa-Singer 1994). Beliefs of what causes cancer may determine what interventions are preferred and appropriate to treat cancer. In more traditional Asian families, cancer is believed to be caused primarily by hereditary defects. This belief can cause the offspring in families with cancer history to be viewed as less "desirable" or "marriageable" (Jenkins and Kagawa-Singer 1994). Others may believe that cancer is a punishment for transgressions in this life or in past lives. These beliefs may cause Asian immigrants who suspect cancer themselves to delay seeking diagnosis and treatment from a physician (Jenkins and Kagawa-Singer 1994). Even after they are diagnosed, they are also less likely to be compliant with treatment recommendations.

Beliefs on past transgressions or cancer as a form of retribution may make traditional Asian families reluctant to admit cancer openly and seek treatment promptly. This reluctance may explain the late stage of diagnosis for cervical cancer among Chinese and Vietnamese women (Jenkins and Kagawa-Singer 1994). Health care providers should keep an open mind and be more aware of the traditions and cultural beliefs of Asian immigrants concerning wellness, health, and diseases. They must include their patients' perception of health in the assessment and delivery of health care. In order to adequately understand and provide health care to the patients, medical providers should be sensitized to their patients' cultural beliefs, health practices, traditional medicine within Asian cultures, and alternative treatment approaches.

## MISCONCEPTIONS REGARDING RISK, VULNERABILITY, SUSCEPTIBILITY TO, AND SERIOUSNESS OF DISEASES

Several studies have explored the perception regarding risk, vulnerability, susceptibility to, and seriousness of cancer among Asian American women (Juon et al. 2004; Taylor et al. 2004; Hoeman et al. 1996). The study results found that these women believed they had a lower risk of breast and cervical cancer than American women and therefore associated the need of preventive health behaviors with American women rather than with themselves. In the 1996 study by Hoeman et al., participants believed that cervical cancer was related to early sexual activities among American women, and because they did not engage in high-risk behaviors, they did not believe themselves to be susceptible to cancer. With regard to perceived seriousness of breast cancer, only one-third of Chinese women in Lu's (1995) study recognized the seriousness of breast cancer, whereas more than 50 percent had no opinion or did not consider breast cancer as a serious problem. The same study also revealed that social and family impact of illness is a major concern among these women, especially when cancer involves the risk of death or interference with the ability to become a mother.

The fear that cancer is fatal prevails in Asian culture (Sun et al. 2005; Mo 1992). For many Asian patients, the initial immediate reaction after discovering cancer is one of shock, disbelief, disregard, resignation, and withdrawal (Jenkins and Kagawa-Singer 1994). Fear of cancer itself, beliefs that thinking about cancer can provoke the onset of cancer, and financial obstacles, are cited as formidable barriers to cancer education and screening in the Asian American group (Sadler et al. 1998). Modesty as a personal factor inhibiting Vietnamese and Chinese women from obtaining Pap smears is also cited as a barrier (Taylor et al. 2004; Hoeman et al. 1996). Based on cultural beliefs on the role of women, their reproductive functions, attention to birthing, as well as other culturally defined role behaviors, fear of exploitation by a health practitioner during Pap smear screening was a factor that prevented Chinese women from seeking preventive gynecological care (Mo 1992). Studies also cited perceived benefits of participating in preventive health behaviors as "the avoidance of transferring bad genes to the next generation, the provision of a sense of being personally safe, and the perception that such behaviors were good for reproductive function" (Hoeman et al. 1996, p. 527), and that cervical cancer is curable if detected earlier (Taylor et al. 2004). In summary, health care organizations need to recognize the ramification of these cultural beliefs on health-seeking behaviors among Asian Americans and their implications on early detection and screening activities in order for their services to reach the target population they intend to serve effectively.

## SOCIOECONOMIC BARRIERS TO PREVENTIVE HEALTH

Socioeconomic status (SES), race, and ethnicity are often studied simplistically in health literature as static variables controlled in epidemiology, or they are treated as the context in health promotion and disease prevention (Pasick 1997). Current health promotion approaches are not derived nor tested adequately on populations of different cultures and SES (Pasick 1997). Researchers and health care professionals need to consider and address these complex issues in order to develop effective preventive health education and screening programs for the medically underserved population. Several studies reported that SES is a major factor affecting quality of health and health disparity (Adams et al. 2003; Adler and Newman 2002; Cutler et al. 2006). Low SES is associated with higher cancer incidence, morbidity, and mortality (Ward et al. 2004;

Kagawa-Singer 1995), and with lower participation in cancer screenings among Asian Americans (Islam et al. 2006; Juon et al. 2004; Lee et al. 2006). The overall five-year survival rate of poor Americans for all cancers combined is 10 percent lower than that of more affluent Americans (Ward et al. 2004). Economic status, regardless of race, acts as a powerful symbol of human conditions and circumstances and explains a higher cancer incidence and lower survival (Freeman 1991). Because SES is an important mediator for quality of health care, studying barriers to health care among Asian Americans cannot be separated from studying disparity in health care due to low socioeconomic status.

Being poor creates economic, social, psychological, access, and information barriers to health care that affect individuals regardless of age, gender, or race (Palos 1994). Identifying these barriers to health promotion may help health care professionals understand why the poor have a lower rate of compliance with recommended health practices. Barriers the poor experience include substandard and overcrowded housing, neighborhood crime, chronic malnutrition, lack of enabling resources, knowledge, and skills, illiteracy and innumeracy, provider cultural insensitivity and lack of awareness on patients' coping styles and belief systems, systemic failure to address patients' lack of insurance, and other nonmedical impediments to quality health care (Langer 1999; Reilly et al. 1998).

Jang and colleagues (1998) studied health-related needs in the low-income San Francisco Chinatown and found that poverty, limited English skills, and noncitizenship status were significant barriers for Chinese residents to access and use health care services. Juon and colleagues (2004) found that employed Korean American women without health insurance had lower rates of mammograms than those employed with insurance. The study by Islam et al. (2006) showed that education and insurance status were factors affecting screening practices of South Asian women living in the New York City area. All these factors create competing priorities in the lives of poor individuals that prevent them from participating in early detection and health screening activities and from actively seeking treatment when diagnosed with diseases. Sadly, the economically disadvantaged and medically underserved often have additional health risk factors. The cumulative effect of chronic malnutrition, substandard housing, unemployment, excessive exposure to environmental pollutants, and chronic stress could damage the primary function of the body and affect its inherent ability to defend itself from internal and external stressors (Underwood and Hoskins 1994). As a result, individuals who are economically disadvantaged become candidates to belong to high-risk groups for certain types of diseases, and they also experience lower survival rates and higher mortality rates as compared with middle-class or affluent Americans (Palos 1994).

Because of great concern over cost, the poor are often discouraged from seeking state-of-the-art diagnostic examinations or treatments

(Bastani et al. 1991), and they experience tremendous difficulties in accessing care and health screening activities. The "inverse care law" (Hart 1971) postulates that the availability of good quality medical care tends to vary inversely with the need of the population served. From birth to adult to old age, the medically underserved population experiences disease, illness, and medical care in a different way than the general population does (Reilly et al. 1998), and they encounter numerous barriers to better health care.

Misconceptions of risk, vulnerability, and susceptibility to certain diseases are also common among the poor. For example, despite their previous family history of cancer, the poor often think that cancer does not affect those who are healthy and young, or those who are afflicted with other chronic diseases, and therefore they may not perceive the need for cancer prevention or early detection of cancer (Underwood and Hoskins 1994). In addition, the poor tend to share a "fatalistic" or "powerless" view (Freeman 1989). This perception of "powerlessness" seems to have a strong influence on their preventive health behavior. The poor often report incidents whereby they are either told by health care professionals not to worry about changes in their bodies or made to feel that those concerns are unwarranted, and that their symptoms are of no consequence. When they are not involved in the decision-making process, or when they perceive themselves as being incapable of making their own health decisions, they feel that their sense of control is taken away. As a result, they may falsely appear to be ignorant. When cancer is diagnosed, their hope of recovery may be replaced with feelings of hopelessness, pessimism, and fatalism (Underwood and Hoskins 1994).

## LIMITED HEALTH KNOWLEDGE AND LOW HEALTH LITERACY

The poor are often described as having less accurate information on cancer prevention, early detection, and treatment (Underwood and Hoskins 1994; Loehrer et al. 1991; Freeman 1989). Loehrer et al. interviewed socioeconomically disadvantaged cancer patients to assess their knowledge on cancer and its treatment and to evaluate their care-seeking behaviors. Although these patients relied primarily on their physicians for cancer information, they had a lot of misinformation regarding cancer. About one-fifth of these patients incorrectly identified the primary site of their cancer, and about one-third of those with metastases identified sites of metastases incorrectly. When asked about how to respond to common cancer-related signs and symptoms, these patients frequently reported inappropriate care-seeking behaviors. This study concluded that when health knowledge of socioeconomically disadvantaged patients was based on incomplete or erroneous information regarding cancer and its treatment, they would seek care inappropriately. Juon et al. (2004) also concurred that lack of knowledge of cancer-screening guidelines was associated with low screening behaviors. In contrast, having greater knowledge on cancer and taking preventive health measures are associated with employment outside the home and more years of education (Phipps et al. 1999).

Studies of Asian immigrant women indicated an association between self-reported cancer-screening behavior and socioeconomic status, educational level, English proficiency level, and the degree of acculturation (McPhee and Nguyen 2000; McPhee et al. 1997; Juon et al. 2004; Islam et al. 2006). Other studies also found a variety of reasons for the low rates of breast and cervical cancer screening among Asian American women (Phipps et al. 1999; McPhee et al. 1997; Hiatt et al. 1996). These reasons include lack of knowledge on risk factors and screening procedures, lack of preventive care orientation, preference of Eastern (traditional) medicine, and modesty. Although Freeman (1991) argued that ethnic differences in cancer is largely secondary to socioeconomic factors and related issues, noneconomic issues such as language, education, and cultural factors are also significant in studying cancer screening and preventive health behaviors of the Asian medically underserved populations.

Schiffman et al. (1991) found that cancer control educational materials are not effectively disseminated to the medically underserved immigrant populations that comprise a large number of low literate adults. Michielutte et al. (1999) reviewed recent studies on the relationship between health literacy and health care experience. They noted that patients with low reading ability have difficulty accessing the health care system as well as understanding instructions and recommended regimens. The required reading levels for many educational pamphlets on prevention, detection, and treatment of breast cancer ranged from ninth to twelfth grade (Michielutte et al. 1999). As a result, many of these printed health education materials are inaccessible to those who are illiterate, or have low reading skills, with an average of fourth-grade reading level or below, and also to many individuals who are defined as having "good" reading ability.

While low literacy among American adults could be a result of lack of education, reading and/or comprehension problems, or specific learning disabilities (Michielutte et al. 1999), low literacy among Asian immigrant groups could often mean reading and comprehension difficulties associated with learning English as a second language as well. Asian women who have an eighth-grade education or less or who do not speak English fluently are less likely to ever have had mammograms than their counterparts who are more educated or speak English more fluently (Centers for Disease Control 1992). Another study confirms that the ability to speak English well is significantly associated with breast–and cervical cancer–screening knowledge and practices (Lee et al. 1996). Therefore, it is important for health care providers to be aware of the low health literacy status of their patients and to explain medical information clearly so that patients can understand it (Lam et al. 2004).

## HEALTH CARE DELIVERY SYSTEM BARRIERS TO PREVENTIVE CARE

Efforts to prevent disease and to reduce morbidity and mortality cannot be effective unless patients adhere to preventive screening guidelines. Gritz et al. (1989) defined noncompliance as encompassing not only the failure of the patient to follow screening guideline as recommended by the physician but also the behavior of the physician, physician-patient interactions, and the health care setting in which the patient and the physician interact. In Asian culture, the physician is an authority figure (Lee 1998), and his recommendations on cancer screening are very important. Patient adherence to cancer-screening guidelines largely depends on the amount of information and support patients receive from their physicians, the physicians' knowledge of cancer-screening guidelines, and their ability to perform screenings or make appropriate referrals. Effective patient–health care provider communication gains the trust of the patient and the family and facilitates the use of health promotion activities (Ulrey and Amason 2001).

Over the past decades, although the American health care system has made major advances in medical and biomedical technology and treatment, the human aspect of care often receives little attention. This is reflected in inadequate communication between patients and health care providers on diagnosis, medical procedures, and pharmacological or surgical treatments. Many traditional Asian patients may not have an adequate understanding of diseases or diagnostic and treatment processes. The health care delivery system and the role of primary care providers versus that of the specialists are all very foreign to these people, who are used to a different medical system in their country of origin. Naturally, they looked to their medical providers for information, advice, and guidance, especially when they had specific health concerns. When that need for information and education was not adequately met, they became frustrated and even distrustful of the provider and the health care system. Effective communication between the physician and the patient is essential in promoting patient adherence to preventive health care (Glasser 2000).

Taira et al. (2001) found that Asians' assessments of the quality of primary care were lower than those of other ethnic and racial groups after adjustment for socioeconomic and other factors. Part of the reason was due to poor quality of communication between physician and patient and the physician's knowledge of the patient. Thus, although Asians were portrayed as better educated, had fewer chronic conditions, and were more likely to be employed in professional or technical occupations than other ethnic groups, they had the lowest primary care performance assessments after adjustments for all of the previously mentioned differences. Case Example 3 illustrates a typical frustrating experience of what an immigrant, who is often poorly informed of his ailment and of the options available to resolve his medical problems.

### Case Example 3—A Quest for Cure That Went Astray

Although prostate problem is common among elderly men and prostate cancer is usually treatable, men who suffer from prostate problem such as prostate enlargement or prostate cancer could lead quite a miserable life. This is because the prostate affects urinary functions, continence, and sexual performance. If symptoms such as frequent urination or urine retention go untreated or are inappropriately addressed, it could greatly affect one's quality of life and normal daily functioning. The following is a story of an elderly man who sought treatment for his prostate problems. He did everything he could, including going along with the doctor's recommendation and went for surgery after surgery, even though sometimes he did not quite understand the rationale behind it. But yet, after several invasive procedures and surgeries, he still ended up with the same symptoms. Although he could be a complicated case of having failures in the whole urological system with involvement in his prostate, bladder, and urethra, it was, however, apparent that he was unclear as to why surgeries were warranted in the first place, and how come after repeated operations, he still experienced the same symptoms! The journey that he went through is sadly a typical experience of what an immigrant, who is often poorly informed of his condition of the options available to resolve his medical problems:

"In the past when I had health benefits from the union, I used to get an annual check up. At some point as I grew old, my prostate became enlarged and I had to urinate more frequently. My PSA level fluctuated. Sometimes it was 6, other times it was 4, and another time it was 8. Then I began to experience urinary retention. Instead of urinating more frequently, I also had difficulties urinating and had blood in my urine. . . . I went for a check-up again, my PSA level was 6. The PSA result was inconclusive for prostate cancer, but I suspected that I might have prostate cancer. So I went to the doctor again for my urine retention problem. The doctor put a catheter in to help me pee. After that he told me to go for surgery because my PSA had increased to 26 . . .

When the doctor did the biopsy, the result was negative for prostate cancer. The surgery was done anyway. That's why I said they exaggerated my PSA results to make a case so as to lure me into surgery . . . They also made a hole in my lower abdomen. I found out that other surgeries could be done on either the urethra or the bladder . . . They operated on my lower bladder . . . Before my first surgery, I used to pee many times during the day. After surgery, I could hold off peeing for more than 3 hours. My condition was better initially after my prostate was removed. A year later, I had a relapse. In the beginning, I did not pay too much attention to it. But suddenly I had difficulties peeing again, then suddenly I became incontinent of urine, and my pants were all wet. I made an emergency visit to the doctor. They put in a foley catheter again to help me pee, and I had yet another surgery. After a year, I had the same old problem again . . . I went for another surgery at a hospital. After the operation, my condition was fine in the beginning. Still my urethra was too small . . . In the same year I had the same old problem of urine retention. Then I had another procedure at a hospital and I had another tube. It was a mess. Most likely my first surgery was not done properly and therefore I had a relapse . . . They did not find the problem. I asked whether I had cancer or not and they said it was not cancer."

In the Maxwell et al. (2000) study, Filipino women were more likely to accept a screening test if recommended by a physician. Other studies with Korean and Vietnamese women also indicated that they would very likely participate in cancer screening if their doctor recommended it (Taylor et al. 2004; Juon et al. 2004). Lack of physician referral is found to be an important factor contributing to the low use of cancer screening among Asian American women (Yu et al. 2001; Lee et al. 1999). One main reason is that physicians often focus on chief complaints presented by the patient rather than on promoting the concept of preventive health (Lee et al. 1999). Alternatively, physicians are less likely to recommend screening tests when the patient comes for an unrelated problem (Lee et al. 1999). If the chief complaints presented are not clearly related to cancer, screening would not be recommended. Reluctance to disrobe, especially among Vietnamese and other Southeast Asian women, and physician deference to the patient's modesty may also contribute to the low referral rate of cancer-screening procedures (Bastani et al. 1991).

Socioeconomically disadvantaged and less educated patients tend to rely heavily on physicians for information on cancer, cancer screening, and treatment (Liang et al. 2004; Loehrer et al. 1991; Yu et al. 2001). In the study by Loehrer et al. (1991), the results indicated that 90 percent of the respondents identified their physician as the primary source of disease-related information. However, only 37 percent reported being less than or only somewhat satisfied with the information they received from their physician, and one-third of them expressed the need to get more information.

From the above studies, we may conclude that the following principles are effective in increasing patients' adherence to early detection and screening activities:

- Demonstrate a genuine interest in the patient's beliefs and attitudes.
- Recognize and understand how the patient's cultural and individual perspectives may affect his or her decisions on health care and preventive behavior.
- Enlist the patient's cooperation in formulating service plans and focus more on the patient's needs and perspectives rather than on the disease.
- Incorporate patient-centered care practices such as sending reminder notices for preventive or follow-up care, providing information from referring

physician promptly, and making medical records/test results readily to patients when needed.

- Be sensitive to the socioeconomic barriers encountered by the patient and understand what social and economic factors may shape the patient's help-seeking behavior.

- Educate the patient on health maintenance and relevant disease management strategies; and teach the patient how to accomplish certain health care goals.

- Be aware of the low health literacy status of the patients and explain medical information clearly to patients.

- Empower the patient to partner with the physician in actively maintaining and improving health and increase patients' feelings of competence in their ability to manage their disease.

## FUTURE OUTLOOK

This chapter is based on the assumption that patterns of health beliefs, health-seeking behavior, and the utilization of preventive health and screening services among Asian Americans are interwoven into their cultural, socioeconomic, and other aspects of daily lives. Access to preventive health services among Asian Americans continues to be a major public health concern. Disparities in preventive health-screening services among Asian Americans are a result of many factors.

This chapter discussed many barriers Asian Americans face in accessing preventive care. These barriers can be best described within the framework of the Systems Model of Clinical Preventive Care (Walsh and McPhee 1992). Cultural beliefs, attitudes, and perceptions are all factors that predispose Asian patients to seek preventive care. Within the Systems Model, patient enabling factors include education, knowledge, skills, and income. Lack of patient-centered and literacy-appropriate health information about health risks and benefits of screening activities were cited as major barriers to preventive health-screening among Asian Americans. Advice and recommendation from a health care provider plays an important role in a patient's decision to adhere to cancer-screening guidelines. Many Asian patients would accept preventive health screening if their physician recommended it to them. Beliefs, attitudes, sensitivity, and personal health practices are factors that predispose physicians to provide preventive care in the model. Factors that enable a provider to promote health-screening behavior include physicians' knowledge of cancer-screening guidelines and their ability to perform screenings or make appropriate referrals. The health care delivery system barriers to preventive care include suboptimal patient-doctor communication, lack of health insurance, and poor coordination between primary care and specialty care. Effective communication between the physician and the patient was listed as a major factor that facilitates the use of health promotion activities among Asian Americans.

**Table 34.2** Strategies to Enhance and Improve Access to Preventive Health

**Educational Materials:**
- Educational brochures on disease and illnesses should be in large print and contain both key health information as well as illustrative diagrams.
- Display health education posters in public areas and community-based locations to maximize the public's access to health information.

**Patient Education and Outreach Activities:**
- Use ethnic mass media, such as newspapers and radio programs, as instrumental and effective means of disseminating health information and reaching a large audience.
- Conduct educational seminars and workshops in a small-group setting, a venue in which participants can ask specific questions on the health topic.
- Conduct workshops, seminars, and community events in the evening and on weekends so as to accommodate working people.
- Conduct community outreach by bringing educational events to the workplace and to communities to target newly arrived immigrants.
- Use the "word of mouth" and "bring your friends" approaches in community outreach.
- Educate the public on patient rights and responsibilities and on proper complaint and grievance channels and procedures so that any allegation of mistreatment or exploitation may be properly addressed and investigated.

**Free or Low-Cost Screening**
- More free and low-cost screening and follow-up services made available for low-income individuals and families.
- No questions asked on participants' immigration status to avoid fear of apprehension and deportation of the undocumented population.
- Send the screening results, whether positive or negative, to patients promptly to minimize unnecessary fear and anxiety on the part of the patient.
- If there is an abnormal finding in a screening result, contact the patient and schedule a clinic visit to discuss with the patient the test result, its implication, as well as any treatment options available.

**Information Hotline and Service Referral Center**
- Establish a comprehensive service center to provide health education, service referral, and health counseling at one central location.
- Host a hotline in patient's language and dialect to answer questions on health issues and provide information on services available based on medical need and geographical locations.

In order to successfully and effectively address these issues, a comprehensive multipronged approach designed to address these issues in diverse Asian American populations is needed. Table 34.2 is a summary of recommendations to enhance and improve access to preventive health care for Asian Americans. All of these strategies are essential in achieving national health objectives and ultimately in reducing health disparities to preventive care in Asian American populations.

# REFERENCES

Adams, P., Hurd, M., McFadden, D., Merrill, A., and Ribeiro, T. (2003). Healthy, wealthy, and wise? Tests for direct causal between health and socioeconomic status. *Journal of Econometrics,* 112: 3–56.

Adler, N. E., and Newman, K. (2002). Socioeconomic disparities in health: Pathways and policies. *Health Affairs,* 21: 60–76.

Ahn, A., Ngo-Metzger, Q., Legedza, A., Massagli, M., Clarridge, B., and Phillips, R. (2006). Complementary and alternative medical therapy use among Chinese and Vietnamese Americans: Prevalence, associated factors, and effects of patient-clinician communication. *American Journal of Public Health,* 96(4): 647–653.

Ashing, K. T., Padilla, G., Tejero, J., and Kagawa-Singer, M. (2003). Understanding the breast cancer experience of Asian American women. *Psycho-Oncology,* 12: 38–58.

Bandura, A. (1977). *Social learning theory.* Englewood Cliffs, NJ: Prentice-Hall.

Basch, C. E. (1987). Focus group interview: An underutilized research technique for improving theory and practice in health education. *Health Education Quarterly,* 14(4): 411–448.

Bandura, A. (2004). Health promotion by social cognitive means. *Health Education & Behavior,* 31(2): 143–164.

Bastani, R., Marcus, A. C., and Hollatz-Brown, A. (1991). Screening mammography rates and barriers to us: A Los Angeles County survey. *Preventive Medicine,* 20: 350–363.

Becker, M. H., Drachman, R. H., and Kirschy, J. P. (1974). A new approach to explaining sick role behavior in low-income populations. *American Journal of Public Health,* 64: 205–216.

Bradley, C., Given, C., and Roberts, C. (2002). Race, socioeconomic status, and breast cancer treatment and survival. *Journal of the National Cancer Institute,* 94(7): 490–496.

Carter, A. R. (1994). *Chinese American: 96.* New York: New Discovery Books.

Chen, A., Lew, R., Thai, V., Ko, K. L., Okahara, L., Hirota, S., Chan, S., Wong, W. F., Saika, G., Folkers, L. F., and Marquez, B. (1992). Behavior risk factor survey of Chinese: California, 1989. *Morbidity and Mortality Weekly Report,* 41(16), 266–270.

Chen, M. S., Jr. (2005). Cancer health disparities among Asian Americans: What we know and what we need to know. *Cancer* (Suppl.), 104(12): 2895–2902.

Chen, Y. L. (1996). Conformity with nature: A theory of Chinese American elders' health promotion and illness prevention processes. *Advances in Nursing Science,* 19: 17–26.

Cutler, D. M., Deaton, A., Lleras-Muney, A. (2006). The determinants of mortality. *Journal of Economic Perspectives,* 20: 97–120.

Dyche, L., and Zayas, L. H. (1995). The value of curiosity and naivete for the cross-cultural psychotherapist. *Family Process,* 34: 389–399.

Engstrom, M. (2006). Physical and mental health: Interactions, assessment, and intervention. In S. Gehlert and T. Browne (eds.), *Handbook of health social work*. Hoboken, NJ: Wiley, pp 194–251.

Freeman, H. P. (1989). Cancer in the economically disadvantaged. *Cancer,* 64(Suppl.): 324–334.

———. (1991). Race, poverty, and cancer. *Journal of the National Cancer Institute,* 83: 526–527.

Gielen, A. C., McDonald, E. M., Gary, T. L., and Bone, L. R. (2008). Using the PRECEDE-PROCEED model to apply health behavior theories. In K. Glanz, B. K. Rimer, and K.Viswanath, (eds.), *Health behavior and health education: Theory, research and practice* (3rd ed.). San Francisco: Jossey-Bass, pp. 407–434.

Glaser, V. (2000). Cancer screening and management. *Patient Care,* (May): 78–92.

Green, L. W., and Kreuter, M. W. (2005). *Health program planning: An educational and ecological approach* (4th ed.). New York: McGraw-Hill.

Gritz, E. R., DiMatteo, M. R., and Hays, R. D. (1989). Methodological issues in adherence in cancer control regimens. *Preventive Medicine,* 18: 711–720.

Hart, J. T. (1971). The inverse law. *Lancet,* 1: 405–412.

Hedeen, A. N., White, E., and Taylor, V. (1999). Ethnicity and birthplace in relation to tumor size and stage in Asian American women with breast cancer. *American Journal of Public Health,* 89: 1248–1252.

Hiatt, R. A., Pasick, R. J., Perez-Stable, E. J., McPhee, S. J., Engelstad, L., and Lee, M., (1996). Pathways to early cancer detection in the multiethnic population of the San Francisco Bay Area, *Health Education Quarterly,* 23 (Suppl.): S10–S27.

Hoeman, S. P., Ku, Y. L., and Ohl, D. R. (1996). Health beliefs and early detection among Chinese women. *Western Journal of Nursing Research,* 18(5): 518–533.

Hopps, J. G., Pinderhughes, E., and Shankar, R. (1995). *The power of care: Clinical practice effectiveness with overwhelmed clients.* New York: Free Press.

Ino, S. M., and Glicken, M. D. (1999). Treating Asian American clients in crisis: A collectivist approach. *Smith College Studies in Social Work,* 69(3): 525–540.

Islam, N., Kwon, S. C., Senie, R., and Kathuria, N. (2006). Breast and cervical cancer screening among South Asian women in New York City. *Journal of Immigrant and Minority Health,* 8(3): 211–221.

Jang, M., Lee, E., and Woo, K. (1998). Income, language, and citizen status: Factors affecting the health care access and utilization of Chinese Americans. *Health & Social Work,* 23(2): 136–145.

Jenkins, C. H., and Kagawa-Singer, M. (1994). Cancer. In N. W. S. Zane, D. T. Takeuchi, and K. N. J. Young (eds.). *Confronting critical health issues of Asian and Pacific Islander Americans.* Thousand Oaks, CA: Sage Publications, pp. 105–147.

Juon, H.-S., Kim, M., Shankar, S., and Han, W. (2004). Predictors of adherence to screening mammography among Korean American women. *Preventive Medicine*, 39: 474–481.

Kagawa-Singer, M. (1995). Socioeconomic and cultural influences on cancer care of women. *Seminars in Oncology Nursing*, 11(2): 109–119.

Kagawa-Singer, M. (1996). Cultural systems. In R. McCorkle, M. Grant, M. Frank-Stromborg, and S. B. Baird (eds.). *Cancer nursing—A comprehensive textbook* (2nd ed.). Philadelphia: W.B. Saunders.

Lam, T., Cheng, Y., and Chan, Y. (2004). Low literacy Chinese patients: How are they affected and how do they cope with health matters? A qualitative study. *BMC Public Health*, 4, 14. http://www.biomedcentral.com/1471-2458/4/14.

Langer, N. (1999). Culturally competent professionals in therapeutic alliances enhance patient compliance. *Journal of Health Care for the Poor and Underserved*, 10(1): 19–26.

Lane, D. S., Zapka, J., Breen, N., Messina, C. R., and Fotheringham, D. J., for the NCI Breast Cancer Screening Consortium (2000). A systems model of clinical preventive care: The case of breast cancer screening among older women. *Preventive Medicine*, 31: 481–493.

Lee, E. E., Fogg, L. F., and Sadler, G. R. (2006). Factors of breast cancer screening among Korean immigrants in the United States. *Journal of Immigrant and Minority Health*, 8(3): 223–233.

Lee, M. (1998). Breast and cervical cancer early detection in Chinese American women. *Asian American Pacific Islander Journal of Health*, 6: 351–357.

Lee, M., Lee, F., and Stewart, S. (1996). Pathways to early breast and cervical detection for Chinese American women. *Health Education Quarterly*, 23(Suppl.): S76–S88.

Lee, M., Lee, F., Stewart, S., and McPhee, S. (1999). Cancer screening practices among primary care physicians serving Chinese Americans in San Francisco. *Western Journal of Medicine*, 170: 148–155.

Liang, W., Yuan, E., Mandelblatt, J. S., and Pasick, R. J. (2004). How do older Chinese women view health and cancer screening? Results from focus groups and implications for interventions. *Ethnicity & Health*, 9(3): 283–304.

Loehrer, P. J., Greger, H. A., Weinberger, M., Musick, B., Miller, M., Nichols, C., Bryan, J., Higgs, D., and Brook, D. (1991). Knowledge and beliefs about cancer in a socioeconomically disadvantaged population. *Cancer*, 68(7): 1665–1671.

Lu, Z.-Y. J. (1995). Variables associated with breast self-examination among Chinese women. *Cancer Nursing*, 18(1), 29–34.

Ma, G. X. (1999). *The culture of health: Asian communities in the United States.* Westport, CT: Bergin & Garvey.

———. (2000). Barriers to the use of health services by Chinese Americans. *Journal of Allied Health*, 29(2): 64–70.

Maxwell, A. E., Bastani, R., and Warda, U. S. (2000). Demographic predictors of cancer screening among Filipino and Korean immigrants in the U.S. *American Journal of Preventive Medicine*, 18(1): 62–68.

McBride, M. R., Pasick, R. J., Stewart, S., Tuason, N., Sabogal, F., and Duenas, G. (1998). Factors associated with cervical cancer screening among Filipino women in California. *Asian American and Pacific Islander Journal of Health,* 6: 358–367.

McPhee, S. J., Bird, J. A., Davis, T., Ha, N., Jenkins, C. N., and Le, B. (1997). Barriers to breast and cervical cancer screening among Vietnamese-American women. *American Journal of Preventive Medicine,* 13: 205–213.

McPhee, S. J., and Nguyen, T. T. (2000). Cancer, cancer risk factors, and community-based cancer control trials in Vietnamese Americans. *Asian American and Pacific Islander Journal of Health,* 8: 19–31.

Michielutte, R., Alciati, M. H., and Arculli, R. (1999). Cancer control research and literacy. *Journal of Health Care for the Poor and Underserved,* 10(3): 281–297.

Mo, B. (1992). Modesty, sexuality, and breast health in Chinese-American women. *Western Journal of Medicine,* 157(3): 260–264.

Murdaugh C. L., and Veranno, J. A. (1987). Theoretical modeling to predict physiological indicants of cardiac preventive behavior. *Nursing Research,* 36: 284–294.

Naleway, A. L., Smith, W. J., and Mullooly, J. P. (2006). Delivering influenza vaccine to pregnant women. *Epidemiologic Reviews,* 28: 47–53.

Olsen, S. J., and Frank-Stromborg, M. (1993). Cancer prevention and early detection in ethnically diverse populations. *Seminars in Oncology Nursing,* 9(3): 198–209.

Palos, G. (1994). Cultural heritage: Cancer screening and early detection. *Seminars in Oncology Nursing,* 10(2): 104–113.

Panos, P., and Panos, A. (2000). A model for a culture-sensitive assessment of patients in health care settings. *Social Work in Health Care,* 31(1): 49–62.

Pasick, R. J. (1997). Socioeconomic and cultural factors in the development and use of theory. In K. Glanz, F. M. Lewis, and B. K. Rimer (eds.). *Health behavior and health education: Theory, research and practice* (2nd ed.). San Francisco: Jossey-Bass, pp. 425–440.

Pasick, R. J., D'Onofrio, C. N., and Otero-Sabogal, R. (1996). Similarities and differences across cultures: Questions to inform a third generation for health promotion research. *Health Education Quarterly,* 23(Suppl.): S142–S161.

Pedersen, P. B., Draguns, J. G., Lonner, W. J., and Trimble, J. E. (2008). *Counseling across Cultures* (6th ed.). Thousand Oaks, CA: Sage.

Phipps, E., Cohen, M. H., Sorn, R., and Braitman, L. E. (1999). A pilot study of cancer knowledge and screening behaviors of Vietnamese and Cambodian women. *Health Care for Women International,* 20: 195–207.

Reilly B., Schiff, G., and Conway, T. (1998). Primary care for the medically underserved: Challenges and opportunities. *Disease a Month,* 44(7): 320–346.

Rosenstock, I. (1974). Historical origins of the health belief model. *Health Education Monographs,* 2(4): 328–335.

Rosenstock, I. M., Strecher, V. J., and Becker, M. H. (1988). Social learning theory and health belief model. *Health Education Quarterly*, 15: 175–183.

Rosenstock I. (1990). The health belief model: Explaining health behavior through expectancies. In K. Glanz, L. F. Marcus., and B. K. Rimer (eds.). *Health behavior and health education: Theory, research, and practice.* San Francisco: Jossey-Bass, pp. 39–62.

Sadler, G. R., Nguyen, F., Doan, Q., Au, H., and Thomas, A. G. (1998). Strategies for reaching Asian Americans with health information. *American Journal of Preventive Medicine*, 14(3): 224–228.

Schiffman, S., Cassileth, B. R., Black, B. L., Buxbaum, J., Celentano, D. D., Corcoran, R. D., Gritz, E.R., Laszlo, J., Lichtenstein, E., Pechacek, T. F., Prochaska, J., and Scholefield, P. G. (1991). Needs and recommendations for behavior research in the prevention and early detection of cancer. *Cancer*, 67(Suppl.): 800–804.

Silberfarb, P. M. (1982). Research in adaptation to illness and psychosocial intervention. *Cancer*, 1(Suppl.): 1921–1925.

Spector, R. E. (2000). *Cultural diversity in health and illness* (5th ed.). Upper Saddle River, NJ: Prentice Hall Health.

Strecher, V. J., and Rosenstock, I. M. (1997). The health belief model. In K. Glanz, F. M. Lewis, and B. K. Rimer (eds.). *Health behavior and health education: Theory, research, and practice.* San Francisco: Jossey-Bass, pp. 41–59.

Sue, D. W., and Sue, D. (2007). *Counseling the culturally diverse: Theory and practice* (5th ed.). Hoboken, NJ: John Wiley.

Sun, A., Wong-Kim, E., Stearman, S., and Chow, E. (2005). Quality of life in Chinese patients with breast cancer. *Cancer* (Suppl.) 104(12): 2952–2954.

Taira, D. A., Safran D. G., Seto, T. B., Rogers, W. H., Inui, T. S., Montgomery, J., and Tarlov, A. R.. (2001). Do patient assessments of primary care differ by patient ethnicity? *Health Services Research*, 36(6): 1059–1071.

Taylor, V. M., Yasui, Y., Burke, N., Nguyen, T., Acorda, E., Thai, H., Qu, P., and Jackson, J.C. (2004). Pap testing adherence among Vietnamese American women. *Cancer Epidemiology, Biomarkers, & Prevention*, 13(4): 613–619.

Uba, L. (1994). *Asian Americans: Personality patterns, identity, and mental health.* New York: Guilford Press.

———. (2002). *A postmodern psychology of Asian Americans—Creating knowledge of a racial minority.* Albany, NY: State University of New York Press.

Ulrey, K., and Amason, P. (2001). Intercultural communication between patients and health care providers: An exploration of intercultural communication effectiveness, cultural sensitivity, stress, and anxiety. *Health Communication*, 13(4): 449–463.

Underwood, S. M., and Hoskins, D. (1994). Increasing nursing involvement in cancer prevention and control among the economically disadvantaged: The nursing challenge. *Seminars in Oncology Nursing*, 10(2), 89–95.

U.S. Department of Health and Human Services. (2001). *Mental health: Culture, race, and ethnicity—A supplement to mental health: A report of the surgeon general.* Rockville, MD: Author.

Walsh, J. M. E., and McPhee, S. J. (1992). A systems model of clinical preventive care: An analysis of factors influencing patient and physician. *Health Education Quarterly,* 19: 157–175.

Ward, E., Jemal, A., Cokkinides, V., Singh, G., Cardinez, C., Ghafoor, A., and Thun, M. . (2004). Cancer disparities by race/ethnicity and socioeconomic status. *CA: A Cancer Journal for Clinicians,* 54(2): 78–93.

Wellisch, D., Kagawa-Singer, M., Reid, S. L., Lin, Y.-J., Nishikawa-Lee, S., and Wellisch, M. (1999). An exploratory study of social support: A Cross-cultural comparison of Chinese-, Japanese-, and Anglo-American breast cancer patients. *Psyhco-Oncology,* 8: 207–219.

Wood, M. E. (2008). Theoretical framework to study exercise motivation for breast cancer risk reduction. *Oncology Nursing Forum,* 35(1): 89–95.

Yu, E., Kim, K., Chen, E., and Brintnall, R. (2001) Breast and cervical cancer screening among Chinese American women. *Cancer Practice,* 9(2): 81–91.

# Chapter 35

# Diet and Health of Asian Americans

## Sally Wong

Disparities in health and disease persist among Asian Americans as well as other minority groups. The five leading causes of death for Asian Americans are cancer, heart disease, stroke, unintentional injuries, and diabetes (APIHF 2006). Theoretically, cultural influences on dietary behaviors and other aspects of health lifestyles could be positive, negative, or neutral (Baranowski et al. 2001). Western dietary habits include higher intakes of red and processed meats; sweets and desserts; and refined grains (Fung et al. 2002; Manson et al. 2004). Among the environmental factors, changes toward a Western type of diet or lifestyle have been found to increase the risk of many lifestyle chronic diseases, such as cardiovascular diseases (CVDs), obesity, diabetes, and cancers among immigrants (Satia-Abouta et al. 2002; Klatsky and Armstrong 1991; Kramer et al. 2004). Evidence suggests that dietary changes may be secondary to various social, cultural, and demographic influences (Archer 2005).

CVDs remain the leading cause of death in the United States, accounting for 34.8 percent of deaths in Asian Americans (Ferdinand 2006). Assessed separately, heart disease and stroke, the major diseases classified as CVDs, are still the second and third leading causes of death for this ethnic group. CVD risk and death rates are higher among Asian Americans partly because of higher rates of obesity, diabetes, and high blood pressure. According to the Centers for Disease Control (CDC), overweight and obesity are both labels for ranges of weight that are greater than what is generally considered healthy for a given height. Overweight and obese individuals are at increased risk for many diseases and health conditions, including diabetes mellitus, cardiovascular disease (CVD), and some forms of cancer.

Asian Americans/Pacific Islander (AAPI) women are the only U.S. population group that experienced an overall increase in cancer mortality for all cancers combined between 1990 and 1995. Between 1980 and 1993, the cancer death rate for AAPI women increased by 240 percent, and the rate for AAPI men increased by 290 percent—the highest for all ethnic/racial groups (NCHS 1995). The incidence of liver cancer in Chinese, Filipino, Japanese, Korean, and Vietnamese populations is 1.7 to 11.3 times higher than rates among white Americans, with Vietnamese men having the highest rate of liver cancer of all racial/ethnic groups, and Korean men experiencing the highest rate of stomach cancer of all racial/ethnic groups, and a fivefold increased rate of stomach cancer over white American men (Miller et al. 1996).

## DIETS OF ASIAN AMERICANS

Asian Americans account for 5 percent of the nation's population. This number represents an increase of 63 percent from the 1990 census, making Asian Americans the fastest growing of all major racial/ethnic groups (U.S. Census, 2000). The following states have the largest Asian American populations: California, New York, Hawaii, Texas, and New Jersey (OMH 2008). They are exceedingly diverse, coming from nearly fifty countries and ethnic groups, each with distinct cultures, traditions, and histories, and they speak over 100 languages and dialects. Asian Americans have immigrated to the United States from different parts of Asia, including Cambodia, China, Hong Kong, India, Japan, Korea, Laos, Pakistan, Bangladesh, Sri Lanka, the Philippines, Thailand, and Vietnam. Two key elements draw the diverse cultures of the Asian region together: the composition of meals, with an emphasis on vegetables and rice, with relatively little meat; and cooking techniques (Chen and Hawks 1995). Eating is a vital part of the social matrix, and Asian American cuisine includes a wide variety of meals, snacks, and desserts for social occasions. Asian food preparation techniques include stir-frying, barbecuing, deep-frying, boiling, and steaming. All ingredients are carefully prepared (chopped, sliced, etc.) prior to starting the cooking process.

Although there are similarities among Asian cuisines, major differences and specific characteristics also exist. Some Asian foods, such as Thai and Filipino food, are generally spicy, hot, and high in sodium, whereas the Japanese are very concerned about both the visual appeal of food and the "separateness" of the foods and tastes. Garlic and hot pepper, commonly used among Asian Americans, are not common in the Japanese cuisine. Korean Americans eat *kimchi* with each meal. Kimchi is cabbage preserved in salted water and layered with peppers and spices in crockery, and left to ferment for a few days. South Asians (people from India, Pakistan, Bangladesh, and Sri Lanka) use spices (e.g., ginger, garlic, fenugreek, cumin, etc.) and condiments in their cuisine.

## Traditional Asian Diets

Good health involves strength, energy, and power, not merely the absence of disease. The boundary between what is considered food and what is considered medicine is not very well defined in Asian culture. Food could be categorized as medicine and medicine categorized as food, which shows very clearly the extent to which food and health are connected in folk thought. Although many Asian cultures share the tradition of family gathering to socialize or celebrate over a big meal, the various cultures of Asia each developed their own ethnic cuisine through the interaction of history, environment, and culture.

The latest food guide pyramid called MyPyramid was released in April 2005 and incorporated recommendations from the 2005 Dietary Guidelines for Americans, released by the U.S. Department of Agriculture and U.S. Department of Health and Human Services in January 2005 (MyPyramid.com, 2008). A traditional Asian American food guide pyramid is also available from the Center for Nutrition Policy and Promotion to reflect food items commonly consumed by Asian Americans.

Asian food is diverse and full of flavor. Culinary historians and anthropologists tend to identify three main categories of Asian dietary cultures that have developed through the centuries (Chen & Hawks, 1995). As with virtually any classification system, there is some overlap, but they roughly represent the three main groups or types of traditional Asian cooking.

### Southeastern Asian Diet

The Southeastern Asian diet generally includes dietary culture from countries in the southern part of Asia. These include Cambodia, Vietnam, Thailand, Indonesia, Laos, Malaysia, and Singapore. The traditional emphasis in the southeastern diet highlights aroma, and it often incorporates a balance of grilling, stir-flying, braising, and frying. The use of discrete spices and herbs are not uncommon, and this may include lemongrass, tamarind, cilantro, basil, mint leaves, and citrus juice. Many of the dishes also call for coconut milk, fish sauce, and chicken broth in their recipes. These ingredients can add additional flavor to the cuisine as they intensify the taste and aroma in the dishes.

### Southwestern Asian Diet

The Southwestern Asian cuisine generally refers to cuisines from India, Pakistan, Sri Lanka, Nepal, Bangladesh, and Burma. Having its roots in the Persian Arabian civilization, the eating of naan (or flat bread) became widespread, along with mutton, kebabs (derived from Turkish cooking), and the use of ghee (a butter oil), hot peppers, black pepper, cloves, and other strong spices.

Indian food is perhaps the best-known cuisine among the Southwestern Asian diet for its richness, color, aroma, and unique taste. Diversity can be found in India's food as well as its culture, geography, and climate (Ling 2002). Spices are at the heart of Indian food to enhance the flavor of a dish. The people of India have adapted their cooking to the erratic climatic conditions. Healthy Indian food tends to contain more vegetables. Rice is the staple diet and forms the basis of every meal for South Indians, whereas a typical North Indian meal would consist of rotis made from wheat flour. South Indian dishes such as dosa (rice pancakes), idli (steamed rice cakes), and vada, which is made of fermented rice, are now popular throughout the country.

### Northeastern Asian Diet

Lastly, the Northeastern Asian cuisine is composed of diets from China, Taiwan, Japan, and Korea. A typical Northeastern Asian diet—which includes a lot of vegetables, fish, and seafood but very little sugar or dessert—is proved to be healthy. Besides stir-frying and deep-frying, this diet uses a wide variety of cooking methods: steaming, boiling, stewing, roasting, baking, and generally avoiding excessive greasy food. Unlike Westerners, Northeastern Asians select live seafood, fresh meats, and seasonal fruits and vegetables local markets to ensure freshness. Food preparation is meticulous, and consumption is ceremonious and deliberate. The majority of Northeastern Asians are not vegetarian. Some may be vegetarian because of personal choice and some because of their religion. Many Buddhists do not refrain from eating meat, except on special occasions such as the first and fifteenth days of each month according to the Lunar calendar.

Chinese cuisine is probably the most prominent cuisine among Asian diets, with several different styles according to the region of China, the most basic difference being between northern and southern China. Most Chinese Americans incorporate fresh food in their cooking. There are several Chinese concepts of healthy eating habits. The most basic one is the balance of yin (feminine) and yang (masculine). Failure to maintain this balance is the root to many illnesses: excessive yin leads to weakness, and excessive yang leads to restlessness manifested in inflammation and ulcers. Yin food includes fruits and vegetables, whereas yang food includes meat. The concept of yin and yang encompasses other dichotomous concepts of cold and hot, soothing and irritating, weakening and strengthening, clearing and contaminating, and so on.

### Asian Diet Comparison

In comparing the three Asian cuisines with each other, it is apparent that curries are very important to the cuisines of the Southeast and Southwest, but less so in the East. Southwestern curries are generally based on yogurt, whereas the curries of the Southeast are generally based on coconut milk. Of course, rice is a staple starch in all three cuisine areas. In addition to rice,

Southwestern cuisines are supplemented with a variety of leavened and unleavened breads, whereas Southeast and Northeast cuisines add noodles made from rice, egg, or potatoes (remember, pasta was invented in China). Garlic and ginger are used in all three cuisine areas, whereas chilies are much more common in the Southwest and Southeast. Table 35.1 shows a comparison of traditional Asian diets for various Asian ethnic groups.

**Table 35.1** Merits and Weaknesses of Traditional Asian Diets

| | Staple Foods | Merits of Diet | Weaknesses of Diet | Common Diseases |
|---|---|---|---|---|
| **Cambodian** | Rice Fish Tea | Low in fat Low in sugar | People often unable to obtain necessary food | Tuberculosis Polio |
| **Chinese** | Rice Vegetables | Reduces risk of heart disease and certain cancers | Iodine deficiency Iron deficiency | Anemia |
| **Filipino** | Rice Vegetables Seafood Fruit | Reduces risk for heart disease and cancers | Protein deficiency Iron deficiency | Anemia Diarrhea Respiratory infections |
| **Hmong** | Rice Vegetables Meat Fish | Low in fat Low in sugar | Lack of fruit Calcium deficiency | |
| **Asian Indian** | Cereals Rice Vegetables | Low in fat Low in sugar | Protein deficiency Iron deficiency Vitamin A deficiency | Respiratory infections Intestinal infections Anemia Protein-energy malnutrition Diabetes |
| **Laotian** | Rice Vegetables Fish | Low in fat Low in sugar | Vitamin A deficiency Iron deficiency | Goiter Anemia |
| **Vietnamese** | Rice Fish Fruit | Low in fat Low in sugar | Iron deficiency | Anemia |

*Sources:* National Library of Medicine. "Asian American Health." Available at http://www.asianamericanhealth.nlm.nih.gov.
Cornell University Science News (1995). "Asian Diet Pyramid Offers Alternative to U.S. Food Guide." Available at http://www.news.cornell.edu/science/Dec95/st.asian.pyramid.html.

In the traditional Asian diet, rice, wheat, and barley are the main crop and dietary staple, forming the base of the Asian American food guide pyramid. For example, rice, noodles, or buns accompanied by an abundance of fruits/vegetables and a moderate amount of meat is generally considered a typical well-balanced meal for most Chinese Americans. That said, the traditional Asian American dietary pattern is generally considered what Americans often call the "prudent pattern," which is high in fruits, vegetables, whole grains, and low in meat and dairy products. However, as acculturation takes place, cereals and bread in the Western diet pattern will gradually replace rice and rice-based food items. A progressive adoption of the "western diet" (Funt et al. 2004)—characterized by high intakes of red and processed meats, refined grains, sweets and desserts, and high-fat dairy product—has been associated with acculturation (Satia-Abouta et al. 2002). Cultural differences in food preparation and cooking methods can affect the nutritional content of a food item. The nutrient intakes vary depending on how the food was produced and the preparation method used—that is, whether it was cooked or not, whether it was broiled or stir-fried, and what was added to the food. In contrast to the American cuisine, traditional Asian dishes rarely calls for deep-frying as dishes are generally sautéed or stir-fried with a moderate amount of oil. Also, Asian American diet consists of dishes of mixed foods cut into small pieces, making estimation of portion sizes extremely difficult. To further complicate matters, Asian "bowls" and "dish plates" reflect a totally different measurement from dishware used in the American mainstream.

Lactose intolerance is common among Asian Americans; thus, Asian Americans generally do not consume large amounts of dairy products, often substituting dairy products with fortified soymilk, tofu, and fish with small bones as sources of protein and calcium. Fish, pork, and poultry are the main sources of animal protein. Significant amounts of nuts and dried beans are also eaten, and they are sources of protein for vegetarians. Rice, bread, noodles are the mainstay of the diet, and they are commonly eaten at every meal among Asian Americans. Lastly, fresh fruits and vegetables make up a large part of food intake, and they are generally included in every meal.

## DIETARY ACCULTURATION

### Definition and Methodology

Dietary acculturation is defined as "the process that occurs when members of a minority group adopt the eating patterns/food choices of the host country" (Satia-Abouta et al. 2002). Immigrants can either retain or modify traditional eating patterns, or incorporate new foods into their diet (Chavez et al. 1994; Satia-Abouta et al. 2002), resulting in healthy or unhealthy dietary changes (Satia-Abouta et al. 2002). Studies have shown that acculturation is related to disease outcomes and to risk factors for chronic diseases (Cantero et al. 1999; Sundquist and Winkleby 2000). Dietary intakes are highly determined by various cultural, social, and demographic influences (Archer 2005). After Asian people immigrate to the United States, they may adopt Western dietary patterns while maintaining traditional Asian eating habits, rather than completely rejecting either one of them (Lv and Cason 2004). Although most of the studies examined reveal negative dietary practices with dietary acculturation, it is important to note that dietary acculturation can be both healthful and unhealthful. First- and second-generation migrants to a new country can retain many aspects of their native cuisine long after migration to the host countries (Hankin et al. 2001). Knowledge of dietary acculturation and dietary pattern among these first- and second-generation Asian immigrants is crucial for the development of culturally sensitive nutrition interventions tailored for this population. Understanding dietary acculturation can assist dietetic professionals working with first- and second-generation Asian Americans to better grasp the complexity of factors affecting their food choices (Satia-Abouta et al. 2002).

Dietary practices are highly related to dietary acculturation (Hankin et al. 2001). The ability to accurately assess dietary acculturation is a vital component of nutrition education, interventions, and research in any ethnic/racial population. Acculturation can be measured in several ways in dietary patterns and acculturation studies. An ideal tool that assesses acculturation should enable one to understand dietary acculturation and offer opportunities to intervene more effectively on diet and health among minority groups in the United States. Yet, there are few tools available to assess dietary acculturation. There are two major single-item, unidimensional measures of general acculturation, and two dietary acculturation scales.

Most studies reviewed use unidimensional measures to assess dietary acculturation. These nonscale measures can be used individually or in combination, and they offer greater flexibility in that they explore the health effects of separate dimensions of acculturation. Among the most frequently used nonscale acculturation measures are length of residency in the host country, migration status, generation, English proficiency, and nativity among immigrants. Specifically, migration status and length of residence are repeatedly cited as "an indirect measure of acculturation" that reflect high levels of validity and reliability (Dixon et al. 2000; Kaplan et al. 2004; Salant and Lauderdale 2003). For the most part, acculturation studies emphasize unidirectional, unidimensional models through their use of temporal indices or lifestyle measures. The use of such nonscale measures often lacked any explicit theoretical model. Moreover, specific indicators demonstrate complex relationships to acculturation and health outcomes among diverse ethnic groups (Salant and Lauderdale 2003).

Therefore, it is not surprising to observe inconsistent findings for studies employing temporal measures.

To effectively address questions about the nature and magnitude of changes in dietary habit, it may be particularly useful to examine how the process of acculturation influences eating pattern (Neuhouser et al. 2004). Recent studies have used qualitative interviews and focus groups to acquire a more in-depth understanding of factors associated with and contributing to acculturation. In fact, qualitative interviews are an excellent tool and can be used prior to developing a dietary acculturation scale to generate rich data that reflect the participants' point of view (Satia 2001). Dietary acculturation scales take into account the multidimensional process of overall adaptation of immigrants to the host society. They provide a means of assessing multiple life dimensions, and their use reflects awareness of the complexity of the acculturative process (Salant and Lauderdale 2003). As an example, Satia et al. and Cuellar et al. developed and validated dietary acculturation scales measuring changes in eating behaviors among Chinese American and Mexican American immigrants, respectively. The Chinese American dietary acculturation scale included a 5-item Chinese dietary acculturation scale and a 10-item Western dietary acculturation scale, which was then coded for analysis purposes, with scores divided into low, intermediate, and high (Satia et al. 2001). Similarly, the Mexican American dietary acculturation scale had 30 items that measured frequency of using the English and Spanish languages, frequency of accessing English and Spanish media, frequency of interacting with Mexicans and Anglos now and as a child, and ethnic identity of self and parents. This scale used a response made on a 5-point Likert scale from 1 to 5, with a final score classified into 1 of the 4 quadrants established by Cuellar et al. (1980). Dietary acculturation scales as such are generally more comprehensive and measure several facets and exposure to the host country and are less likely to misclassify a person's level of acculturation (Archer 2005; Satia-Abouta et al. 2002). Acculturation scales can be used to assess changes in eating patterns, and they can also be used along with other instruments that assess acculturation (Archer 2005). They are also similar in that they combine their items into a composite score. Although some argue that the combined score may cause blurring of potentially variable effects of different acculturation dimensions (Salant and Lauderdale 2003), acculturation scales can be particularly useful in quantitative studies as they are able to provide quantifiable data.

## Dietary Acculturation among Asian Americans

According to the report *Unequal Treatment: Confronting Racial and Ethnic Disparities in Healthcare,* by the Institute of Medicine, ethnicity, as a concept, is more useful than race to distinguish people who share a culture, way of life, language, folkway, religion, and material culture such as food, music, clothing, literature, and art (IOM 2002). The role of immigration as a factor for changing food intake and altering the risk of certain diseases and nutritional status of Asian Americans has received limited attention. As previously noted, acculturation to mainstream U.S. society among immigrants might be associated with both good and bad health indices.

Populations that have migrated from one part of the world to another provide a unique opportunity for assessing the relative contributions of genetics and environmental factors to disease (Langseth 1996). Migration to a new country can represent substantial shift in a person's lifestyle and environment, and these changes can result in modifications in chronic disease risk factors. Studies have shown that migrant groups eventually acquire the disease patterns of their new countries, but that the change occurs more rapidly for some diseases than for others. With the remarkable growth in the U.S. immigrant population, the health status of racial and ethnic minorities has become an increasingly important public health issue (Satia-Abouta et al. 2002).

Changes toward a Western type of diet or lifestyle have been found to increase the risk of many lifestyle chronic diseases, such as obesity, hypertension, diabetes mellitus, cardiovascular diseases, and cancers among immigrants (Satia-Abouta et al. 2002). Compared to the Chinese living in Asia, those living in the United States have high rates of chronic disease attributable to poor diet and health (Campbell et al. 1998; LeMarchand et al. 1997). Acculturation to the United States has been associated with shifts from traditional diets of vegetables, meats, and whole grains to the more processed, high-fat, and sugary foods that are popular and easily available in the United States (Unger et al. 2004). A study of 56 Chinese American females in California reported consuming about 34 percent of energy from total fat (Schultz et al 1994), comparable to the high amount of fat consumed in the typical American diet (Fung et al. 2004). Similarly, a study of 244 Chinese American females found significant associations between Western acculturation and fat-related dietary habits as well as increased fruit and vegetable intake since immigration (Satia et al. 2001). Some studies also found that the amount of food consumed greatly increases after immigration to the United States. For example, more than half (62%) of 71 Asian American immigrant college students reported weight gain after immigrating to the United States, accompanied by a significant increase in the consumption of fats, sweets, and dairy products, whereas their vegetable consumption significant decreases after immigration to the United States (Pan et al. 1999). A cross-sectional study of 619 Asian American and 1385 Hispanic adolescents in Southern California suggests that acculturation is significantly associated with a lower frequency of physical activity and a higher frequency of fast-food consumption (Unger et al. 2004). Another cross-sectional study with 399 first-generation Chinese Americans in Pennsylvania found that the consumption frequency of food items from all seven food groups in the food guide pyramid increased after they had immigrated to the United States. Specifically, the study noted that grain products had the highest level of consumption frequency, followed by dairy products, fats/sweets, beverages, fruits, vegetables, and meat/meat alternatives (Lv and Cason 2004).

Based on these results, Asian Americans may be at a higher risk of developing lifestyle diseases as a result of changes in dietary patterns. The increase in the consumption frequency of meat/meat alternatives and fats/sweets by Asian American immigrants may be explained by greater access to the mainstream culture (Lv and Cason 2004). The increase in the consumption of dairy products and fat may contribute to the overall increase in caloric and fat intake, especially if low-fat or fat-free substitute had not been used. This major shift represents dietary acculturation as a result of Westernization of eating patterns.

With the exposure to a new food supply, changes can occur in food consumption and preparation (Satia-Abouta et al. 2002). Dietary variety generally increases significantly as foods are more readily available year-round in American supermarkets compared to other parts of the world. In a cross-sectional study of 239 American-born and foreign-born Chinese adolescents residing in New York City and Chinese adolescents in China, the intake of complex carbohydrate was highest among native Chinese students, followed by foreign-born Chinese Americans and U.S.-born Chinese Americans (Sun and Wu 1997). The study noted that native Chinese students consumed the lowest amount of saturated fat when compared to foreign- and U.S.-born Chinese Americans. A case-control study among 1665 Chinese Americans found that an increase in carbohydrate consumption is associated with a higher risk of colorectal cancer in both men and women (Borugian et al. 2002).

Cultural differences in food preparation and cooking methods can affect the nutritional content of a food item. Nutritional values vary depending on how the food was produced and the preparation method used—that is, whether it was cooked or not, whether it was broiled or stir-fried, and what was added to the food. In contrast to the American cuisine, traditional Chinese dishes rarely call for deep-frying as dishes are generally sautéed or stir-fried with a moderate amount of oil. Cooking oil is generally vegetable oil such as corn, peanut, and soybean oil, with practically no butter or cream.

## DIETARY SUPPLEMENT USE AMONG ASIAN AMERICANS

After the passage of the Dietary Supplement Health and Education Act in 1994 (DSHEA), which deregulated the supplement industry, there was an explosion in the types of supplements and possible combinations of vitamin, minerals, and herbal products available to consumers (Satia-Abouta et al. 2002). As much as $1.3 to $1.7 billion are spent annually on vitamin and mineral supplements in the United States (Balluz et al. 2000).

The DSHEA broadens the traditional definition of dietary supplements, which had previously encompassed only essential dietary nutrients. It expanded the definition to include ingredients not known to be required for human nutrition. The DSHEA defines dietary supplement as "a product, other than tobacco, taken by mouth that contains a dietary ingredient intended to supplement the diet" (DSHEA 1994). According to the DSHEA, a dietary supplement is a product that is labeled as a dietary supplement and is not represented for use as a conventional food or as a sole item of a meal or the diet. The DSHEA's definition of dietary supplements expanded beyond vitamin and mineral combinations to include products that are nonvitamin and nonmineral. Nonvitamin nonmineral (NVNM) supplements include, but are not exclusive to, nontraditional, nonprescriptive ingredients such as herbs, botanicals, amino acids, concentrates, extracts, or a combination of these (Wold et al. 2005). Dietary ingredients may include vitamins, minerals, herbs or other botanicals, amino acids, and substances such as enzymes, organ tissues, and metabolites.

The awareness of dietary supplement use among Asian Americans is important as they contribute to total vitamin and mineral intake. In general, Asian immigrants are more likely to use dietary supplements as a "tonic" for their medical conditions because this is a common practice in Asia (Anderson and Anderson 1974). However, a cross-sectional study of female Asian elders age sixty-five and older showed that use of any type of dietary supplements, use of vitamins and minerals, or use of dietary supplements other than multivitamins and calcium was not different than their white non-Hispanic counterparts (Gordon and Schaffer 2005). In another cross-sectional study of ethnic elders, 36 percent of Asian American adults age sixty-five and older reported using some form of dietary supplements for pain, health maintenance, and blood pressure (Najm et al. 2003), compared to the national average of 34 percent reported by the 2000 NHIS (Millen et al. 2004) and the national average of 36 percent American adults reported by the Center for Complementary and Alternative Medicine in 2004 (NCCAM 2004). In contrast, a recent cross-sectional study from eleven community health centers in the United States of a Chinese American population with a mean age of 51.4 years found that approximately 62 percent of Cantonese-speaking Chinese Americans and 48 percent of Mandarin-speaking Chinese Americans used dietary herbal medicines in the past (Ahn et al. 2006).

Recent studies also reveal that many elderly and ethnic minorities are using dietary and NVNM supplements in combination with over-the-counter medications and/or prescribed drugs (Wold et al. 2005; Archer 2005). Several studies have examined lifestyle and demographic associations with dietary and NVNM supplement use in the United States, finding that users are more likely to have been diagnosed with a disease (Jasti et al. 2003; Najm et al. 2003; Gordon and Schaffer 2005), more likely to be on some type of diet (Jasti et al. 2003), more likely to be older (Archer et al.

2005; Radimer et al. 2000; Wold et al. 2005), and more likely to be non-white (Radimer et al. 2000). Dietary differences including lower fat consumption and higher fiber intake have been found among dietary supplement users compared to nonusers (Foote et al. 2003). A cross-sectional, multiethnic cohort study in Hawaii and Los Angeles, California, found that of the 100,196 participants, Asian Americans (n = 16,060) and whites (n = 15,979) reported substantially more long-term use of supplements compared to other ethnic groups. A cross-sectional study of 3109 participants in northern California found that Asians and Pacific Islanders (n = 222) did not significantly differ in vitamin and mineral supplement use when compared to white, non-Hispanic participants, but they were significantly less likely to use NVNM supplements (Gordon and Schaffer 2005).

Ethnic minorities, specifically Asian Americans, are highly likely to use dietary and NVNM supplements. This has important implications for health practitioners, as one must take into account dietary and NVNM supplements when evaluating the nutritional status of Asian Americans. Dietary supplements can contribute to the vitamin and mineral intake of an individual; thus they cannot be ignored when assessing the dietary intake of an individual or group. In addition, because many dietary and NVNM supplements may interact with prescribed medications, it is important that we understand the prevalence of such supplements among Asian Americans so that physicians, pharmacists, and dietitians can address any potential side effects they may have.

## DIET ASSESSMENT METHODS

There are major disparities in the nutrition and health status between many foreign-born persons in the United States and native-born Americans. This includes difficulties in assessing dietary intake of ethnic minorities.

For individual-based studies, an accurate method of assessing dietary intake is crucial. The 24-hour dietary recall is highly recommended as a resource for nutrition professionals who rely on accurate dietary recalls to meet their objectives. The 24-hour dietary recall method is easy to administer, economical, and is not dependent on the literacy of the respondent. This dietary assessment method relies primarily on episodic memory of all actual events in the very recent past. Therefore, it is appropriate for studies where the researcher is trying to obtain information on the present diet rather than on diet in the distant past (Langseth 1996). Furthermore, dietary recalls and records are used as the primary comparison method in questionnaire validation studies because this method is open ended, it does not depend on memory or perception of portion sizes, and it enables details of food to be recorded directly (Willett 2003). Participants are usually asked open-ended questions regarding their usual dietary intake, which requires the subjects to make judgments about their food habits. The interviewer generally prompts a respondent to recall and describe all foods and beverages consumed over the past twenty-four hours (Langseth 1996). Food models, measuring cups and spoons, and other tools are often used to get a rough estimate of portion sizes when using dietary recalls. Consequently, an experienced, trained interviewer may be able to attain an objective, nonbiased diet history. One of the drawbacks of this dietary assessment method is that participants may under- or overreport their total food consumption (Dwyer 1999; Thompson and Subar 2001). Thus, the answers may reflect what the subjects think they have eaten rather than what they have actually eaten. Furthermore, data may not accurately reflect differences in intake on weekdays versus the weekend and from season to season. Therefore, the gold standard is generally to obtain a minimum of three dietary recalls, two days during the week and one day during the weekend. Nonconsecutive days are preferable to capture more of the variability in an individual's diet, because eating behaviors on consecutive days are often correlated (Thompson and Subar 2001).

Food Frequency Questionnaires (FFQs) are commonly used to rank or group study subjects for the purpose of assessing the association between dietary intake and disease risk, such as in case-control or cohort studies (Dwyer 1999; Subar et al. 2001). They are the most commonly used dietary assessment method in nutrition epidemiology (Block 2001). FFQs provide a reasonable measure for both the past or present intake. Participants can either complete an interview-administered or self-administered FFQ that asks how frequently they consume a certain food item. Also, specific information about nutrients can be obtained if food sources of nutrients are confined to a few sources. Generally, FFQs provide a quantitative food description of how often foods are eaten in a specific time period, and they are extremely useful for describing food intake patterns for diet and meal planning, for studying the association of types of food and disease, and for developing nutrition intervention programs (Block 2001). Compared with other approaches, such as 24-hour dietary recalls and food records, FFQs usually collect less detailed information regarding the foods consumed, cooking methods, and portion sizes (Subar et al. 2001). Therefore, a major drawback of this dietary assessment method is that it provides limited information about energy and selected nutrient intakes because portion sizes usually are not obtained (Langseth 1996). To combat this problem, some FFQs include photographs of small, medium, and large portion sizes of foods to assist with estimating portion sizes of foods. Another drawback of FFQs is that they require numerous cognitive skills related to comprehension. This method requires respondents to remember and characterize food intake accurately and may present more complex cognitive tasks than are required in 24-hour dietary recalls.

Short dietary assessment tools can include abbreviated FFQs, food checklists, and questionnaires on specific eating patterns (Dwyer 1999). They are generally designed to capture information about a single nutrient or a specific eating behavior, so the entire diet cannot be assessed. This simple instrument can be used to give health care providers a preliminary look at people's diets and other health behaviors to know whether a more extensive nutrition workup is needed. Short dietary assessment method falls in the middle between a screening tool and a comprehensive dietary assessment method. A limitation of this methodology is that it does not provide quantitative accuracy as with other dietary assessment methods; nor does it provide quantitative estimates of more than a few nutrients or food groups (Thompson and Subar 2001). Therefore, estimates of dietary intake for the population cannot be made. The method, however, has the advantages of easy administration by both dietetic professional and nondietetic professionals, short duration for completion, and it may be useful for nutrition education (Dwyer 1999). It can also be used in a community and population level, whereby people can assess their own intake in order to improve their own diets (Block 2001). A comparison of the various dietary assessment methods is shown in Table 35.2.

## Dietary Assessment among Asian Americans

Currently, there is a lack of comprehensive food composition tables and assessment tools appropriate for the analysis of Asian American diets. The lack of an available "gold standard" in dietary assessment tool for the Asian American diet presents a major dilemma for assessment of dietary patterns in this population. With the increasing number of Asian Americans in the United States, it is imperative to have access to dietary assessment tools to study the dietary patterns of this population in relation to health issues. Cultural differences in food preparation and cooking methods can, to a great extent, affect the nutritional content of a food item. The nutrient intakes vary depending on when or how the food was produced—that is, whether it was cooked or not, whether it was broiled or stir-fried, and what was added to the food. Consequently, an ethnically sensitive and portion-sensitive (good portion estimation) tool that can capture the differences between the American diet and the typical Asian American diet is essential.

*Asian Assist* is a computer-based, picture-prompted, and self-reported dietary assessment tool designed to improve data collection in terms of both quality and efficiency. This method can capture accurate dietary information in a reasonable amount of time. This software has been shown to have content validity with respect to culturally specific patterns of food intake in the Chinese American population. This is because it includes ethnic food items in addition to the American food, and recipes are included in the software. The current version (third in series)

**Table 35.2** Comparison of Common Diet Assessment Methodologies in Nutrition Studies

| Dietary Assessment Methods | Description | Strengths | Weaknesses |
|---|---|---|---|
| Food Frequency Questionnaire | Food questionnaire used to rank or group-study subjects for the purpose of assessing the association between dietary intake and disease risk, such as case-control or cohort studies | • Economical<br>• Time efficient<br>• Good in showing association of diet and disease<br>• Can be used to measure past and present intake | • Limited information about energy and certain nutrients<br>• Requires numerous cognitive skills related to comprehension<br>• May result in recall bias |
| 24-Hour Dietary Recall | The interviewer generally prompts a respondent to recall and describe all foods and beverages consumed over the previous 24 hours | • Provides detailed information on energy and nutrients<br>• Ideal for collection of detailed nutrient profile<br>• Used as questionnaire validation studies<br>• Does not depend on the participants' literacy level<br>• Easy to administer | • Labor intensive<br>• Time consuming<br>• Can result in over- or underreporting<br>• Requires experienced or trained interviewers<br>• May require more than one day of data for validity |
| Short Dietary Assessment Tools (e.g., Abbreviated Food Frequency Questionnaire, Food Checklist) | Short abbreviated dietary method used to capture information about a single nutrient or a specific eating behavior, so the entire diet cannot be assessed | • Easily administered<br>• Economical<br>• Time efficient<br>• Can be used on a community level with limited staff/budget<br>• Participants can assess their own intake | • Entire diet cannot be assessed<br>• Does not provide quantitative estimates of more than a few nutrients or food groups |

comprises all the USDA nutrient databases and about 300 culturally specific recipes of Chinese dishes that were developed for the program using these databases. The program is both text and picture prompted and is also bilingual (Chinese and English). Food consumption data collected by the program are stored and can be retrieved later for statistical analysis. This bilingual dietary assessment program represents a major milestone in the assessment of dietary pattern in the Chinese American population.

There is a tremendous need for an Asian American dietary assessment method to be developed in this population. The method will allow health care professionals and researchers to better understand the health and medical aspects of nutrition in this ever-growing population.

## CONCLUSION

The diets of Asian Americans have a strong influence on health, and they vary widely according to country of origin, use of supplements, cooking techniques, and Westernization of dietary practices. The methods to assess this variation are very limited. This limits both our ability to learn about Asian American nutrition and to improve it. With the rapid growth of the Asian American community, this is an important public health issue.

## REFERENCES

Ahn, A.C., Ngo-Metzger, Q., Legedza, A.T.R., Massagli M.P., Clarridge B.R., Phillips R.S.. (2006). Complementary and alternative medical therapy use among Chinese and Vietnamese Americans: Prevalence, associated factors, and effects of patient clinical communication. *American Journal of Public Health* 96:647–653.

Centers for Disease Control: Office of Minority Health & Health Disparities. Accessed February 20, 2008. Available at: http://www.cdc.gov/omhd /Populations/AsianAm/AsianAm.htm.

Chen, M.S., Jr., and Hawks, B.L. (1995). A debunking of the myth of healthy Asian Americans and Pacific Islanders. *American Journal of Health Promotion* 9:261–268.

Deurenberg, P., Yap, M., and Van Staveren, W.A. (1998). Body mass index and percent body fat: A meta-analysis among different ethnic groups. *International Journal of Obesity Related Metabolism Disorder* 22:1164–1171.

Dixon, L.B., Cronin, F.J., and Krebs-Smith, S.M. (2001). Let the pyramid guide your food choices: Capturing the total diet concept. *Journal of Nutrition* 131:461S–472S.

Ferdinand, K.C. (2006) Coronary artery disease in minority racial and ethnic groups in the United States. *American Journal of Cardiology* 97:12A–19A.

Foote, J.A., Murphy, S.P., Wilkens, L.R. Hankin, J.H., Henderson, B.E., Kolonel, L.N.. (2003). Factors associated with dietary supplement use among healthy adults of five ethnicities. *American Journal of Epidemiology* 157:888–897.

Fung, T.T., Schulze, M., Manson, J.E., Willett, W.C., and Hu, F.B. (2004). Dietary patterns, meat intake, and the risk of type 2 diabetes in women. *Archives of Internal Medicine* 164:2235–2240.

Gordon, N.P., and Schaffer, D.M. (2005). Use of dietary supplements by female seniors in a large northern California health plan. *BMC Geriatric* 5:1–10.

Klatsky, A.L., and Armstrong, M.A. (1991). Cardiovascular risk factors among Asian Americans living in northern California. *American Journal of Public Health* 81:1423–1428.

Ko, G.T.C., Chan, J.C.N., Cockram, C.S., Woo, J.(1999). Prediction of hypertension, diabetes, dyslipidemia or albuminuria using simple anthropometric indexes in Hong Kong Chinese. *International Journal of Obesity Related Metabolism Disorder* 23:1136–1142.

Lin, Kathy (November 2000). "Chinese Food Cultural Profile." Harborview Medical Center, University of Washington. Available at: http://www.ethnomed.org.

Ling, Kong Foong (2002). *The food of Asia: Authentic recipes from China, India, Indonesia, Japan, Singapore, Malaysia, Thailand, and Vietnam.* Boston, MA: Perplus Editions.

Miller, B.A., Kolonel, L.N., Bernstein, L., and Young, J.L., Jr. (1996). Racial/ethnic patterns of cancer in the United States 1988–1992. Bethesda, MD: National Cancer Institute [NIH Publication No. 96-4104].

Nan, L.V., and Cason, K.L. (2004). Dietary pattern change and acculturation of Chinese Americans in Pennsylvania. *Journal of the American Dietetic Association* 104:771–778.

National Center for Health Statistics. Health, United States, 1995. Hyattsville, MD: Public Health Service, 1996.

Pan, Y.L., Dixon, Z., Himburg, S., and Huffman, F. (1999). Asian students change their eating patterns after living in the United States. *Journal of the American Dietetic Association* 99:54–57.

Park, Y.W., Allison, D.B., Heymesfield, S.B., and Gallagher, D. (2001). Larger amounts of visceral adipose tissue in Asian Americans. *Obesity Research* 9:381–387.

Satia, J.A., Patterson, R.E., Kristal, A.R., Hislop, T.G., Yasui, Y., and Taylor, V.M. (2001). Development of dietary acculturation scales among Chinese Americans and Chinese Canadians. *Journal of the American Dietetic Association* 101:548–553.

Satia-About, J., Patterson, R.E., Neuhouser, M.L., and Elder, J. (2002). Dietary acculturation: Applications to nutrition research and dietetics. *Journal of the American Dietetic Association* 102:1105–1118.

Sun, W.Y., Wu, J.S.. (1997). Comparsion of dietary efficacy and behavior among American-born and foreign-born Chinese adolescents residing in NYC and Chinese adolescents in Guangzhou, China. *Journal of the American College Nutrition* 16(2):127–133.

Unger, J.B., Reynolds, K., Shakib, S., Spruijt-Metz, D., Sun, P., and Johnson, A. (2004). Acculturation, physical activity, and fast food consumption among

Asian American and Hispanic adolescents. *Journal of Community Health* 29:467–481.

U.S. Census 2000. The Asian Population 2000. Washington, DC: U.S. Census, February 2002.

Wildman, R.P., Gu, D., Reynolds, K., Duan, X., and He, J. (2004). Appropriate body mass index and waist circumference cutoffs for categorization of overweight and central adiposity among Chinese adults. *American Journal of Clinical Nutrition* 80:1129–1136.

Wildman, R.P., Gu, D., Reynolds, K., Duan, X., Wu, X., and He, J. (2005). Are waist circumference and body mass index independently associated with cardiovascular disease risk in Chinese adults? *American Journal of Clinical Nutrition* 82:1195–1202.

Willett, W.C. (2003). Invited commentary: OPEN questions. *American Journal of Epidemiology* 158:22–24.

Wold, R.S., Lopez, S.T., Yau, C.L., Butler, L.M., Pareo-Tubbeh, S.L., Waters, D.L., Garry, P.J., Baumgartner, R.N. (2005). Increasing trends in elderly persons' use of nonvitamin, nonmineral dietary supplements and concurrent use of medications. *Journal of the American Dietetic Association*105:54–63.

# Chapter 36

# Traditional Medical Practices of Asian Americans and the Influence of Traditional Medicine in the United States

*Lixin Zhang, Tony V. Lu, and Thomas Tsang*

"聖人不治已病治未病, 夫病已成而後藥之, 亂已成而後治之,

亂已成而後治之, 譬猶渴而穿井, 鬥而鑄兵, 不亦晚乎?"

— 黃帝內經

"Treating an illness after it has begun is like suppressing revolt after it has broken out. If someone digs a well when thirsty or forges weapons after becoming engaged in battle, one can't help but ask: are not these actions too late?"
—*Yellow Emperor's Internal Classics*

## A BRIEF OVERVIEW OF THE TRADITIONAL ASIAN MEDICINE (TAM) SYSTEM

The concept of disease prevention and health maintenance is ingrained in the development of traditional Asian medicine (TAM). TAM emphasizes the interconnection of the individual and his or her surrounding natural and societal environment, the inseparability of mental and spiritual health from physical well-being, and the importance of disease prevention, health maintenance, and health promotion. TAM traces its root to two of the most ancient and yet living traditions in the world: traditional Chinese medicine (TCM) and Ayurveda, traditional Indian medicine.

## Traditional Chinese Medicine (TCM)

The development of TCM has been embedded in Chinese culture and evolved from the influence of philosophy, religion, and natural science. The origin of the development of TCM is often attributed to Shen Nong, the father and originator of Chinese herbal medicine, who is believed to have lived in the period between 2838 to 2698 BCE. A later classic TCM text, the *Divine Husbandman's Classic of the Materia Medica (Shen Nong Ben Cao Jing)*, was named after him to signify the importance of his contribution. The *Yellow Emperor's Internal Classics (Huang Di Nei Jing)*, a seminal classic, laid the foundation for the development and advancement of TCM.

One of most essential elements in TCM is the concept of wholeness. An extensive and unified medical system, TCM emphasizes the interconnection, inseparability, and unification within parts of the human body and between human beings and the universe. The external organs and internal structures, the outward manifestations and inward substances, the physical and mental functions are interconnected as parts of the whole. Individuals are also considered inseparable from the spiritual, natural, and societal world in which they live. The three parts, "heaven," "earth," and "human beings," form a unified system.

Ancient Asian philosophical doctrines—qi, yin and yang, and the five elements—contribute significantly to the TCM foundations. Qi, "the breath" (literally translated), the most basic element constituting the world, is the life-sustaining and life-preserving substance for human beings. Formed from the inherited essence, nutrients and breath, qi circulates throughout the body and functions by warming, protecting, propelling, controlling, and generating.

The notion of the unity of the opposite, yin and yang, classifies the nature of every phenomena as two polarizing yet connecting and complementing aspects. When yin and yang are harmonized, the person is healthy and not susceptible for the invasion of pathogens. Diseases result from the loss of the balance between the two components. The five elements in the natural world (wood, fire, earth, metal, and water) and their characteristics, changes, and interactions are used to illustrate the five systems or phrases observed in every phenomenon in nature, society, and the human body. Applied to TCM, the five elements classify the structure and function of the human body into five organ-viscera systems (liver-gall bladder, heart-small intestine, spleen-stomach, lung-large intestine, and kidney-bladder).

The channels and collaterals are the pathway of qi, blood, essence, and fluids connecting the exterior and interior, the organs and viscera, and the limbs, joints and orifices together. Diseases occur when qi is weak and when external pathogens, extreme emotions, irregular diet and lifestyle, injuries, or inherited factors disturb the balance between yin and yang, qi, and blood, and the functions of organ-viscera and channel-collateral system. The process of the battle between the influencing factors and qi determines the transition, transformation, and prognosis of the diseases.

TCM practitioners collect information via inspecting, listening, inquiring, palpitation, and feeling the pulse to decide the cause, nature, and location of the imbalance. TCM therapies are then applied according to their respective mechanisms to correct the imbalance based on the formulated diagnoses.

## Ayurveda

Ayurveda, meaning "life" and "knowledge," is the traditional Indian medical system. Like TCM, the fundamental principle of Ayurveda is the interconnection between the microcosm and macrocosm. As miniatures of the surrounding world, human beings and the outside world form an integrated system. Interruptions of the system and imbalance of basic physiological principles of the body cause physical manifestations of diseases. Ayurveda theory emphasizes the influence of mind on health, particularly the connection between stress and unhealthy lifestyle.

According to Ayurveda, the universe consists of five basic interconnected and interacting elements: earth, air, fire, water, and space. The human body is made up from three forces (*doshas*), seven body constituents (*dhatus*), and three wastes (*malas*). In addition, three types of enzymes (*agnis*) help digest and assimilate food. The three doshas—wind (*vata*), bile (*pitta*), and phlegm (*kapha*)—regulate body functions. Disease (*ama*) results from suboptimal levels of enzyme activity or blockage of channels or vessels of the body (*srotas*), through which all substances flow.

Ayurveda practitioners employ a detailed system of diagnosis using observation, touch, interrogation, pulse examination, urine examination, and examination of body parts to formulate preliminary diagnoses. In addition, further differentiation of etiology, early and manifested signs and symptoms, together with eighteen different experiments using drugs, diet, and regimens and a six-step process determining pathogenesis are carried on to acquire a comprehensive understanding of the illness.

Ayurveda emphasizes on disease prevention and health preservation based on lifestyle approaches including diet, sleep and exercise programs, and pharmaceutical and purification therapies. Ayurvedic practitioners commonly use meditation, relaxation therapies, and Yoga to improve physical and mental health. Purification and alleviation therapies, such as emetic and purgative therapies, enemas, and medicinal oil massage, are used individually or together to cleanse and remove accumulated toxins and eliminate *dosha* imbalance.

**Table 36.1** Summary of TAMP

| | Procedure | TAM Systems | Administering Type | Main Practicing Groups | Clinical Studies |
|---|---|---|---|---|---|
| Herbal Medicine 中药 | Herbs, minerals, animal parts are prepared in the forms of soups, powders, pills, or tincture | TCM, Ayurveda, folk therapy | Provider–administered (P-A), Self-administered (S-A) | Almost every Asian subgroup | HIV infection,[75] hepatitis B,[76] menopausal symptoms,[77] SARS,[78,79] liver fibrosis,[80] diabetes,[81] senile advanced nonsmall cell lung cancer,[82] asthma,[83] epilepsy,[84] chronic headache,[85] dermatology,[86] stroke,[87] irritable bowel syndrome[88] |
| Acupuncture 针 | A fine needle is inserted into the skin based on acupuncture points along the channels and meridians | TCM | P-A | Chinese, Japanese, Korean, | migraine, headache,[89–91] hypertension,[92] insomnia,[93,94] nausea and vomiting,[95] depression,[96–98] low back pain,[99] asthma,[100] obesity,[101] ulcerative colitis,[102] ankylosing spondylitis,[103,104] chronic prostatitis,[105] Parkinson's disease,[106] cervicogenic headache[107], osteoarthritis[1,108,109] |

| Practice | Description | System | Category | Ethnic groups | Conditions |
|---|---|---|---|---|---|
| Moxibustion 灸 | Dried or powdered leaves of *artemesia vulgaris* (ai ye) in the form of (chopped) sticks are applied on or in proximity to the skin | TCM | P-A | Chinese, Korean | Poststroke urinary symptoms,[110] cervical vertigo[111] Bell's palsy[112] systemic lupus erythematosus,[113] ulcerative colitis,[102] ankylosing spondylitis,[103,104] chronic prostatitis[105] |
| Massage (*tui na, acupressure, shiatsu*) 按摩 按摩 按摩(推拿,指压) | A complex series of hand movements such as pressing, rubbing, rolling, kneading, and grasping are used on specific points or body areas to accomplish desired effects | TCM, Ayurveda, folk therapy | P-A, S-A | Chinese, Indian, Japanese, Korean | Fibromyalgia,[114] Parkinson's disease,[106] cervicogenic headache,[107] insomnia,[94] dementia,[115] smoking cessation,[116] dysmenorrhea[117] |
| Cupping 拔罐 | A bamboo or glass cup is overturned and placed onto certain points or areas in the body after the inside air is warmed to create vacuum | TCM, folk medicine | P-A, S-A | Chinese, Vietnamese, Korean | obesity,[118] chronic fatigue syndrome,[119] health maintenance,[120] cough and asthma,[121] acute eczema[122] |

**Table 36.1** (Continued)

| | Procedure | TAM Systems | Administering Type | Main Practicing Groups | Clinical Studies |
|---|---|---|---|---|---|
| Yoga 瑜珈 | Using postures, breathing techniques and meditation to achieve physical, mental and spiritual health | Ayurveda | P-A, S-A | Indian, Sri Lankan | fibromyalgia,[114] diabetes,[123,124] cancer,[120] hypertension,[125] arthritis,[126] pain,[127,128] cardiac health,[129,130] anxiety,[131] depression,[132] multiple sclerosis[133] |
| Dietary therapy 食疗 | Foods are selected based on their characteristics and properties to achieve remedial effect according to individuals' TAM diagnoses | TCM, Ayurveda, folk therapy | P-A, S-A | Chinese, Indian, Hmong, Japanese | atopic dermatitis[134] |
| Bloodletting 放血 | Blood (drops to less than 350ml) on acu-points, channels, or veins is let out to treat certain refractory diseases | TCM, Ayurveda, folk therapy | P-A, S-A | Chinese, Indian, Vietnamese | herpes zoster,[135] cough and asthma,[121] acute eczema[122] |

| Practice | Description | | | Ethnic groups | Evidence/conditions |
|---|---|---|---|---|---|
| Coin-rubbing (Gua Sha) 刮痧 | Objects with smooth edges (e.g. coins, spoons) are used to apply in strokes with repetitive pressure on surface of the body or meridians | Folk therapy, TCM | S-A | Vietnamese, Cambodian, Thai, Indonesian, Korean, South Chinese | headache[136] |
| Skin-pinching 捏皮 | Parts of skin (e.g. along the spine) are repetitively and rapidly pinched until they become slightly red | Folk therapy, TCM | S-A | Vietnamese, Chinese | no study has been found |
| Tai chi 太极 | An ancient martial art with gentle and relaxed movement for balance and strength | Folk therapy, TCM | S-A | Chinese | hypertension,[137] diabetes,[138] prevention of falls,[139] rheumatoid arthritis[140] |
| Qi gong 气功 | Using breath, movement, and meditation to cleanse, strengthen, and circulate the vital like energy and blood | Folk therapy, TCM | S-A, P-A | Chinese | Parkinson's disease,[106] hypertension,[141] cancer,[142] multiple sclerosis[143] |

## A BRIEF INTRODUCTION TO TRADITIONAL ASIAN MEDICAL PRACTICES (TAMP)

Table 36.1 lists the therapies commonly used by TCM and Ayurveda practitioners, as well as folk therapies practiced by people of some Asian Pacific Islanders (API) groups. The practice of these therapies is guided or influenced by TCM and Ayurveda principles. After formulating a diagnosis, the TAM provider chooses the therapies deemed necessary and appropriate to correct excess or insufficiency and restore balance.

Depending on the nature of the condition, TAMP were used individually or together to achieve the desired result. For example, A TCM doctor could diagnose a patient having symptoms of persistent early morning diarrhea as deficiency of the spleen and kidney yang. Consequently, he or she may prescribe herbal medicine to strengthen the two organ systems, moxibustion to warm the spleen and kidney, and massage (*tui na*) to alleviate the symptoms of the upset stomach. An Ayurveda practitioner may advise patients on lifestyle changes, proper diet, yoga, meditation, or administration of cleansing programs. Likewise, agents or elements of individual therapies are worked together to enhance the benefits and reduce adverse reactions to other treatments. For example, different herbs are selected based on their properties, characteristics, and running channels in a formula to fend off pathogen, unblock stagnation, invigorate blood, tonify qi, and benefit yin.

Since the development of the TAM was deeply rooted in the nature, culture, and society in which people lived, self-administered TAMP are widespread, even though people continue seeking advices and instructions from providers. Many of the self-administered TAMP are employed as health promotion tools as well as first-contact intervention. The images of the elderly practicing tai chi and vendors selling raw herbs at bazaars are not unfamiliar to people in the United States.

Dietary therapy is based on the concept that food and drug shares a common source and acknowledgement of the importance of food and diet in causing and treating diseases. Just as herbs have difference properties and characteristics, food also varies in its medicinal functions. Considering individuals' constitution and seasonal changes, providers and individuals choose or avoid certain food based on their functions to prevent and treat diseases.

Some TAMP were derived from certain techniques or methods of provider-administered therapies. They are also used as self-administered practices among certain API groups. For example, bloodletting had been a fairly routine acupuncture practice in early TCM history and is still being used by TCM, Ayurveda, and Tibetan medical practitioners today. Skin-pinching (*bat gio, nie ji*), one of the massage (*tui na*) techniques, and coin-rubbing (*cao gio, gua sha*), another ancient treatment technique, are widely used by Vietnamese, Cambodians, Thai, Indonesians, Koreans, and Southern Chinese.

The last column of Table 36.1 includes lists of clinical studies documenting the efficacy of the respective TAMP in treating specific conditions. Among the listed TAMP, acupuncture is one of the most thoroughly researched and documented therapies. Numerous clinical trials on the treatment of a variety of conditions have shown compelling, if not statistically conclusive, evidence for the effectiveness of acupuncture. A consensus reached by the NIH development panel on acupuncture concludes that acupuncture is effective for postoperative and chemotherapy-induced nausea and vomiting, postoperative pain, and dental pain.[1] Promising evidence also suggests that acupuncture can be cost effective.[2, 3]

Though studies on other TAMP show promising results, only preliminary conclusions can be drawn about their efficacy and effectiveness for several reasons. First, some of the original works published in languages other than English are difficult to translate into standard analyses and methods considered acceptable or gold standard for of biomedical research in the United States. Second, the application of standardized biomedical research methods to the study of many TAMP, which employs a holistic and individualistic approach to health and illness, can be a challenge. Third, many of the published research findings either lack appropriate and rigorous research design, are unclear in the sampling strategy, or insufficiently describe and report the data.[4] Lastly, the mechanism of certain TAM Modalities is not fully understood and, as a result, it is more difficult to design an ideal placebo to use for comparison.

Research has also been published on the adverse reactions of some TAMP, especially herbal medicine. Certain herbal products, especially patent herbs, have been reported to contain toxic ingredients, such as heavy metal, prescription drugs, or unapproved agents. Many of the ingredients may or may not be identified in the label. Herbal products that are taken without supervision may exceed the limits of safe dose and thus cause toxic effect. Additionally, interactions between herbs and drugs may occur, especially when they are taken simultaneously. There is an urgent need for further research on the benefits and adverse effects of the wide range of herbs, and the development and enforcement of regulations in the production, preparation, and distribution of herbal products.

## PRACTICE OF TAMP IN THE GENERAL POPULATION

TAMP in the United States could probably be traced back to the time when the first Filipino sailors settled in California in 1750 and when Chinese, Indian, Japanese, Korean, and Filipino workers were recruited to work in gold mines, fields, and farms in California and Hawaii in the 1800s. However, many of the TAMP have not been well known outside of the Asian American communities until 1971 when Jame Reston's highly publicized report of appendectomy with acupuncture anesthesia and postoperative care led to substantial public interest in TCM and attention to TAMP.

The rise in interest in TAMP took place during the period in which the increasing prevalence of complementary and alternative medicine (CAM) was noticed. In 1991, Eisenberg and colleagues conducted the first national representative telephone survey documenting the use of CAM in the United States. They found that one third of the population used at least one of sixteen CAM therapies in 1990. Their follow-up survey in 1997 indicated a 42 percent increase in the prevalence of the use of CAM.[5,6] A later study based on the 2002 National Health Interview Survey (NHIS) shows that 62% of the adults used some type of CAM therapies during the previous 12 months if health-related prayers were included.[7]

CAM is defined as consisting of a broad group of systems, practices, and products that are not presently considered to be part of the conventional biomedical therapies. As the traditional or "conventional" form of medical care belonging to coherent and cohesive systems in many parts of Asian countries, TAMP are included under the broad umbrella term of CAM and represented across five groups of modalities categorized by National Center for Complementary and Alternative Medicine (NCCAM): alternative medical systems, biologically based therapies, manipulative and body-based therapies, mind-body therapies, and energy medicine.

Though some TAMP therapies, such as acupuncture, Ayurveda, yoga, tai chi, and qi gong, have distinctive roots in Asia, other TAMP have also been practiced in different culture and ethnic groups, though the forms and procedures may vary. For example, herbal medicine and massage therapy are the most ancient and yet still widely practiced therapies in various parts of the world. Originating from oriental religious practice, particularly from India, China, and Japan, meditation is practiced in different regions. Various forms of folk medicine have ancient roots in Africa (e.g., rootwork), Europe (e.g., powwowing), and Latin America (e.g., *curanderismo*), in addition to Asia. Without specifying the origin and tradition of these practices, it is difficult to find the true prevalence of the use of TAMP in the general population.

Unfortunately, the only available national survey about CAM that was conducted more recently, the 2002 NHIS, did not ask TAMP-specific questions in the questionnaire. It found that among the nine TAMP surveyed, herbal medicine (biologically based therapies) was used most frequently (19%) among the adult population in the United States, followed by meditation (7.6%), yoga (5.1%) (mind-body therapies), massage (5.0%) (manipulative and body-based therapies) and acupuncture (1.1%). Extrapolating to the entire population, it was found that more than 10 million practiced yoga and 2.13 million people used acupuncture during the previous twelve months. Studies focusing on certain regions, demographic characteristics, and illness types also indicated high levels of the use of herbal medicine, mind-body therapies, and manipulative and body-based therapies, and among cancer patients.[8-34]

In general, women, people of middle age, people with higher education, mid- to higher-income people, and those who live in the West were more likely to use CAM.[7] Similar demographic profiles were found among users of TAMP. A survey of TCM users of eight clinics across the United States found the sample consisted of middle-aged, well-educated, employed, and mid-income patients.[35] It has been documented that the use of CAM varies among race and ethnicity. Hispanics were less likely than non-Hispanics overall to use CAM;[36] Black adults were found to be more likely than Whites or Asians to use mind-body therapies, including prayers for health reasons; Asian adults were more likely than Whites or Blacks to use CAM if prayers were excluded; Whites were more likely to use manipulative and body-based therapies than Asian or black adults.[7]

The top reasons respondents sought TAMP were improving mental health, maintaining good health, and relieving pain.[35] Other explanations of why people use TAMP include belief in the efficacy of combined treatment of CAM conventional medicine, holistic health philosophy, transformational life experiences, interests in alternative life styles, desires in taking control of own health, mistrust of health care system, being cynical about biomedicine, dissatisfied by doctor-patient relationships, recommendation from conventional health professional, and cost of conventional medicine.[11, 37-44]

## PRACTICES OF TAMP AMONG ASIANS AND PACIFIC ISLANDERS (API) IN THE UNITED STATES

As the increasing practice of acupuncture, yoga, meditation and relaxation therapies continue to be documented among the general population in the United States, the reasons and factors for the use of TAMP among APIs, particularly at the national level, have been relatively less known. Several factors might have contributed to the gap in the literature. First, the latest national survey including questions about CAM use was conducted seven years ago, and thus the current prevalence of TAMP use is not available. Second, the reported prevalence of CAM use among APIs has been based on NCCAM categories rather than individual TAMP. Third, the majority of surveys based on the general population were conducted in English, excluding immigrants with limited English proficiency, the cohort of people who might be the most active users of TAMP. Lastly, the lack of information about the use of specific TAMP among different API subgroups is also evident.

Despite of the aforementioned limitations, results from national surveys and studies of certain regions or specific therapies, and ethnic groups may suggest high prevalence of TAMP among APIs. We conducted analyses

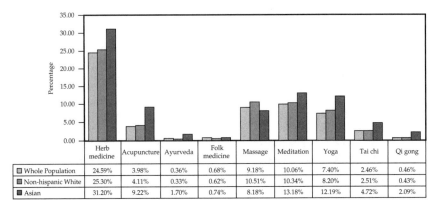

**Figure 36.1** Percentage of Use of TAMP by APIs Based on the 2002 NHIS.

|  | Herb medicine | Acupuncture | Ayurveda | Folk medicine | Massage | Meditation | Yoga | Tai chi | Qi gong |
|---|---|---|---|---|---|---|---|---|---|
| Whole Population | 24.59% | 3.98% | 0.36% | 0.68% | 9.18% | 10.06% | 7.40% | 2.46% | 0.46% |
| Non-hispanic White | 25.30% | 4.11% | 0.33% | 0.62% | 10.51% | 10.34% | 8.20% | 2.51% | 0.43% |
| Asian | 31.20% | 9.22% | 1.70% | 0.74% | 8.18% | 13.18% | 12.19% | 4.72% | 2.09% |

based on the 2002 NHIS and calculated the TAMP-specific prevalence rate among APIs. The results (Figure 36.1) indicate that the proportions of TAMP used by APIs in the United States were significantly higher than that of the White and other racial/ethnic groups for herbal medicine, acupuncture, Ayurveda, folk medicine, meditation, yoga, tai chi and qi gong.[45] The actual prevalence of TAMP use among APIs could be even higher if non-English speaking immigrants were surveyed.

APIs are heterogeneous groups consisting of ethnically and linguistically diverse populations. Just as the use of CAM varies by race and ethnicity, the uses of TAMP also vary among different API ethnic subgroups as documented in regional and ethnic-specific studies. Based on the 2002 NHIS, Mehta et al found that Indians were more likely to use mind-body therapies than Chinese.[46] The results from the 2001 California Health Interview Survey show that Japanese Americans (29%) and South Asians (30%) were most likely to use mind-body treatments, and Chinese (10%) were the least likely to use these therapies. However, the prevalence of the use of biologically-based therapies (herbs/supplements) among Chinese was the highest (83%).[47] A survey of Chinese and Vietnamese who visited one of eleven community health centers across the United States found that herbal medicine and acupuncture were used more often by Chinese, but cupping, coining, and massage were used mostly by Vietnamese.[48]

## FACTORS ASSOCIATING WITH TAMP USE AMONG THE APIS

### Immigration and Diversity

APIs are one of the fastest growing racial and ethnic groups in the United States, projected to grow 213 percent by 2050 to 33.4 million with a doubled increase of the nation's population share. The majority of the population growth of APIs will be caused by immigration.[49] Coming from diverse ethnic and cultural backgrounds, many of the API immigrants share common beliefs and values about health. Though a rich medical and cultural anthropology literature on cultural beliefs points to its relationship with perceptions of health and illnesses and treatment choices, studies of health beliefs, behaviors, and practices among API populations, especially immigrants, are rather limited.[50-53]

One study documented the health beliefs and practices of Southeast Asian refugees in Franklin County, Ohio, composed of Vietnamese, Laotian, Cambodian, and Hmong ethnic groups who had resettled in the United States since 1975. The study found that the concept of imbalance and a naturalist view toward disease and treatment as influenced by TCM and Ayurveda were part of the predominant belief system among Cambodian and Vietnamese refugees. While Hmong attribute many illnesses to supernatural causes, the health beliefs of Laotian refugees are a combination of natural and supernatural elements, with the former predominating. Though TAMP were the first treatment options among Vietnamese and Hmongs, Cambodians showed no preferences for TAMP or biomedicine, and very few Laotians reported consulting a TAM practitioner or using TAMP since arrival in the United States.[54]

The results of another study of 119 Laotian refugees from Laos in Richmond, California, showed that home remedies, herbal medicine, and healing ceremonies were commonly used together with biomedical services and that health beliefs determined the treatment choices.[55] A study of another cohort of 80 Southeast Asian refugees including Laotians, Mien (a tribal people with distinctly separate culture living in Mountain regions of Laos), Cambodian, and Chinese in a primary care clinic in Washington found that TAMP were commonly used among the participants with variations among different ethnic groups. Coining was the most frequently reported therapy used by Cambodian (70%), Chinese (35%), and Laotian (10%). Cupping was used only by Cambodians and Mien, and moxibustion and healing ceremonies were only practiced almost exclusively by Mien.[56]

A more recent study conducted at two community health centers in California serving immigrant Chinese found that almost 100 percent of 198 patients interviewed used TCM.[57] Several studies also indicate that API immigrants, especially those with limited English and who have lived in North America for a shorter period of time, used TAMP commonly.[47, 58, 59] Though further research is needed to examine the relations between the health beliefs and TAMP use among APIs, the available literature seem to suggest that TAMP are commonly used by API immigrants.

## Acculturation

Levels of acculturation may also influence the use of TAMP among APIs. As immigrants stay in the United States longer and become more acculturated, they may become less likely to use TAMP. However, survey research has not found evidence of the negative association between acculturation and the use of TAMP. Based on the 2001 California Health Interview Survey (CHIS), though it found that Chinese Americans with limited English proficiency were more likely to use CAM, those who immigrated more than ten years ago were less likely than the U.S.-born Chinese Americans to use CAM. No association was found between levels of acculturation and the use of any CAM therapies among Pilipino Americans, Japanese Americans, South Asians, and other Asians.[47] Another survey of Chinese and Vietnamese Americans of eleven community health centers throughout the United States did not find the levels of English proficiency and number of years in the United States related to the use of any of the six TAMP, including herbal medicine, acupuncture, coining, cupping, tai chi or qi gong, and massage.[48]

The results of a cross-sectional survey of 143 Korean Americans in New York show that younger, well educated individuals with high levels of acculturation levels, but who had stayed in the United States for a relatively shorter period of time were more likely to use herbal medicine, chiropractic, megavitamins, acupuncture, or acupressure.[60] A survey of patients visiting an emergency department indicates that the use of TCM was common for both the first and second generation Chinese, with prevalence rates of 44 and 42 percent respectively.[61] An analysis based on the 2002 NHIS found that as immigrants stay longer in the United States and become more proficient in English, their use of CAM actually increases, gradually approaching the level of CAM used by those born in the United States in the general population.[62]

Without distinguishing TAMP from other CAM therapies, the positive association between levels of acculturation and CAM use found in the above studies does not necessarily indicate increased use of TAMP with increased levels of acculturation among APIs. However, the high prevalence of TAMP among both new and longer-term immigrants and APIs born in the United States seems to be evident.

## Biomedicine and Access to Conventional Care

In certain regions of Asia and Africa where access to biomedical health services is limited, traditional medical practices serve as the primary or "conventional" source of care. In some Asian societies, such as China, Korea, and Vietnam, TAMP integrate with biomedicine to provide preventive and curative care.[63] In America, TAMP are increasingly used as complementary or alternative health care options to biomedicine.

The results based on the analysis of the 1996 and 1998 Medical Expenditure Panel Survey suggest that the substitution and complementariness between biomedicine and TAMP varies by race-ethnicity and specific therapies. Acupuncture was found to be complementary for non-Hispanic Whites and Blacks, massage was complementary for Asians and

Blacks, and herbal medicine was complementary for Asian but alternative for American Indians.[64] Bonafede and colleagues analyzed managed care insurance claims data consisting of 1,688 acupuncture users and 16,282 nonusers. Acupuncture was found to be a statistically significant substitute for primary care, surgery, outpatient care, pathology services, and gastrointestinal medicines, but not a complement for any therapies after controlling for unobserved characteristics.[65]

In addition to cultural background, health beliefs, and effectiveness of therapies, another important factor to consider in understanding the use of health care services is cost and access. TAMP are not commonly covered by insurance, except for acupuncture, which is often covered with limitations (e.g., pain management with a referral requirement, restrictions in the number of visits).[66] Thus, the substitution of and complementariness between biomedical services and TAMP is also determined by the cost and availability of conventional health care. For those who have health insurance and a regular source of care, the use of TAMP, especially provider-administered therapies, would bring additional out-of-pocket cost to the insured. But for those without health insurance coverage or who could not afford conventional health care, TAMP may provide a less expensive and alternative option, considering the fact that TAMP generally cost less than conventional health care.

Based on the 2002 NHIS, Pagan and Pauly found that adults with unmet or delayed health care needs because of cost were more likely than other adults to use TAMP, including herbal medicine, message, acupuncture, yoga, tai chi, qi gong, and relaxation techniques, except Ayurveda.[67, 68] Analyzing the associating factors to the use of herbal medicine specifically, Gardiner et al. confirmed that those without health insurance and who considered conventional medical treatments too expensive were more likely to use herbal medicine.[11]

However, studies of the association between access to care and use of TAMP among API populations have been rare. Hsiao et al. analyzed a representative survey of 9187 California adults of four Asian population subgroups. They did not find any significant relationship between health care access and any CAM use except for other Asians.[69] As we discussed before, the use of any CAM does not represent the use of TAMP-specific therapies. But unfortunately, there have not been conclusive findings regarding the access to conventional health services and the use of TAMP among the APIs due to lack of information.

## COMMUNICATION AND ADHERENCE

Despite the common use, communications between conventional health care providers and users is extremely low, and Asians were found less likely to talk with providers about the use of CAM.46 Based on the aforementioned survey of eleven community health centers, less

718 Praeger Handbook of Asian American Health

than one in ten patients (7.6%) discussed their use with clinicians, despite the fact that two thirds of the respondents used TAMP.[48] A study of immigrant Chinese patients seeking emergency room care found that only 5 percent of the providers asked about the use of TCM.[61]

Providers' lack of understanding of cultural beliefs and health care practices can result in miscommunication and distrust, dissatisfaction with care, reduced levels of adherence to treatment, and unintended consequences from the misuse of TAMP. API patients, especially immigrants, regardless of social position or education, are reluctant to talk with providers when they sense that their concept of health care and practices of TAM would be ignored or dismissed. The resulting barriers to open communication and full trust, coupled with language difficulty, low literacy levels, and unfamiliarity with the health care system, may lead to frustration, poor compliance, and suboptimal medical care.[62]

A study conducted in an emergency department in India indicated that lack of knowledge about the need to take medicine regularly and the use of TAMP were associated with noncompliance-related hospital admissions.[70] However, this study was conducted outside of the United States and the cross-sectional nature of the dataset does not allow for any conclusion about whether TAMP poss barriers to the adherence to conventional medications. But no study has been found assessing the influence of the use of TAMP on the adherence to conventional medications among the API populations, especially among immigrants.[71-74]

It is evident that lack of adherence to medications affects health care outcomes directly and results in financial and resource loss, but the reasons for the lack of adherence are not so evident. It would be simplistic and unrealistic to attribute the causes of nonadherence to a lack of knowledge or ignorance. In fact, many API patients with chronic and incurable diseases make the conscious decision to adhere or not adhere to biomedicine or TAMP. Even though the reasons behind these decisions have not been understood well, one of the key determinants of effective care for APIs, especially immigrants, lie in open communications between providers and the patient about TAMP.

## SUMMARY AND CONCLUSION

Belonging to two ancient, living and thriving systems of TCM and Ayurveda, TAMP may offer effective and culturally valuable care to APIs in the United States. As included in the broader category of CAM, TAMP is being used widely and increasingly in the United States, and APIs are in general more likely than other population groups to use TAMP. When examining the factors influencing the use of TAMP among APIs, we need to take culture, immigration, variations among subgroups, and access to conventional health care into consideration.

However, the results from the literature review suggest that research about traditional health care practices among APIs is rather limited, and the unknowns probably far exceed what has been known. The fact that available studies offer inconclusive, inconsistent, and even contradictory findings points to the clear needs in this area of research. As TAMP use is prevalent and increasing in the United States, whose population is projected to become ever more diverse in the next fifty years, understanding these traditional, alternative, or complementary health care practices has a far-reaching effect for improving the health and care of the people in the nation.

While proven evidence has clearly shown the efficacy, effectiveness, and cost-effectiveness of several TAMP, conclusive statements are not available for other TAMP due to lack of appropriate research method, paucity of high quality clinical studies, and insufficiency of research funds. Moreover, the seriousness of the safety issues caused by the adulteration, adverse effects, side effects, toxicity, and unsupervised use of herbs and herb-drug interaction demands adequate regulatory mechanisms, sufficient knowledge and trainings of conventional health professionals, and open communications between providers and patients.

## REFERENCES

1. Anonymous. NIH Consensus Conference. Acupuncture. *JAMA*. Nov 4 1998;280(17):1518–1524.

2. Vickers AJ, Rees RW, Zollman CE, et al. Acupuncture of chronic headache disorders in primary care: randomised controlled trial and economic analysis. *Health Technology Assessment (Winchester, England)*. Nov 2004;8(48):iii.

3. Witt CM, Jena S, Selim D, et al. Pragmatic randomized trial evaluating the clinical and economic effectiveness of acupuncture for chronic low back pain. *American Journal of Epidemiology*. Sep 1 2006;164(5):487–496.

4. Lao L. [Recommendations for enhancing the quality of traditional Chinese medicine clinical research reporting.] *Zhong Xi Yi Jie He Xue Bao*. Nov 2004;2(6):402-4-06.

5. Eisenberg DM, Kessler RC, Foster C, Norlock FE, Calkins DR, Delbanco TL. Unconventional medicine in the United States. Prevalence, costs, and patterns of use. [See comment.] *New England Journal of Medicine*. 1993;328(4):246–252.

6. Eisenberg DM, Davis RB, Ettner SL, et al. Trends in alternative medicine use in the United States, 1990–1997: results of a follow-up national survey. [See comment.] *JAMA*. 1998;280(18):1569–1575.

7. Barnes PM, Powell-Griner E, McFann K, Nahin RL. Complementary and alternative medicine use among adults: United States, 2002. *Advance Data*. 2004;343:1–19.

8. Upchurch DM, Chyu L, Greendale GA, et al. Complementary and alternative medicine use among American women: findings from The National Health Interview Survey, 2002. *Journal of Women's Health*. Jan–Feb 2007;16(1): 102–113.

9. Gold EB, Bair Y, Zhang G, et al. Cross-sectional analysis of specific complementary and alternative medicine (CAM) use by racial/ethnic group and menopausal status: the Study of Women's Health Across the Nation (SWAN). [See comment.] *Menopause*. Jul–Aug 2007;14(4):612–623.

10. Gardiner P, Kemper KJ, Legedza A, et al. Factors associated with herb and dietary supplement use by young adults in the United States. *BMC Complementary & Alternative Medicine*. 2007;7:39.

11. Gardiner P, Graham R, Legedza AT, et al. Factors associated with herbal therapy use by adults in the United States. *Alternative Therapies in Health & Medicine*. Mar–Apr 2007;13(2):22–29.

12. Shaw A, Noble A, Salisbury C, et al. Predictors of complementary therapy use among asthma patients: results of a primary care survey. *Health & Social Care in the Community*. Mar 2008;16(2):155–164.

13. Pakzad K, Boucher BA, Kreiger N, et al. The use of herbal and other non-vitamin, non-mineral supplements among pre- and post-menopausal women in Ontario. *Canadian Journal of Public Health Revue Canadienne de Sante Publique*. Sep–Oct 2007;98(5):383–388.

14. Weyl Ben Arush M, Geva H, Ofir R, et al. Prevalence and characteristics of complementary medicine used by pediatric cancer patients in a mixed western and middle-eastern population. *Journal of Pediatric Hematology/Oncology*. Mar 2006;28(3):141–146.

15. Rossi P, Di Lorenzo G, Malpezzi MG, et al. Prevalence, pattern and predictors of use of complementary and alternative medicine (CAM) in migraine patients attending a headache clinic in Italy. *Cephalalgia*. Jul 2005;25(7):493–506.

16. Kennedy J. Herb and supplement use in the US adult population. [See comment.] *Clinical Therapeutics*. Nov 2005;27(11):1847–1858.

17. Akyuz A, Dede M, Cetinturk A, et al. Self-application of complementary and alternative medicine by patients with gynecologic cancer. *Gynecologic & Obstetric Investigation*. 2007;64(2):75–81.

18. Boon H, Stewart M, Kennard MA, et al. Use of complementary/alternative medicine by breast cancer survivors in Ontario: prevalence and perceptions. [See comment.] *Journal of Clinical Oncology*. Jul 2000;18(13):2515–2521.

19. Boon HS, Olatunde F, Zick SM, Boon HS, Olatunde F, Zick SM. Trends in complementary/alternative medicine use by breast cancer survivors: comparing survey data from 1998 and 2005. *BMC Women's Health*. 2007;7:4.

20. Bower JE, Woolery A, Sternlieb B, et al. Yoga for cancer patients and survivors. *Cancer Control*. Jul 2005;12(3):165–171.

21. Chan JM, Elkin EP, Silva SJ, Broering JM, Latini DM, Carroll PR. Total and specific complementary and alternative medicine use in a large cohort of men with prostate cancer. *Urology*. Dec 2005;66(6):1223–1228.

22. Fasching PA, Thiel F, Nicolaisen-Murmann K, et al. Association of complementary methods with quality of life and life satisfaction in patients with
gynecologic and breast malignancies. *Supportive Care in Cancer.* Nov
2007;15(11):1277–1284.

23. Humpel N, Jones SC. Gaining insight into the what, why and where of complementary and alternative medicine use by cancer patients and survivors.
*European Journal of Cancer Care.* Sep 2006;15(4):362–368.

24. Klein J, Griffiths P. Acupressure for nausea and vomiting in cancer patients
receiving chemotherapy. *British Journal of Community Nursing.* Sep
2004;9(9):383–388.

25. Lawsin C, DuHamel K, Itzkowitz SH, et al. Demographic, medical, and psychosocial correlates to CAM use among survivors of colorectal cancer. *Supportive Care in Cancer.* May 2007;15(5):557–564.

26. Lee MM, Lin SS, Wrensch MR, Adler SR, Eisenberg D. Alternative therapies
used by women with breast cancer in four ethnic populations. *Journal of the
National Cancer Institute.* Jan 5 2000;92(1):42–47.

27. Lee MS, Pittler MH, Ernst E. Is Tai Chi an effective adjunct in cancer care? A
systematic review of controlled clinical trials. *Supportive Care in Cancer.* Jun
2007;15(6):597–601.

28. Mansky P, Sannes T, Wallerstedt D, et al. Tai chi chuan: mind-body practice or
exercise intervention? Studying the benefit for cancer survivors. *Integrative
Cancer Therapies.* Sep 2006;5(3):192–201.

29. Maskarinec G, Shumay DM, Kakai H, Gotay CC. Ethnic differences in complementary and alternative medicine use among cancer patients. *Journal of
Alternative & Complementary Medicine.* Dec 2000;6(6):531–538.

30. Mustian KM, Katula JA, Gill DL, et al. Tai Chi Chuan, health-related quality
of life and self-esteem: a randomized trial with breast cancer survivors. *Supportive Care in Cancer.* Dec 2004;12(12):871–876.

31. Mustian KM, Katula JA, Zhao H. A pilot study to assess the influence of tai chi
chuan on functional capacity among breast cancer survivors. *The Journal of
Supportive Oncology.* Mar 2006;4(3):139–145.

32. Smith JE, Richardson J, Hoffman C, et al. Mindfulness-Based Stress Reduction
as supportive therapy in cancer care: systematic review.[erratum appears in J
Adv Nurs. 2006 Mar;53(5):618]. *Journal of Advanced Nursing.* Nov
2005;52(3):315–327.

33. Wong-Kim E, Merighi JR. Complementary and alternative medicine for pain
management in U.S.- and foreign-born Chinese women with breast cancer.
*Journal of Health Care for the Poor & Underserved.* Nov 2007;18(4 Suppl):118–129.

34. Yoshimura K, Ueda N, Ichioka K, et al. Use of complementary and alternative
medicine by patients with urologic cancer: a prospective study at a single Japanese institution. [See comment.] *Supportive Care in Cancer.* Sep 2005;13(9):685–690.

35. Cassidy CM. Chinese medicine users in the United States. Part I: Utilization,
satisfaction, medical plurality. *Journal of Alternative and Complementary Medicine.* Spring 1998;4(1):17–27.

36. Ni H, Simile C, Hardy AM. Utilization of complementary and alternative medicine by United States adults: results from the 1999 national health interview survey. *Medical Care*. 2002;40(4):353–358.

37. Astin JA. Why patients use alternative medicine: results of a national study. [See comment.] *JAMA*. 1998;279(19):1548–1553.

38. Furnham A, Forey J. The attitudes, behaviors and beliefs of patients of conventional vs. complementary (alternative) medicine. *Journal of Clinical Psychology*. 1994;50(3):458–469.

39. Furnham A, Smith C. Choosing alternative medicine: a comparison of the beliefs of patients visiting a general practitioner and a homoeopath. *Social Science & Medicine*. 1988;26(7):685–689.

40. Kelner M, Wellman B. Who seeks alternative health care? A profile of the users of five modes of treatment. [See comment.] *Journal of Alternative & Complementary Medicine*. 1997;3(2):127–140.

41. Sharma U. *Complementary Medicine Today: Practitioners and Patients*. Routledge: London; 1992.

42. Siahpush M. Why do people favour alternative medicine? *Australian & New Zealand Journal of Public Health*. 1999;23(3):266–271.

43. Sirois FM, Gick ML. An investigation of the health beliefs and motivations of complementary medicine clients. *Social Science & Medicine*. 2002;55(6):1025–1037.

44. Votova K, Wister AV. Self-care dimensions of complementary and alternative medicine use among older adults. *Gerontology*. 2007;53(1):21–27.

45. Zhang L. A Closer Look at the Use of Asian Traditional Medical Practices among Asians Based on 2002 National Health Interview Survey *Author's analysis, unpublished*. San Francisco; 2008.

46. Mehta DH, Phillips RS, Davis RB, et al. Use of complementary and alternative therapies by Asian Americans. Results from the National Health Interview Survey. *Journal of General Internal Medicine*. Jun 2007;22(6):762–767.

47. Hsiao A-F, Wong MD, Goldstein MS, Becerra LS, Cheng EM, Wenger NS. Complementary and alternative medicine use among Asian-American subgroups: prevalence, predictors, and lack of relationship to acculturation and access to conventional health care. *Journal of Alternative & Complementary Medicine*. Dec 2006;12(10):1003–1010.

48. Ahn AC, Ngo-Metzger Q, Legedza ATR, Massagli MP, Clarridge BR, Phillips RS. Complementary and alternative medical therapy use among Chinese and Vietnamese Americans: prevalence, associated factors, and effects of patient-clinician communication. *American Journal of Public Health*. Apr 2006;96(4):647–653.

49. Bergman M. Census bureau projects tripling of Hispanic and Asian populations in 50 Years; Non-Hispanic Whites may drop to half of total population In: Commerce UDo, ed. Washington DC; 2004.

50. Pachter LM. Culture and clinical care. Folk illness beliefs and behaviors and their implications for health care delivery. *JAMA*. 1994;271(9):690–694.

51. Meleis AI, Lipson JG, Paul SM. Ethnicity and health among five Middle Eastern immigrant groups. *Nursing Research.* 1992;41(2):98–103.

52. Nilchaikovit T, Hill JM, Holland JC. The effects of culture on illness behavior and medical care. Asian and American differences. *General Hospital Psychiatry.* 1993;15(1):41–50.

53. Caralis PV, Davis B, Wright K, Marcial E. The influence of ethnicity and race on attitudes toward advance directives, life-prolonging treatments, and euthanasia. *Journal of Clinical Ethics.* 1993;4(2):155–165.

54. Brainard J, Zaharlick A. Changing health beliefs and behaviors of resettled Laotian refugees: ethnic variation in adaptation. *Social Science & Medicine.* 1989;29(7):845–852.

55. Gilman SC, Justice J, Saepharn K, Charles G. Use of traditional and modern health services by Laotian refugees. *Western Journal of Medicine.* Sep 1992;157(3):310–315.

56. Buchwald D, Panwala S, Hooton TM. Use of traditional health practices by Southeast Asian refugees in a primary care clinic. *Western Journal of Medicine.* May 1992;156(5):507–511.

57. Wu APW, Burke A, LeBaron S. Use of traditional medicine by immigrant Chinese patients. [See comment.] *Family Medicine.* Mar 2007;39(3):195–200.

58. Jenkins CN, Le T, McPhee SJ, Stewart S, Ha NT. Health care access and preventive care among Vietnamese immigrants: do traditional beliefs and practices pose barriers? *Social Science & Medicine.* Oct 1996;43(7):1049–1056.

59. Ferro MA, Leis A, Doll R, et al. The impact of acculturation on the use of traditional Chinese medicine in newly diagnosed Chinese cancer patients. *Supportive Care in Cancer.* Aug 2007;15(8):985–992.

60. Kim J, Chan MM. Factors influencing preferences for alternative medicine by Korean Americans. *American Journal of Chinese Medicine.* 2004;32(2):321–329.

61. Pearl WS, Leo P, Tsang WO. Use of Chinese therapies among Chinese patients seeking emergency department care. *Annals of Emergency Medicine.* Dec 1995;26(6):735–738.

62. Su D, Li L, Pagan JA. Acculturation and the use of complementary and alternative medicine. *Social Science & Medicine.* Jan 2008;66(2):439–453.

63. Holliday I. Traditional medicines in modern societies: an exploration of integrationist options through East Asian experience. *Journal of Medicine and Philosophy.* Jun 2003;28(3):373–389.

64. Farrell TW. The complementarity and substitution between unconventional and mainstream medicine among racial and ethnic groups in the United States. *Health Services Research.* Apr 2007;42(2):811–826.

65. Bonafede M, Dick A, Noyes K, et al. The effect of acupuncture utilization on healthcare utilization. *Medical Care.* Jan 2008;46(1):41–48.

66. Weeks J. Comment on Cleary-Guida et al.: CAM coverage. Survey outcomes pose more critical questions.[comment]. *Journal of Alternative & Complementary Medicine.* 2001;7(3):275–276.

67. Pagan JA, Pauly MV. Access to conventional medical care and the use of complementary and alternative medicine. *Health Affairs*. 2005;24(1):255–262.

68. Pagan JA, Pauly MV. Complementary and alternative medicine: personal preference or low cost option? *LDI Issue Brief*. 2004;10(4):1–4.

69. Jose VM, Bhalla A, Sharma N, Hota D, Sivaprasad S, Pandhi P. Study of association between use of complementary and alternative medicine and noncompliance with modern medicine in patients presenting to the emergency department. [See comment.] *Journal of Postgraduate Medicine*. Apr–Jun 2007;53(2):96–101.

70. Tilburt JC, Dy SM, Weeks K, et al. Associations between home remedy use and a validated self-reported adherence measure in an urban African-American population with poorly controlled hypertension. *Journal of the National Medical Association*. Jan 2008;100(1):91–97.

71. Liu C, Lerch V, Weber K, et al. Association between complementary and alternative medicine use and adherence to highly active antiretroviral therapy in the Women's Interagency HIV Study. *Journal of Alternative & Complementary Medicine*. Dec 2007;13(10):1053–1056.

72. Wutoh AK, Brown CM, Kumoji EK, et al. Antiretroviral adherence and use of alternative therapies among older HIV-infected adults. *Journal of the National Medical Association*. Jul–Aug 2001;93(7–8):243–250.

73. O'Donnell DC, Brown CM, Piziak VK. Alternative therapy use and adherence to antihyperlipidemic drugs in a lipid clinic. *American Journal of Health-System Pharmacy*. Jun 1 2001;58(11):1017–1021.

74. Liu J. The use of herbal medicines in early drug development for the treatment of HIV infections and AIDS. *Expert Opinion on Investigational Drugs*. Sep 2007;16(9):1355–1364.

75. Li Z, Li LJ, Sun Y, Li J. Identification of natural compounds with anti-hepatitis B virus activity from Rheum palmatum L. ethanol extract. *Chemotherapy*. 2007;53(5):320–326.

76. Kwee SH, Tan HH, Marsman A, Wauters C. The effect of Chinese herbal medicines (CHM) on menopausal symptoms compared to hormone replacement therapy (HRT) and placebo. *Maturitas*. Sep 20 2007;58(1):83–90.

77. Hsu CH, Hwang KC, Chao CL, et al. The lesson of supplementary treatment with Chinese medicine on severe laboratory-confirmed SARS patients. *American Journal of Chinese Medicine*. 2006;34(6):927–935.

78. Liu J, Manheimer E, Shi Y, Gluud C. Chinese herbal medicine for severe acute respiratory syndrome: a systematic review and meta-analysis. *Journal of Alternative and Complementary Medicine*. Dec 2004;10(6):1041–1051.

79. Liu P, Hu YY, Liu C, et al. Multicenter clinical study on Fuzhenghuayu capsule against liver fibrosis due to chronic hepatitis B. *World Journal of Gastroenterology*. May 21 2005;11(19):2892–2899.

80. Li WL, Zheng HC, Bukuru J, De Kimpe N. Natural medicines used in the traditional Chinese medical system for therapy of diabetes mellitus. *Journal of Ethnopharmacology*. May 2004;92(1):1–21.

81. Cheng JH, Liu WS, Li ZM, Wang ZG. A clinical study on global TCM therapy in treating senile advanced non-small cell lung cancer. *Chinese Journal of Integrative Medicine*. Dec 2007;13(4):269–274.

82. Li XM, Srivastava K. Traditional Chinese medicine for the therapy of allergic disorders. *Current Opinion in Otolaryngology & Head and Neck Surgery*. Jun 2006;14(3):191–196.

83. Hijikata Y, Yasuhara A, Yoshida Y, Sento S. Traditional Chinese medicine treatment of epilepsy. *Journal of Alternative and Complementary Medicine*. Sep 2006;12(7):673–677.

84. Melchart D, Hager S, Hager U, Liao J, Weidenhammer W, Linde K. Treatment of patients with chronic headaches in a hospital for traditional Chinese medicine in Germany. A randomised, waiting-list-controlled trial. *Complementary Therapies in Medicine*. Jun–Sep 2004;12(2–3):71–78.

85. Koo J, Desai R. Traditional Chinese medicine in dermatology. *Dermatology Therapy*. 2003;16(2):98–105.

86. Gong X, Sucher NJ. Stroke therapy in traditional Chinese medicine (TCM): prospects for drug discovery and development. *Phytomedicine*. Jul 2002;9(5):478–484.

87. Bensoussan A. Establishing evidence for Chinese medicine: a case example of irritable bowel syndrome. *Zhonghua Yi Xue Za Zhi (Taipei)*. Sep 2001;64(9):487–492.

88. Facco E, Liguori A, Petti F, et al. Traditional acupuncture in migraine: a controlled, randomized study. *Headache*. Mar 2008;48(3):398–407.

89. Alecrim-Andrade J, Maciel-Junior JA, Carne X, Severino Vasconcelos GM, Correa-Filho HR. Acupuncture in migraine prevention: a randomized sham controlled study with 6-months posttreatment follow-up. *The Clinical Journal of Pain*. Feb 2008;24(2):98–105.

90. Endres HG, Bowing G, Diener HC, et al. Acupuncture for tension-type headache: a multicentre, sham-controlled, patient-and observer-blinded, randomised trial. *The Journal of Headache and Pain*. Oct 2007;8(5):306–314.

91. Flachskampf FA, Gallasch J, Gefeller O, et al. Randomized trial of acupuncture to lower blood pressure. *Circulation*. Jun 19 2007;115(24):3121–3129.

92. Chen HY, Shi Y, Ng CS, Chan SM, Yung KK, Zhang QL. Auricular acupuncture treatment for insomnia: a systematic review. *Journal of Alternative and Complementary Medicine*. Jul–Aug 2007;13(6):669–676.

93. Zhong ZG, Cai H, Li XL, et al. [Effect of acupuncture combined with massage of sole on sleeping quality of the patient with insomnia]. *Zhongguo Zhenjiu*. Jun 2008;28(6):411–413.

94. Ezzo J, Streitberger K, Schneider A. Cochrane systematic reviews examine P6 acupuncture-point stimulation for nausea and vomiting. *Journal of Alternative and Complementary Medicine*. Jun 2006;12(5):489–495.

95. Allen JJ, Schnyer RN, Chambers AS, Hitt SK, Moreno FA, Manber R. Acupuncture for depression: a randomized controlled trial. *Journal of Clinical Psychiatry*. Nov 2006;67(11):1665–1673.

96. MacPherson H, Thorpe L, Thomas K, Geddes D. Acupuncture for depression: first steps toward a clinical evaluation. *Journal of Alternative and Complementary Medicine.* Dec 2004;10(6):1083–1091.

97. Luo H, Meng F, Jia Y, Zhao X. Clinical research on the therapeutic effect of the electro-acupuncture treatment in patients with depression. *Psychiatry and Clinical Neurosciences.* Dec 1998;52 Suppl:S338–340.

98. MacPherson H, Gould AJ, Fitter M. Acupuncture for low back pain: results of a pilot study for a randomized controlled trial. *Complementary Therapies in Medicine.* Jun 1999;7(2):83–90.

99. Feng JT, Hu CP, Li XZ. Dorsal root ganglion: the target of acupuncture in the treatment of asthma. *Advances in Therapy.* May–Jun 2007;24(3):598–602.

100. Bai YP, Fu JY. [Clinical observation on the regularity of acupuncture-induced body-reduction in excess-heat-type obesity patients ]. *Zhen Ci Yan Jiu.* Apr 2007;32(2):128–131.

101. Joos S, Wildau N, Kohnen R, et al. Acupuncture and moxibustion in the treatment of ulcerative colitis: a randomized controlled study. *Scandinavian Journal of Gastroenterology.* Sep 2006;41(9):1056–1063.

102. Jia J, Wang Q, Zhang T, et al. Treatment of ankylosing spondylitis with medicated moxibustion plus salicylazosulfapyridine and methotrexate—a report of 30 cases. *Journal of Traditional Chinese Medicine.* Mar 2006;26(1):26–28.

103. Chen D, Luo LP, Hong YB, et al. [Controlled study on needle-pricking therapy combined with spinal massage for treatment of ankylosing spondylitis]. *Zhongguo Zhenjiu.* Mar 2008;28(3):163–166.

104. Yu Y, Kang J. Clinical studies on treatment of chronic prostatitis with acupuncture and mild moxibustion. *Journal of Traditional Chinese Medicine.* Sep 2005;25(3):177–181.

105. Eng ML, Lyons KE, Greene MS, et al. Open-label trial regarding the use of acupuncture and yin tui na in Parkinson's disease outpatients: a pilot study on efficacy, tolerability, and quality of life. *Journal of Alternative & Complementary Medicine.* May 2006;12(4):395–399.

106. Hu WQ, Xu SW. Clinical observation on treatment of cervicogenic headache with tui na and acupuncture. *Zhong Xi Yi Jie He Xue Bao/Journal of Chinese Integrative Medicine.* Jul 2005;3(4):310–311.

107. Ernst E. Complementary or alternative therapies for osteoarthritis. *Nature Clinical Practice Rheumatology.* Feb 2006;2(2):74–80.

108. Qin XY, Li XX, Berghea F, et al. [Comparative study on Chinese medicine and western medicine for treatment of osteoarthritis of the knee in Caucasian patients]. *Zhongguo Zhenjiu.* Jun 2008;28(6):459–462.

109. Yun SP, Jung WS, Park SU, et al. Effects of moxibustion on the recovery of post-stroke urinary symptoms. *American Journal of Chinese Medicine.* 2007;35(6):947–954.

110. Xiaoxiang Z. Jinger moxibustion for treatment of cervical vertigo –a report of 40 cases. *Journal of Traditional Chinese Medicine.* Mar 2006;26(1):17–18.

111. Liang F, Li Y, Yu S, et al. A multicentral randomized control study on clinical acupuncture treatment of Bell's palsy. *Journal of Traditional Chinese Medicine.* Mar 2006;26(1):3–7.

112. Kung YY, Chen FP, Hwang SJ. The different immunomodulation of indirect moxibustion on normal subjects and patients with systemic lupus erythematosus. *American Journal of Chinese Medicine.* 2006;34(1):47–56.

113. da Silva GD, Lorenzi-Filho G, Lage LV. Effects of yoga and the addition of tui na in patients with fibromyalgia. *Journal of Alternative & Complementary Medicine.* Dec 2007;13(10):1107–1113.

114. Yang MH, Wu SC, Lin JG, et al. The efficacy of acupressure for decreasing agitated behaviour in dementia: a pilot study. *Journal of Clinical Nursing.* Feb 2007;16(2):308–315.

115. White AR, Moody RC, Campbell JL. Acupressure for smoking cessation–a pilot study. *BMC Complementary & Alternative Medicine.* 2007;7:8.

116. Jun EM, Chang S, Kang DH, et al. Effects of acupressure on dysmenorrhea and skin temperature changes in college students: a non-randomized controlled trial. *International Journal of Nursing Studies.* Aug 2007;44(6):973–981.

117. Bu TW, Tian XL, Wang SJ, et al. [Comparison and analysis of therapeutic effects of different therapies on simple obesity]. *Zhongguo Zhenjiu.* May 2007;27(5):337–340.

118. Chen GL, Xiao GM, Zheng XL. [Observation on therapeutic effect of multiple cupping at back-shu points on chronic fatigue syndrome]. *Zhongguo Zhenjiu.* Jun 2008;28(6):405–407.

119. Huang YL. [Cupping-bloodletting therapy of Saudi Arabia and its clinical application]. *Zhongguo Zhenjiu.* May 2008;28(5):375–377.

120. Lu YY, Liu LG. [Treatment of cough and asthma with blood-letting puncturing and cupping: a report of 3 cases]. *Zhong Xi Yi Jie He Xue Bao/Journal of Chinese Integrative Medicine.* 2004 Jul 2004;2(4):244.

121. Yao J, Li NF. [Clinical observation on pricking and blood-letting and cupping with a three-edge needle for treatment of acute eczema]. *Zhongguo Zhenjiu.* Jun 2007;27(6):424–426.

122. Alexander GK, Taylor AG, Innes KE, et al. Contextualizing the effects of yoga therapy on diabetes management: a review of the social determinants of physical activity. *Family & Community Health.* Jul–Sep 2008;31(3):228–239.

123. Elder C. Ayurveda for diabetes mellitus: a review of the biomedical literature. *Alternative Therapies in Health & Medicine.* Jan–Feb 2004;10(1):44–50.

124. Cohen D, Townsend RR. Yoga and hypertension. *Journal of Clinical Hypertension.* Oct 2007;9(10):800–801.

125. Garfinkel M, Schumacher HR, Jr. Yoga. *Rheumatic Diseases Clinics of North America.* 2000 Feb 2000;26(1):125–132.

126. Graves N, Krepcho M, Mayo HG, et al. Clinical inquiries. Does yoga speed healing for patients with low back pain? *Journal of Family Practice.* Aug 2004;53(8):661–662.

127. Nespor K. Pain management and yoga. *International Journal of Psychosomatics.* 1991;38(1–4):76–81.

128. Jayasinghe SR. Yoga in cardiac health (a review). *European Journal of Cardiovascular Prevention & Rehabilitation.* Oct 2004;11(5):369–375.

129. Mamtani R. Ayurveda and yoga in cardiovascular diseases. *Cardiology in Review.* May–Jun 2005;13(3):155–162.

130. Kirkwood G, Rampes H, Tuffrey V, Richardson J, Pilkington K. Yoga for anxiety: a systematic review of the research evidence. *British Journal of Sports Medicine.* Dec 2005;39(12):884–891; discussion 891.

131. Pilkington K, Kirkwood G, Rampes H, et al. Yoga for depression: the research evidence. *Journal of Affective Disorders.* Dec 2005;89(1–3):13–24.

132. Yadav V, Bourdette D. Complementary and alternative medicine: is there a role in multiple sclerosis? *Current Neurology & Neuroscience Reports.* May 2006;6(3):259–267.

133. Kobayashi H, Mizuno N, Teramae H, et al. Diet instruction for Japanese traditional food in therapy for atopic dermatitis. *Advances in Experimental Medicine & Biology.* 2004;546:281–296.

134. Huo HM, Yang XP. [Observation on therapeutic effect of pricking blood therapy combined with acupuncture on herpes zoster]. *Zhongguo Zhenjiu.* Oct 2007;27(10):729–730.

135. Schwickert ME, Saha FJ, Braun M, et al. [Gua Sha for migraine in inpatient withdrawal therapy of headache due to medication overuse]. *Forschende Komplementarmedizin (2006).* Oct 2007;14(5):297–300.

136. Yeh GY, Wang C, Wayne PM, et al. The effect of tai chi exercise on blood pressure: a systematic review. *Preventive Cardiology.* 2008;11(2):82–89.

137. Lee MS, Pittler MH, Kim MS, Ernst E. Tai chi for Type 2 diabetes: a systematic review. *Diabetic Medicine.* Feb 2008;25(2):240–241.

138. Voukelatos A, Cumming RG, Lord SR, et al. A randomized, controlled trial of tai chi for the prevention of falls: the Central Sydney tai chi trial. [See comment.] *Journal of the American Geriatrics Society.* Aug 2007;55(8):1185–1191.

139. Lee MS, Pittler MH, Ernst E. Tai chi for rheumatoid arthritis: systematic review. *Rheumatology.* Nov 2007;46(11):1648–1651.

140. Guo X, Zhou B, Nishimura T, Teramukai S, Fukushima M. Clinical effect of qigong practice on essential hypertension: a meta-analysis of randomized controlled trials. *Journal of Alternative and Complementary Medicine.* Jan–Feb 2008;14(1):27–37.

141. Lee MS, Chen KW, Sancier KM, Ernst E. Qigong for cancer treatment: a systematic review of controlled clinical trials. *Acta Oncologia.* 2007;46(6):717–722.

142. Husted C, Pham L, Hekking A, Niederman R. Improving quality of life for people with chronic conditions: the example of t'ai chi and multiple sclerosis. *Alternative Therapies in Health and Medicine.* Sep 1999;5(5):70–74.

# Chapter 37

# Addressing the Impact of Tobacco on Asian Americans: A Model for Change

*Rod Lew*

## BACKGROUND

Tobacco has had a deep and resounding impact on many communities within the United States, including Asian Americans, Native Hawaiians and Pacific Islanders (AANHPIs). From its sacred use among American Indians to its commercialization and eventual globalization, tobacco has had a long, complex relationship and history with the United States, particularly for communities of color (Task Force on Advancing Parity 2002). Tobacco played a critical historical role in changing the status of Africans from that of indentured servants to slaves in the seventeenth century (Headen 2001), and later it led to the employment of African Americans in tobacco manufacturing plants, often with poor working conditions (Korstad 2007). The tobacco industry's targeted marketing of Asian Americans and other communities of color has also had tremendous impact. Combined with the high prevalence of tobacco use among some AANHPI subgroups, Asian Americans, Native Hawaiians, and Pacific Islanders are disproportionately impacted by tobacco.

Tobacco is the only product that, when used as intended, is harmful to humans. Tobacco is the single most preventable cause of death for Asian Americans. Tobacco use is highly ingrained in Asian American communities, where it is considered socially and culturally acceptable. The exceptionally diverse AANHPI population, composed of more than fifty different ethnicities and more than 100 different languages and dialects, reside in the fifty U.S. states and six U.S.-associated Pacific Island jurisdictions (U.S. Census 2000). Among some Asian American ethnic subgroups, tobacco prevalence is very high, and is often associated with very high poverty levels. This has served to facilitate the tobacco industry's efforts to recruit new Asian American smokers by creating a pervasive advertising presence in many Asian American neighborhoods, especially low-income environments.

When faced with the challenge of countering tobacco influences, the Asian American community, like other priority populations,[1] have had fewer resources and lack of community-tailored approaches to combat tobacco than the mainstream population. The disproportionately greater impact of tobacco on Asian Americans and other priority populations and the tobacco control resource inequities underscore tobacco's role as a "social justice" or "health justice" issue that requires a new framework for tobacco control. Tobacco's impact on Asian Americans must be addressed through a comprehensive and strategic approach that includes not only community-tailored tobacco prevention and cessation strategies but also capacity-building efforts to develop community infrastructure, community leadership development and a multi-prong policy change approach.

This chapter will explore how tobacco has created an inequitable burden of tobacco-related disease and death for Asian Americans and present a comprehensive framework that integrates critical components, principles, and strategies for addressing tobacco disparities within the diverse Asian American community.

## HISTORY OF TOBACCO FOR ASIANS AND ASIAN AMERICANS

Tobacco has had a long, storied history throughout many parts of Asia and the Pacific. In the seventeenth century, tobacco was introduced to Asia by the Portuguese (U.S. DHHS 1994). Soon after its introduction, tobacco became widely distributed throughout much of Asia and parts of the Pacific. Tobacco took on multiple forms such as cigarettes (including clove flavored), pipes, tobacco mixed with betel nut, smokeless tobacco, bidis, and hookahs. These various forms of tobacco use have become particularly important in twentieth- and twenty-first-century tobacco industry strategies to recruit new smokers, particularly youth, in the United States and other parts of the world.

As tobacco spread across Asia and the Pacific, its use became ingrained in Asian cultures, particularly among men. Tobacco was not traditionally used in Native Hawaiian and Pacific Islander communities. But the commercialization of tobacco led to a high prevalence of tobacco use among both Pacific Islander men and women. In some Asian cultures, tobacco was used as a medicine and also as a protection against mosquitoes. In addition, tobacco had unique historical significance in Southeast Asia during wartime. During the Vietnam War, Hmong soldiers, recruited by the CIA to fight for the United States, were sometimes offered payment for their services in cigarettes. During the genocide of Cambodians during the 1970s, prisoners of the Khmer Rouge were offered cigarettes as a way to stem hunger. Tobacco was also offered as gifts during weddings and some religious ceremonies. As a consequence of the permeation of tobacco within many parts of Asia, Asians came to the United States as immigrants or refugees, with tobacco use already very much a part of their lives.

These factors helped to promote and encourage tobacco use within a cultural and community context that results in a high prevalence of tobacco use among certain Asian American groups and, consequently, in exposure to tobacco-related diseases.

## Tobacco Industry Targeting

Internal tobacco industry documents have provided evidence that the industry actively targeted Asian American communities with the marketing of their tobacco products (Muggli 2002). One example of a comprehensive marketing campaign, representative of other tobacco companies, was Philip Morris' strategic action plan involving the three initiatives of PUSH, PULL, and CORPORATE GOODWILL, developed by the marketing firm FraserSmith. The PUSH strategy recognized the high number of Asian retailers and their potential role in promoting tobacco products. Ironically, this strategy included a "cultural sensitivity program" and the important "Asian objective" of first forming relationships in a business environment. The PULL strategy aimed at increasing the number of Asian American consumers of tobacco through promotional events (the first being the Nisei Week Japanese Festival in Los Angeles), specific brand targeting (particularly Marlboro cigarettes), and cultural sensitivity advertising (as during Chinese New Years). The third strategy, CORPORATE GOODWILL, focused on building a positive image for the tobacco companies, by nurturing relationships with Asian American community leaders and donating monies to community organizations and events.

During the 1980s and 1990s, the tobacco companies recognized the opportunity to increase their consumer base in the Asian American community through these and other strategies. The tobacco industry also recognized the importance of tailoring and targeting their market strategy for Asian immigrants compared to later generations of Asian Americans. "First Generation Asians are important because they represent potential new smokers. However, they are the most difficult to reach due to a language and cultural factors. Later generations are more assimilated and easier to reach by mainstream brand marketing and media approaches" (Muggli 2002).

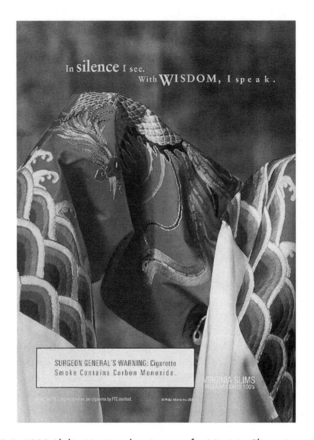

**Figure 37.1** 1999 Philip Morris advertisement for Virginia Slims cigarettes.

Not surprisingly then, studies have shown that Asian American neighborhoods had some of the highest concentration of cigarette billboards, and one of the most "tobacco supportive" environments among all ethnic neighborhoods (Wildey 1992). And when you consider that many Asian American immigrants are exposed to targeted marketing of tobacco products both in their home countries and in the United States, a double dose of targeted marketing or "double targeting" effect is experienced (Lew 1999).

The tobacco industry also saw the potential of recruiting new smokers from a segment of the Asian American community that had not previously had high smoking rates—Asian women and Asian youth. A 1990 Lorillard memo highlighted this strategy, "Investigate the possibility of utilizing men and women and targeting youth in advertising strategies . . . The literature suggests that Asian-American women are

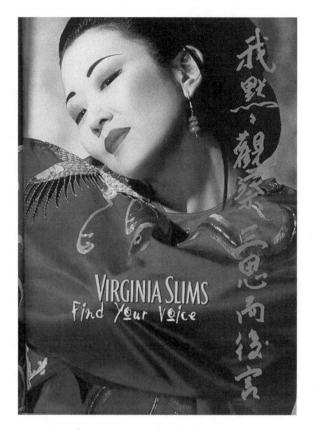

我默，觀察，息而後言

**Figure 37.1** *(Continued)*

smoking more as they believe they should enjoy the same freedom as men" (Muggli 2002).

Even after the 1998 Masters Settlement Agreement (MSA)—an agreement between the attorneys general of forty-six states and the tobacco industry—was reached, supposedly to limit the industry's blatant advertising and promotion tactics, it could not change the predictive impact of the Lorillard memo. In 1999, Philip Morris launched a $40 million Virginia Slims campaign targeting ethnic minority women (including Asian American women), ironically called "Find Your Voice" (see Figure 36.1). Philip Morris also hired corporate goodwill "ambassadors" in priority populations, including the Asian American community, to offer tobacco industry sponsorship and funds in exchange for legitimacy in diverse communities. These campaigns and activities are a few of the many tobacco industry strategies to culturally tailor their targeted marketing to Asian Americans over the past three decades.

## TOBACCO USE AMONG ASIAN AMERICANS

### Smoking Prevalence

Although national tobacco use data is often presented to show that smoking prevalence in the United States is lowest among Asian Americans (16%) of all ethnic groups, this aggregated figure masks startlingly high rates in certain Asian American subgroups. When the data is disaggregated by ethnicity, gender, and immigration status, local community studies (see Table 36.1) have shown that males among certain Asian American ethnic subgroups have some of the *highest* smoking prevalence in the United States, with a range between 48–72 percent among Laotian and 39–71 percent among Cambodian men, for example (Lew 2003), well above the Healthy People 2010 Objectives of 12 percent adult smoking prevalence. Laotian and Cambodian communities also have some of the highest rates of poverty among Asians and in the nation.

Although smoking prevalence among Asian American females has traditionally been low, it is on the rise, perhaps a result of increased targeting of Asian women and girls by the tobacco industry. Additionally, non-smoking females are likely to be affected by secondhand smoke because of high rates of smoking among males in their communities. As Asian American immigrants become more acculturated, their smoking prevalence may approximate that of the general population, with the high prevalence of Asian American immigrant males decreasing somewhat and that of Asian American females increasing. For Asian American women that issue is particularly critical to monitor in terms of future trends and targeted campaigns by the tobacco industry.

Aggregation of tobacco use data for AANHPIs masks the high prevalence of tobacco use among Native Hawaiians and other Pacific Islanders as well. As a result, there is a critical need to analyze tobacco's impact for Native Hawaiians and Pacific Islanders separately from that of Asian Americans. Native Hawaiians have a high prevalence of tobacco use among both males and females (Kaholokula 2005). In other Pacific Islands, tobacco use (particularly mixed with betel nut) is rampant among both males and females. In 2001 Guam, one of the U.S.-associated jurisdictions with a predominant Pacific Islander and Asian population, had the second highest prevalence of adult smoking in the United States and its territories.

### Health Consequences

Tobacco results in multiple adverse health impacts and consequences on those who use it as well as on those exposed to secondhand smoke. For Cambodian, Korean, Laotian, and Vietnamese men, the highest cancer incidence is from lung cancer (Miller 2008). Heart disease and stroke are rated as the second and third leading causes of mortality for Asian

**Table 37.1** Current Adult Smokers by Gender for Selected Asian American Populations Disaggregated by Ethnic Subgroup

|  | Men (%) | Women (%) | Place and Sampling Frame |
|---|---|---|---|
| **Cambodian** | | | |
| (1985) Rumbaut et al., 1989 | 70.7 | 12.9 | San Diego County, CA |
| (1989) CDC, 1992b | 32.8 | — | Washington State, clinic-based |
| (1995) Chen, 2001 | 38.8 | 21.5 | Franklin County, OH, pop-based survey |
| **Chinese** | | | |
| (1989-90) CDC, 1992a | 28.1 | 1.2 | Oakland Chinatown, pop-based survey |
| (1996) Thridandam, 1998 | 16.5 | 2.6 | California, pop-based survey |
| (1997) Yu et al., 2002 | 33.6 | 2.1 | Chicago Chinatown, pop-based survey |
| (2000) Ma et al., 2002 | 31.8 | 15.3 | PA and New Jersey, com-based |
| (2000) Fu et al., 2003 | 25.0 | 3.0 | Philadelphia, PA, clinic-based |
| (2001) Maxwell et al., 2005 | 14.3 | 2.6 | California, pop-based survey |
| (2003) CHIS 2005 | 14.4 | 2.1 | California, pop-based survey |
| (2004) Shelley et al., 2004 | 29.0 | 4.0 | New York City, pop-based survey |
| **Chinese-Vietnamese** | | | |
| (1985) Rumbaut et al., 1989 | 54.5 | 1.7 | San Diego County, CA |
| **Filipino** | | | |
| (2001) Maxwell et al., 2005 | 24.2 | 10.6 | California, pop-based survey |
| (2003) CHIS, 2005 | 25.3 | — | California, pop-based survey |
| **Hmong** | | | |
| (1985) Rumbaut et al., 1989 | 26.0 | 1.7 | San Diego County, CA |
| **Korean** | | | |
| (1989) CDC, 1992b | 38.5 | — | Washington State, clinic-based |
| (1994–95) Lew et al., 2001 | 38.7 | 6.0 | Alameda County, CA, pop-based survey |
| (1998) Juon et al., 2003 | 26.1 | — | Maryland, community-based |
| (1998) Kim et al., 2000 | 38.52 | 6.9 | Chicago, IL, pop-based survey |
| Lee et al., 2000 | 6.9 | 8.5 | Greater New York |

**Table 37.1** (Continued)

|  | Men (%) | Women (%) | Place and Sampling Frame |
|---|---|---|---|
| (2000) Ma et al., 2002 | 41.5 | 11.3 | Pennsylvania and New Jersey, com-based |
| (2001) Hofstetter et al., 2004 | 31.2 | 3.7 | California, pop-based survey |
| (2003) CHIS, 2005 | 36.5 | 8.3 | California, pop-based survey |
| Laotian |  |  |  |
| (1987) Levin et al., 1988 | 72.0 | – | Cook County, IL, pop-based survey |
| (1989) CDC, 1992b | 51.2 | – | Washington State, clinic-based |
| (1995) Chen, 2001 | 48.2 | 10.8 | Franklin County, Ohio, pop-based survey |
| South Asians (2001) * | 26.0 | – | NY taxi drivers, nonprobability sample |
| Vietnamese |  |  |  |
| (1985) Rumbaut et al., 1989 | 64.7 | 0.0 | San Diego County, CA |
| (1987) Jenkins et al., 1990 | 56.0 | 9.0 | Oakland, San Francisco, CA, pop-based |
| (1989) Jenkins et al., 1995 | 39.1 | 2.3 | SF Bay Area, Los Angeles, CA, pop-based |
| (1989) CDC, 1992b | 41.7 | – | Washington State, clinic-based |
| (1991) CDC, 1992a | 34.7 | 0.4 | California, pop-based survey |
| (1994) Wiecha et al, 1998 | 43.2 | – | Massachusetts, pop-based survey |
| (1995) Chen, 2001 | 43.3 | 9.3 | Franklin County, OH, pop-based survey |
| (2000) Ma et al., 2002 | 50.8 | 18.8 | Pennsylvania and New Jersey, com-based |
| (2003) CHIS, 2005 | 29.9 | 2.4 | California, pop-based survey |
| (2005) Xu et al., 2005 | 39.3 | 2.1 | Alabama, community-based |

This table is adapted from Lew R and Tanjasiri SP. Slowing the epidemic of tobacco use among Asian Americans and Pacific Islanders. *American Journal of Public Health* 2003;93:764–768; and from Kim SS et al. Tobacco use and dependence in Asian Americans: A review of the literature. *Nicotine & Tobacco Research* 2007;9(2):169–184.
* From unpublished data

Americans as a whole. For those who use smokeless tobacco, connection with oral cancers is strong although data are not readily available for specific Asian American groups.

## Secondhand Smoke

It is estimated that 50,000 Americans die from secondhand smoke each year. The limited data available suggests that 23 percent of children in Asian American households are exposed to tobacco smoke. This is more than twice the goal for the United States of under 10 percent. A large percentage of Asian Americans also work in the service industry in jobs that have traditionally been known as having high exposure to secondhand smoke. These jobs include restaurant workers, hotel employees, and even casino workers. Although some clean indoor air policies have been successfully implemented in hotels and restaurants, other cities and states in which Asian Americans work and live may not successfully enforce smoke-free policies. And other states such as Nevada have continued to resist approving smoke-free casinos.

## Other Forms of Tobacco

Tobacco use among Asian Americans is more than just cigarette smoking. Tobacco mixed with betel nut has become a major health issue in some parts of the Pacific. Betel nut—traditionally used by peoples in the Pacific, Southeast Asia, and South Asia—has been an easy habit to add tobacco to, an integration of the old and the new. In some places, such as Palau, the prevalence of tobacco use mixed with betel nut is more than 50 percent for both women and men (58.3 percent for men and 67.2 percent for women) (Ysaol 1996).

Other forms of tobacco use inherent in parts of Asia have also risen to a high level in the United States not just among Asian Americans but also among other segments of the population, such as young people. Bidis, small sticks of cheap tobacco originally popular in India, have skyrocketed among youth in the United States. The use of hookahs, traditional in parts of Asia and the Middle East, has risen as well as the number of hookah bars.

## Tobacco Initiation and Tobacco Use among Asian American Youth

Most American smokers start smoking before the age of eighteen. The 2000 National Youth Tobacco Survey (NYTS) showed that Asian American youth face the highest increase of smoking prevalence of all ethnic groups from seventh to twelfth grades (Appleyard 2001). Some Pacific Islander groups, such as Native Hawaiian girls, have the highest smoking prevalence among all ethnic groups in middle school.

In addition, the 2000 NYTS showed that Asian American youth had the second-highest rate of menthol use, second only to African American youth. This is significant in terms of both choice of cigarettes but also perhaps in how the tobacco industry's advertising targets or impacts Asian American youth. The influence of tobacco industry targeting on the "hip hop" generation, such as the Kool Mixx campaign, and its impact on Asian Americans needs to be further studied.

Although there is growing literature about tobacco initiation among Asian American youth, most research has not disaggregated the data by gender, ethnicity, and acculturation. Tobacco initiation has been associated with alcohol use prevalence, sexual activity, and even performance in school. Another study has argued that Asian American youth are likely to have less media receptivity to tobacco industry marketing compared to other ethnic groups (Chen 2003). While this may represent a key protective factor in the early teens, the impact on later years (later high school and early college years) still needs further analysis.

## LACK OF INCLUSION IN THE TOBACCO CONTROL MOVEMENT

Tobacco control has been described as one of public health's major achievements of the second half of the twentieth century. Instrumental to the success of tobacco control has been the "paradigm shift" from individual behavioral change to an environmental or policy approach to public health. For nearly half a century, this mainstream tobacco control policy approach ranging from Surgeon General's reports, federal and state tax on tobacco products, clean indoor air legislation and limitations on cigarette advertising on television have resulted in major declines in both cigarette per capita consumption and smoking prevalence. However, even with these recognized landmarks in tobacco control, Asian Americans and priority populations are still disproportionately impacted by tobacco, and tobacco inequities still exist. Although the 1998 Masters Settlement Agreement (MSA) led to some restrictions on tobacco industry advertising and promotions and to some new funding and resources for addressing tobacco issues for priority populations—most notably through the American Legacy Foundation—its long term, sustainable impact remains to be seen. A survey of how states spent their MSA monies dedicated to tobacco control showed very limited funding for Asian Americans, other communities of color, and lesbian, gay, bisexual, and transgender (LGBT) communities to address tobacco (Themba-Nixon 2002). The findings of this study reflect only one recent example of a much longer, historical lack of inclusion and lack of parity for priority populations in the tobacco control movement.

Although the passage of Proposition 99, a 1988 California tobacco tax initiative, resulted initially in the funding of several Asian American community organizations to implement local tobacco control programs, there were very few tobacco control efforts tailored for Asian Americans in other parts of the country during the early 1990s (Lew 1996). Later in that decade, other states began to support local and regional tobacco control efforts for Asian Americans and other priority populations, but the disparities in funding, resources, and initiatives continued in many states and regions. And even in some cases, where there was early support for funding for tailored approaches to tobacco control for Asian Americans, this changed over time based on changing priorities, budgets, and leadership within state and local tobacco control programs. For example, the California Tobacco Control Section, initially a pioneer and champion for addressing priority populations in tobacco control, drastically reduced funding for local tobacco control programs and statewide networks tailored for Asian Americans and other priority populations. The lack of inclusion within the tobacco control movement and inequities in funding and resources underscore the need for a new framework or paradigm—one that includes components of capacity building, leadership development, parity in resources, and multi-prong policy initiatives tailored for Asian Americans and other priority populations.

## A STRATEGIC FRAMEWORK FOR TOBACCO CONTROL AMONG ASIAN AMERICANS

In 1994, Asian Pacific Partners for Empowerment, Advocacy and Leadership (APPEAL) was founded as a national network to provide support for Asian American, Native Hawaiian, and Pacific Islander tobacco control and other health justice efforts with funding from the Centers for Disease Control and Prevention, Office on Smoking and Health. Over the past fifteen years, APPEAL has helped to build a national tobacco control movement focusing on the priority areas of Capacity building, Leadership development, Education, Advocacy and Network development (CLEAN). Some significant accomplishments include the strategic assessment of the impact of tobacco on Asian American, Native Hawaiian, and Pacific Islander communities through a community readiness model; the training of nearly 600 community advocates through the cross cultural leadership development model; the development of promising and proven practices on capacity building and tobacco prevention and control; and the launching of major tobacco control policy initiatives using a four-prong policy change model.

With the complex history of tobacco and the historical lack of inclusion in the mainstream tobacco control movement, a new framework is needed

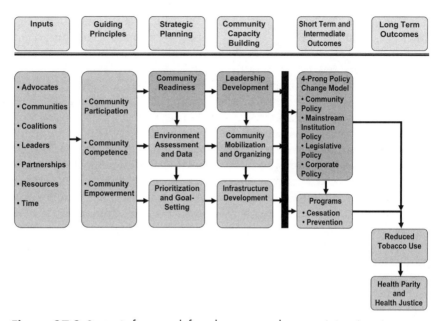

**Figure 37.2** Strategic framework for tobacco control among Asian Americans.

to address tobacco issues effectively and strategically for Asian Americans and other priority populations (Figure 36.2). A singular, mainstream approach to tobacco control for Asian Americans is mostly ineffective in addressing the diversity and complexity of the community and the root causes of tobacco initiation and use. Furthermore, singular, mainstream approaches can even lead to a negative impact on priority populations by diverting critical community resources away from necessary tailored approaches to capacity building and tobacco control. Integral to this new framework are components of key community principles, community readiness, leadership development, and multi-prong policy change models that can help move communities toward health parity and justice.

## Principles

Underlying this strategic framework for tobacco control are key principles of community participation, community competence, and community empowerment. Community participation, which hopefully can lead to community organizing efforts, is important in actively involving community leaders and members to ensure that communities have an investment (and eventually ownership) in their own health status. One of the goals for community participation in tobacco control is to strive for long-term, sustainable, collaborative, and equitable relationships with the communities that are being served. Developing and nurturing these collaborative relationships can contribute to the building of trust, an element that is critical for addressing tobacco control and other health justice issues.

The diversity of the Asian American communities requires a tailored approach to tobacco control. Central to this tailored approach is the principle of community competence that takes into consideration the full complexities of each community (Robinson 2005). Whereas cultural competency focuses on the cultural aspects of an Asian American ethnic group, community competency focuses on multiple factors of history, culture, language, context, and geography. For example, designing a smoking cessation program for Vietnamese Americans in California may vary from designing cessation programs for Vietnamese Americans in Virginia. Community competency involves not only adapting a cessation program culturally (e.g., linguistically and ethnically), but in recognizing a community's geography and history and the community's readiness to engage in smoking cessation or tobacco control. As a state, California has had a much longer history of successful tobacco control policy norm change, whereas Virginia has had a long history as a tobacco-growing state, making any tobacco control efforts much more difficult. Furthermore, a stronger infrastructure of Asian American community organizations in California may make it easier to mobilize communities on tobacco issues and implement successful tobacco control programs compared to a region or state where there are only a few Asian American serving organizations.

Integrating these key community principles can result in the development of promising practices and proven practices for tobacco control. Promising and proven practices are strategies that have been shown to be effective in addressing tobacco issues and can be replicated to create positive change for Asian American communities and other priority populations. Rather than focusing on a deficit model, tobacco control efforts should also build on the many assets of Asian American communities. Building on community assets while implementing tobacco control promising and proven practices can contribute to the empowering of communities. Because tobacco is only one of many priority issues that Asian Americans face, integrating these key community principles can also help address other critical health issues, and perhaps more importantly, the root causes for these health disparities.

## Community Assessment—Community Readiness Model

One of the first steps in developing any tobacco control or public health intervention is to conduct a community assessment. The APPEAL

Community Readiness Model is a promising practice tool for assessing a community's stage of readiness and current ability to respond to tobacco issues (Lew 2001). Adapted from Prochaska and DiClemente's individually based Transtheoretical Model (Prochaska 1983) for smoking cessation, the Community Readiness Model adapted similar measures (precontemplation, contemplation, preparation, action, and maintenance) for assessing community readiness. Using this model, communities can assess their readiness levels on comprehensive areas of tobacco control, including research and data, infrastructure, programs, and policy. The Community Readiness Model highlights the critical importance of community capacity building and infrastructural development.

The significance of this community assessment tool is that designing effective programmatic and policy interventions will vary depending on a community's readiness level. A community that has little exposure to tobacco control may not be ready to engage in comprehensive tobacco control or even tobacco control policy change. Although the model is not prescriptive in terms of interventions, it does provide some guidelines on initial steps and types of technical assistance that help move a community toward readiness to do tobacco control. For example, in Washington State, the Community Readiness Model helped Asian American tobacco control advocates realize the importance of considering tobacco in a broader community context and the need to develop more leaders to address tobacco in the community. This led to the critical formation of the Asian Pacific Islander Coalition Against Tobacco, now a very active community coalition (APPEAL 2006).

## Leadership Development Model

Community leadership can be defined as "the ability to move individuals, communities and systems toward positive social change" (Lew 2007). A second promising practice is a community leadership development model called the APPEAL Leadership Model, initially funded through The Robert Wood Johnson Foundation and implemented with the Asian American and Native Hawaiian and Pacific Islander communities, and then adapted for other priority populations. During the late 1990s, there was a realization that although the mainstream tobacco control movement had leaders advocating for tobacco-free communities, the Asian American community in many parts of the United States had limited leadership dedicated to addressing tobacco issues. The goal of the APPEAL Leadership Model was to develop a core of community leaders to build community capacity for tobacco control by framing tobacco as a social justice issue and advocating for tobacco control for Asian Americans.

Unlike other mainstream leadership programs, the APPEAL Leadership Model is specifically developed by and designed for diverse priority populations to incorporate and address the complexities and challenges of tobacco within the context of each community. The critical elements of the APPEAL Leadership Model include developing an equitable learning environment or "learning community," respecting the diversity of the participants and their learning styles, creating experiential and advocacy-based trainings and leadership opportunities, and applying learnings to real life situations in the community.

The APPEAL Leadership Model has been used to develop over 600 leaders through trainings and programs including the Washington Cross Cultural Leadership Institute, the Guam Leadership Institute, and the First Hispanic/Latino Tobacco Control Leadership Program. The APPEAL Leadership Model has led to many successful tobacco control interventions and policy initiatives for Asian Americans and other priority populations. APPEAL has developed a national youth leadership program for Asian Americans that has been replicated in states such as Ohio.

One of the leadership development highlights has been the LAAMPP Institute, designed for priority populations in Minnesota (Lew 2008). Based on the APPEAL Leadership Model, the Leadership and Advocacy Institute to Advance Minnesota's Parity for Priority Populations (LAAMPP Institute) was convened to effectively respond to tobacco issues impacting Minnesota's diverse priority populations. Thirty-two LAAMPP Fellows from five priority population groups—African/African American; American Indian; Asian American; Latino; and Lesbian, Gay, Bisexual and Transgender (LGBT)—successfully completed the program in August 2007. Adapted from the APPEAL Leadership Model, the LAAMPP Institute was designed to help participants develop leadership skills and to create cross-cultural opportunities to collaboratively address tobacco disparities in Minnesota.

Based on extensive evaluation findings, LAAMPP was successful in facilitating positive change and leadership development on multiple levels, including individual, community, systems, and cross-cultural levels. The following two examples describe the impact of LAAMPP on the Fellows on the systems and cross-cultural levels, respectively (Lew 2008):

I have used my experiences in LAAMPP to have priority populations included in the implementation of our new statewide (smokefree) law. This is something that mainstream has not done at all. Now we have priority populations sitting on two of the committees in charge of implementation of our new statewide law participating in a real and meaningful way. I was part of making this happen.

I will no longer only work with my community, but also work with peers from other ethnic groups. This is something beautiful that I learned from LAAMPP. It was important to understand that we were all there to work with our communities and to realize we were after the same goals.

The APPEAL Leadership Model underscores the importance of cross-cultural collaboration. The common factors of tobacco as a high impact community issue, being targeted by the tobacco industry and institutional inequities provides a unique opportunity for collaboration across priority populations. In some states and regions, the population of Asian Americans and other communities of color may be small relative to the mainstream population and joining forces and collaborating can provide a more powerful "voice" in advocating for tobacco control for all priority populations. Cross cultural collaboration can also lead to the sharing of lessons learned and promising practices without "reinventing the wheel" or diluting the need for community-tailored approaches to tobacco control. Because priority populations share common issues and challenges, adapting promising practices from one priority population to another may require less tailoring than adapting from a mainstream approach. And it is community leadership development and cross cultural collaborative leadership that can lead to successful policy change in tobacco control.

### Four-Prong Policy Change Model

A third promising practice has been the APPEAL Four-Prong Policy Change model. Much has been written about making the paradigm shift from individual behavioral change to environmental policy change, particularly following policy advocacy strategies in tobacco control. Tobacco control policy advocacy demonstrates the potential of public health, and its success has been published and documented widely. However, whereas a major part of the policy advocacy work in the mainstream tobacco control movement is focused on clean indoor air legislation and excise tax increases, there is a need to expand that policy approach for diverse communities.

While Asian American communities, particularly those at early stages of readiness, may need to first build capacity to do tobacco control and engage in individual level activities such as workshops, health fairs, and cessation, the long term strategy should move towards policy and systems level change. Policy level change ultimately has greater impact on a larger part of the community and usually is more sustainable.

APPEAL's four levels of policy change include (1) policies within Asian American communities and other priority populations where tobacco is not always a high priority; (2) policies with mainstream institutions where Asian Americans have not been the priority; (3) policies with legislators where neither Asian Americans nor tobacco control is a priority; and (4) policies against the tobacco industry where Asian Americans and other priority populations *have been* the priority (Lew 2003). In some cases, policy change can occur at more than one of the four levels.

Tobacco control policy change within Asian American communities focus on creating community norm change. Community organizing is a primary strategy for policy change at the community level with the intention of impacting large groups of community members. Some examples of successful community policy approaches include developing clean indoor air policies among low-income apartment complexes where Asian Americans and other communities of color reside and gettting Asian American community organizations to refuse tobacco industry sponsorship. Another community level policy change is a youth-led advocacy campaign to encourage Asian American merchants and restaurant owners to comply with local clean indoor air ordinances.

The second level of tobacco control policy change is with mainstream tobacco control institutions where Asian Americans and other communities of color have not been a high priority. A key word in addressing this level of policy change is parity. Parity in tobacco control can be defined as "being equal in the process, as well as the outcomes attained in tobacco control" (Task Force on Advancing Parity 2002). The concept of parity recognizes that there are institutional inequities built into our political, socioeconomic, and health care systems that still permeate our society and into the tobacco control movement that can negatively impact priority populations. Although in some mainstream institutions, parity in tobacco control has improved over the past decade, the historical lack of inclusion and absence of community-tailored tobacco control programs has created a distinct disadvantage for Asian Americans and other priority populations. A necessary environment to achieve parity is one conducive to equitable allocation of resources and involvement of priority populations as equal partners in priority setting and other critical decision-making opportunities. In order to achieve equitable change in tobacco control for all communities and to achieve the fullest health potential, parity efforts for priority populations must be integrated into all aspects of the tobacco control movement whether in local, state, or national tobacco control institutions.

Tobacco control policy change at the mainstream institution level can include advocating for parity in funding for priority populations and inclusion on boards of directors and other decision-making bodies; leadership development; and other community development opportunities to build the capacity of priority populations to respond to tobacco. One example of policy change at the mainstream level is when the Parity Alliance, a national independent coalition of tobacco control advocates from priority populations formed in 2001, was successful in getting parity adopted as the theme of the 2002 National Conference on Tobacco or Health.

The third level of policy change is with legislators or governmental policymakers. Throughout the history of successful tobacco control policy, national, state, and local legislators have been one of the key elements in creating and implementing mainstream tobacco control policies. However, legislative efforts to specifically address tobacco's impact on Asian Americans and other priority populations and that lead to significant policy change have been lacking. Although there have been some successful efforts, most notably, by the Praxis Project's Policy Advocacy on Tobacco or Health (PATH) initiative sponsored by the Robert Wood Johnson Foundation to link community organizers with potential policy advocacy on multiple policy change levels, more legislative efforts are needed to advance tobacco control efforts for Asian Americans and other priority populations. In addition, mainstream tobacco control institutions need to better involve and integrate representatives from priority populations at the earliest stages of any policy change efforts involving the legislative level.

The final level of policy change is on the corporate level. Getting the tobacco industry to voluntarily adopt policy change that restricts their marketing tactics targeted at Asian Americans and other priority populations is difficult to nearly impossible for the obvious reasons. The tobacco industry has been proactive in countering most efforts to introduce and pass legislation that would limit their corporate ability to freely advertise and promote tobacco products. The 1998 MSA between the states attorneys general and the tobacco industry has been one isolated example of a successful tobacco control policy change at the corporate level. In hindsight, though, the MSA is a limited success story because most of the states eventually diverted funds away from tobacco control and other health interventions.

However, the international stage offers some hope with the passage of the Framework Convention on Tobacco Control (FCTC)—the first global public health treaty—intended to address tobacco industry marketing campaigns and cigarette smuggling. The FCTC, ratified by 164 countries, potentially impacts 86 percent of the world's population. Ironically, the United States, a pioneer in making the paradigm shift to tobacco control policy change, remains one of the few countries that has not ratified the treaty. The FCTC is an example of a policy change measure that can positively impact not only priority populations in the United States but communities worldwide.

## Global Tobacco

Any discussion about tobacco use among Asian Americans in the United States must also consider the impact of tobacco use in Asia and the Pacific. By the year 2025, it is estimated that 10 million people will die from tobacco use each year in China alone. Because the majority of Asian Americans are born outside of the United States, tobacco plays a unique role for Asian American immigrants in terms of "double targeting" both in the United States and their home countries. Furthermore, tobacco control advocates surmise that the tobacco industry may have used the industry's targeting of Asian Americans to develop similar strategies in Asia. Simon Chapman, former editor of Tobacco Control stated that "in the tobacco industry, strategies that successfully boost sales in one country are quickly globalized. What works targeting Asian Americans and Pacific Islanders in the United States today may well be used in Asia and the Pacific tomorrow" (Burton 2002). A focus on transnational tobacco control interventions may begin to provide a necessary bridge in addressing both tobacco use in Asian American communities and the growing global tobacco epidemic.

## Cessation

Finally, although the focus of any major tobacco control strategy must include a core component on policy change at one or more of the four levels, one cannot focus on policy change without addressing the need for culturally and linguistically tailored tobacco cessation services. This is particularly the case for limited-English speaking Asian Americans, a multicultural community that has not benefited from mainstream cessation efforts. Not only do tobacco users need the necessary services to stop their addiction, but any successful policy change initiatives will ultimately result in scores of smokers who will be encouraged to quit.

A literature review of published tobacco cessation studies for Asian Americans has revealed only two clusters of controlled studies and one uncontrolled smoking cessation intervention study (Chen 2007). The Vietnamese Community Health Promotion Project (Suc Khoe la Vang), through the University of California, San Francisco, conducted cessation studies in the mid-1990s using media campaigns as a primary intervention strategy. Chen and associates used a lay health worker approach to assess smoking prevalence and conduct cessation among Cambodians, Laotians, and Vietnamese in Ohio. A one-group, uncontrolled intervention was conducted through Temple University among several Asian American groups.

In addition, other tobacco cessation promising practices for Asian Americans, Native Hawaiians and Pacific Islanders have been documented in the APPEAL toolkit on community approaches to cessation (APPEAL 2006). Although the few smoking cessation studies and promising practices provide important guidance in designing cessation programs for the diverse Asian American community, more studies are needed to better understand cessation issues on integration within community health centers, use of nicotine replacement therapy, and smokeless tobacco.

Since 1992, the California Smokers' Helpline has been successful in providing cessation services in four Asian languages—Cantonese, Korean, Mandarin, and Vietnamese. However, in many cases, Asian-language quitlines require parallel promotional and media campaigns to promote the quitline services and trained bilingual staff to respond to calls by limited-English speaking smokers and their relatives (proxy calls). Certainly, a cessation or quitline program alone cannot be an effective strategy in addressing norm changes on tobacco in Asian American communities, but it can provide a complementary service as part of a more comprehensive tobacco control framework.

## CONCLUSION

It is clear that tobacco will continue to have a deep, lasting impact on Asian Americans and other priority populations for many years. Although individual behavioral change tobacco control strategies may contribute initially to creating awareness about tobacco, long-term, sustainable community norm change can only result from a comprehensive policy change approach that includes community capacity building, leadership development, and multi-prong policy initiatives. Key principles of community participation, community readiness, and community competence are critical for developing effective tobacco control interventions. This can lead to the development of community-tailored promising and proven practices and policy change strategies. If successful, these efforts may foster the empowering of communities and eventually lead to the addressing of some of the root causes of health disparities. Only then will Asian Americans and other priority populations in the United States begin to realize the vision of a healthy and tobacco-free community and achieve health parity and justice.

## NOTES

1. In this article, priority populations include African Americans and African immigrants; American Indians and Alaskan Natives; Asian Americans; Native Hawaiians and Pacific Islanders; Hispanics/Latinos; Lesbian, Gay, Bisexual, and Transgenders (LGBTs).

## REFERENCES

APPEAL. Implementing a Community Readiness Approach to Tobacco Control, 2006.

APPEAL. Tobacco cessation among Asian Americans and Pacific Islanders: A community approach, 2006.

Appleyard, J., Messeri, P., and Haviland, M.L. Smoking among Asian American and Hawaiian/Pacific Islander youth: New data from the 2000 National Youth Tobacco Survey. *Asian American and Pacific Islander Journal of Health*, 9, no. 1 (Winter-Spring, 2001): 6–14.

Chen, M., and Tang, H. Review of smoking cessation research among Asian Americans: The state of the research. *Nicotine and Tobacco Research* 9, no. 3 (2007): S485–S493.

Headen, S., and Robinson, R.G. Tobacco: From slavery to addiction. In *Health Issues in the Black Community*. 2nd Edition, ed. R.L. Braithwaite and S.E. Taylor, 347–383, San Francisco, California, Jossey-Bass, 2001.

Kaholokula, J.K., Braun, K.L., Kana'iaupuni, S., and Grandinetti, A. Ethnic-by-gender differences in cigarette smoking among Asian and Pacific Islanders. *Nicotine & Tobacco Research,* 8 no. 2 (April 2006): 275–286.

Korstad, R.R. *Civil Rights Unionism: Tobacco Workers and the Struggle for Democracy in the Mid-Twentieth-Century South,* Chapel Hill, North Carolina, University of North Carolina Press, 2007.

Muggli, M., Pollay, R.W., Lew, R., and Joseph, A.M. Targeting of Asian Americans and Pacific Islanders by the tobacco industry: Results from the Minnesota Tobacco Document Depository. *Tobacco Control* 11 (2002):201–209.

Lew, R., and Tanjasiri, S.P. Slowing the epidemic of tobacco use among Asian Americans and Pacific Islanders. *American Journal of Public Health* 93, no. 5 (2003):764–768.

Lew, R. APPEAL Leadership Model. Presented at the APACHLI Institute, New York, 2007.

Lew, R., Baezconde-Garbanati, L., Portugal, C., and Honma, J. Assessing the impact of the Leadership and Advocacy Institute to Advance Minnesota's Parity for Priority Populations (LAAMPP Institute): A Final Evaluation Report, March 2008.

Prochaska, J.O., and DiClemente, C.C. Stages and processes of self-change in smoking: Toward an integrative model of change. *Journal of Consulting and Clinical Psychology,* 51, (1983):390–395.

Robinson, R.G. Community development model for public health applications: Overview of a model to eliminate population disparities. *Health Promotion Practice* 6, no. 3, (2005): 338–346.

Task Force on Advancing Parity and Leadership for Priority Populations. Moving toward health: Achieving parity through tobacco control for all communities. 2002. www.appealforcommunities.org.

Themba-Nixon, M., Sutton, C., Shorty, L., and Lew, R. More money, more motivation? Master Settlement Agreement and tobacco control funding in communities of Color. *Health Promotion Practice* 5, no. 3 Suppl., 113S–128S, 2004.

U.S. Census Bureau 2000.

U.S. Department of Health and Human Services. 1998 Surgeon General's Report: Tobacco Use among U.S. Racial/Ethnic Minority Groups, 1998.

U.S. Department of Health and Human Services. Healthy People 2010 National Health Promotion and Disease Prevention Objectives on Tobacco. Washington, DC: DHHS.

Wildey, M.B., Young, R.L., Elder, J.P., Demoor, C., Wold, K.R., and Fiske, K.E. Cigarette point of advertising in ethnic neighborhoods in San Diego, California. *Health Values* 16, no. 1 (1992): 23–28.

Ysaol, J., Chilton, J.I., and Callaghan, P. In *ISLA: A Journal of Micronesian Studies* 4, no. 1, (Rainy Season 1996): 244–255.

# Chapter 38

# Voices of the Community
## East Meets West: A Dialogue in the Pursuit of Longevity

### Daniel Chen and Ira Frankel

"Man thinks."

—Spinoza
*Ethics*

"At fifteen I thought only of study; at thirty I began playing my role; at forty I was sure of myself; at fifty I was conscious of my position in the universe; at sixty I was no longer argumentative; and now at seventy I can follow my heart's desire without violating custom."

—Confucius
*The Sayings of Confucius*

This chapter will, first, discuss longevity from Western and Eastern perspectives; and, second, it will describe Flushing Hospital Medical Center's model of successful aging through Life Style Medicine. The model integrates alternative and complementary biopsychosocial practices from the East with standard biomedical and biopsychosocial practices from the West to destigmatize mental illness and promote longevity.

## BACKGROUND

Dr. Chen is a physician, psychiatrist, and assistant chairman of psychiatry at Flushing Hospital Medical Center, located in Queens County, New York, one of the largest Asian communities in America. He was born in Shanghai, China. He has been trained in both Eastern and Western medical paradigms.

Dr. Frankel has a PhD in Human Relations, and he is a clinical behavior analyst and an administrator of psychiatry at Flushing Hospital Medical Center in Queens. He was born in Brooklyn, New York.

Drs. Chen and Frankel became colleagues several years ago. They immediately embarked on a dialogue that focused on the pursuit of successful aging and longevity. Their goal became to create and sustain an environment of successful aging for each other, their colleagues, and the patients in the Flushing community. Drs. Chen and Frankel have collaborated on a Geriatric Physical Health–Mental Health Integration Grant Project, and they continue to submit other grant proposals to integrate physical and mental health throughout the life span. Their long-term goal is to create the Center for Integrated Eastern-Western Life Style Medicine, which will promote mental and physical health through lifestyle medicine toward successful aging and longevity in the transcultural Flushing community. The present chapter is one product of their ongoing dialogue.

## THE WESTERN PERSPECTIVE

Confucius's thinking man reaches across centuries and continents to Spinoza's thinking man, who looks back as both complement each other's rational edifice for longevity, in which behavioral *logos* is a unifying element. The behavioral *logos* is the formal and informal behavioral experimentation that takes place in the Eastern and Western cultures, the outcomes of which select behaviors leading to longevity.

Western medicine has struggled with the tension between the biomedical paradigm, which focuses on specific systems and subsystems, and the biopsychosocial paradigm, which focuses on the behavior of total organism (Engel 1977; Foucault 1994). A similar tension has existed between the Eastern and Western paradigms.

The *Oxford English Dictionary* (2002) defines medicine as "the art of restoring and preserving the health of human beings by the administration of remedial substances and the regulation of diet, habits, and the conditions of life." This definition reinforces the idea that medicine has biomedical elements with the administration of remedial substances and biopsychosocial elements with modification of lifestyle behaviors as key ingredients to successful aging and longevity.

Hippocrates (400 BC), the founder of Western medicine, wrote, "The physician must not only be prepared to do what is right himself, but also to make the patient, the attendants, and the externals cooperate." This statement points to the behavior-changing role that the physician plays in creating a health-promoting lifestyle and environment around the patient, first as he becomes an example by modeling the necessary behavior; second, by helping others to become examples to each other of successful aging; and, third, by engaging in face-to-face behavior modification to help the patient change toward successful aging, too.

The MacArthur Foundation Study of Aging in America (Rowe and Kahn 1998) determined that the basic ingredients of successful aging are behaviorally based. The ingredients are diet, exercise, the pursuit of mental challenges, self-efficacy, and social support. To live long, a person must have a proper diet and a regular exercise routine. Both of these behaviors are mentally challenging. Achieving self-control of these behaviors produces self-efficacy; that is, the feeling that "I can do it!" An important mental challenge is novelty. A willingness to put oneself in novel situations to solve novel problems, the outcomes of which are uncertain, but to persevere despite obstacles, strengthens self-efficacy and the ability to continue persevering. Finally, engaging in these activities with another person through social support makes each person more likely to successfully engage in these behaviors and live longer.

The MacArthur Foundation's findings on successful aging support the data from the U.S. Centers for Disease Control's Healthy People 2010 initiative (Healthy People 2010). The Healthy People 2010 database shows that access to medical care is affected by many variables including ethnicity, race, age, immigration status, socioeconomic status, insurance, and degrees of similarity between a group's traditional medical practices and alternative practices.

Foucault (1986) summarized the biopsychosocial core of the Western perspective. He wrote, "It [Medicine] was also supposed to define, in the form of a corpus of knowledge and rules, a way of living, a reflective mode of relation to oneself, to one's body, to food, to wakefulness and sleep, to the various activities, and to the environment. Medicine was expected to propose, in the form of a regimen, a *voluntary and rational structure of conduct* [emphasis ours]." That is, the end product of medicine is to help individuals live properly, which is the most difficult mental challenge of all.

Western medicine continues struggling with the tension between the biomedical and the biopsychosocial paradigms, with the biopsychosocial paradigm currently making a resurgence.

## THE EASTERN PERSPECTIVE

Eastern medicine, of which Chinese medicine is an example, is currently in a more philosophical or biopsychosocial mode than is Western medicine, which is in a more evidence-based or biomedical mode. Chinese medicine views and treats a person as a whole unit; it is holistic, with an emphasis on the balance and harmony (yin and yang) of the entire, or various parts of the body. Although there are many differences between the biomedical and biopsychosocial paradigms, the final goal is the same: to heal the sick and keep the healthy healthy.

Therefore, we need to *Qiu Tong Cun Yi*, that is, we need to cast aside differences and focus on this ultimate common goal by adopting healthy lifestyles to prevent and manage diseases, which in turn promotes longevity with good fortune, wealth, and enjoyment—in Chinese, *Fu Lu Shou Xi*. In fact, the old Chinese wisdom of longevity is very similar to the Western principles of longevity, which include good nutrition, physical activity, rest, mental balance, self-efficacy, and social support (Harrison et al. 2005).

Regarding the use of Western and Eastern medicine, researchers have surveyed participants of various ethnic backgrounds, and the findings have been encouraging. For instance, Ma (1999) found that Chinese immigrants believe Western medicine to be more effective for acute complaints, whereas Chinese medicine is better for chronic problems and health promotion in general. In terms of health promotion, participants told Ma that Chinese medicine enhances immune functioning, has antiviral and anti-inflammatory effects, balances mind and body, relieves aches and pains, and reduces cholesterol. Western-trained and traditionally trained Chinese practitioners agree that healing herbs, acupuncture, massage or health exercises can play a vital role in prevention, treatment, and rehabilitation even though the illness might require Western medicine. Furthermore, alternative healing practices offer a range of care choices for the whole person, with a broad perspective on their social, mental, emotional, and spiritual well-being. Ma believes that alternative medicine deserves more attention in the biomedical-oriented Western health care system, and that the incorporation of alternative medicine into this system should be viewed as complementary rather than competitive.

In another study, Mackenzie and colleagues (2003) found that all ethnic groups—including whites, African Americans, Latinos, Asians, and Native American—were equally likely to use at least one alternative method. The authors believe that if alternative medicine were integrated into the existing biomedical paradigm, people of different ethnic backgrounds would be better served.

The findings from the literature are consistent with Dr. Frankel's observation from the Western point of the view and Dr. Chen's experience from both Eastern and Western systems. Both Drs. Chen and Frankel agree that although it is important to respect the unique aspects of each culture, it is equally important to identify those common aspects, so that everyone, regardless of cultural background, can benefit from an integration of Eastern and Western paradigms. At Flushing Hospital Medical Center, Drs. Chen and Frankel have incorporated both Eastern and Western medicine into their routine practice. They adopted the concept of Life Style Medicine (Murphy 2007) because they believe it best reflects the common ground between Eastern and Western medicine. According to Murphy, Life Style Medicine is a specialty that utilizes lifestyle modifications in order to prevent and manage diseases, with or without medication.

Flushing Hospital Medical Center's model of Life Style Medicine was established based on the concept that pursuing longevity and the pathways to it are universal goals: healthy diet, physical and mental activity, rest, and social support.

*Case Example: A Survivor of the Chinese Cultural Revolution*

Mr. X is a 77-year-old married Chinese male who attends Flushing's Ambulatory Care Clinic for treatment of medical conditions. As all patients over 65 are, Mr. X was screened for depression with a Chinese version of the PHQ-9 that was administered by a Chinese-speaking Behavioral Health Clinician. While he didn't screen positive for depression, he described symptoms of Post-Traumatic Stress Disorder when he started telling his story of being sent to a labor and correction camp for many years during the Cultural Revolution because he was a teacher, intellectual, and writer.

The Chinese-speaking clinician engaged him in verbal therapy and encouraged him to write. In addition, she helped him to mindfully meditate at home so that he could increasingly tolerate the images of the horror of the labor re-education camp, engaged him in Tai Chi to help him reduce bodily tension that was related to his hypertension, discussed the traditional herbal products that he used so that their use would not adversely affect the Western medication that he was taking, and promoted a healthy diet and proper sleep habits to help fortify him. With the use of the integrated life style modification techniques, the clinician helped reduce his PTSD and hypertension symptoms, promote a healthier relationship with his wife, reduce his suspicions of the Chinese Community so he could participate more fully in it, and develop integrity and avoid despair as he approached the end of his life. Mr. X would have continued to live his life in despairing isolation if he hadn't been noticed and engaged by the East-West integration project.

## THE FLUSHING HOSPITAL: MODEL OF SUCCESSFUL AGING THROUGH LIFE STYLE MEDICINE

As is illustrated in the case example, the purpose of this section is to describe the integrated model of successful aging through Life Style Medicine, a model that Drs. Chen and Frankel have been implementing at Flushing Hospital Medical Center. This model has evolved since 2001, when Drs. Chen and Frankel started their dialogue. The quotes from Spinoza and Confucius are a small sample of Drs. Chen and Frankel's East-West dialogue that guided the Life Style Medicine integration project and placed behavioral *logos* at its center.

As part of its long-range planning, Flushing Hospital's Department of Psychiatry and Addiction Services initiated annual behavioral health conferences in 2001. The purpose of these conferences was to present the general narrative of successful aging throughout the life span and to set the stage for gradually implementing parts of the physical health–mental health integration model throughout the Medical Center. The topics included

Cultural Factors in Behavioral Health (2002), Child Psychiatry (2002), Successful Aging (2003), the Challenge of Overweight and Obesity (2005), Suicide Prevention (2006), the Challenge of the Addictions (2007), and the Challenge of Integrating Physical and Mental Health through Life Style Medicine (2008).

Each topic initiated practical Life Style Medicine projects within the department and throughout Flushing Hospital. The New York State Office of Mental Health's Wellness Self-Management Project is bringing behavioral self-management approaches for physical conditions into the Mental Health Clinic. The elements of successful aging became a part of everyone's vocabulary throughout the Flushing Hospital. Depression screening and suicide detection and prevention were implemented in both outpatient and inpatient settings. Nicotine patches and smoking cessation counseling were offered to patients, employees, and community residents. The smoking cessation program has been offering these services for more than ten years. In 2004, the Flushing Hospital developed a partnership with the New York City Department of Health and Mental Hygiene to expand the program, distribute free nicotine patches, and include additional lifestyle modification practices. The program became a Center of Excellence and was recognized as such by the commissioner of the New York City Department of Health and Mental Hygiene.

With Dr. Chen's initiative and the leadership of the chairman of Ambulatory Care, the Medical Center helped cosponsor the Get-Fit-Flushing weight control program through integrated lifestyle modification with a Chinese owned pharmacy chain that is dedicated to integrated lifestyle modification and the Flushing Chinese Business Association, developed partnerships with the American Cancer Society's Asian Unit, offered educational lectures through radio, TV, written media, and many Chinese organizations, and presented physical and mental health promotion activities at local symposia.

A current outcome of the dialogue occurred when Drs. Chen and Frankel, along with the chairman of Ambulatory Care, successfully secured a New York State Office of Mental Health Geriatric Physical Health–Mental Health Integration Demonstration Grant. The grant's purpose is to destigmatize mental illness by integrating mental health services into physical health practice in the primary care clinics, teaching the primary care physician Life Style Medical practices, and integrating alternative and complementary biopsychosocial practices from the East with standard care from the West.

The behavioral health team consists of a psychiatrist consultant-educator, a nurse practitioner, behavioral health clinicians, and a patient care coordinator. The team is culturally competent in English, Chinese, Korean, and Spanish. The behavioral health team educates the primary care team to destigmatize mental illness by thinking about it as a problem of successful aging and lifestyle medical practice; that is, as a problem about mental challenges such as diet, exercise, self-efficacy, and social support. Administrators, attending physicians, resident physicians, nurses, nursing assistants, and clerical staff are educated about these ideas in weekly meetings and monthly lectures.

The psychiatrist consultant-educator engages all staff by bringing the concept of the communicative dialogue into the primary care encounters with patients from all cultures. The communicative dialogue emphasizes the face-to-face, interpersonal aspects of medical care, which highlight the Eastern concept of holistic medicine. Within this context that teaches practitioners to look and see, every patient is screened at every primary care visit using culturally validated screening scales such as the Patient Health Questionnaire-9 for depression, the Generalized Anxiety Disorder-7 for anxiety, the CAGE for substance abuse, and the Min-Cog and Mini-Mental Status Examination for cognitive impairment and dementia. These devices set the stage for practitioners to enter a dialogue with patients that focuses on the patient, the doctor, and their relationship.

The integration steps are woven into the fabric of the primary care processes by resolving daily obstacles. A nursing assistant begins the process by taking vital signs and making sure that the patient completes the mental health screenings. The adult nurse practitioner makes sure at discharge that the patient has successfully completed the communicative dialogues with the resident physician, attending physician, nurses, behavioral health clinicians, and clerical staff.

The nurse practitioner coordinates the results of the mental health screenings, assessments, and treatment plans with the resident and attending physicians, behavioral health clinicians, and nurses. The two major treatment approaches are Western biomedical medications and psychosocial therapies, and Eastern meditative practices such as tai chi and yoga. Other forms of exercises and lifestyle modifications are also offered. The psychosocial therapies include individual and group support, education, cognitive therapy, interpersonal therapy, lifestyle behavioral self-management, and other behavior modification approaches. Integrated East-West diet, exercise, mental challenges, self-efficacy, and social support are used as destigmatizing ideas for mental illness.

Culturally congruent techniques are used to enhance the complementary integration of specific cultural groups into the behavior change program. This reflects Ma's observation (1999) that healing herbs, acupuncture, massage, and health exercises play a vital role in prevention, treatment, and rehabilitation. These practices offer a wide range of choices to patients, and tend to care for the whole person, with a broad perspective on their social, mental, emotional, and spiritual well-being. Therefore, Ma urges that these techniques be incorporated into Western biomedical practices.

The nurse practitioner conducts individual and small-group instruction in these techniques to Asian and non-Asian patients alike.

Yoga, tai chi, and other meditative exercises are practiced, thereby promoting the integration of exercise from different cultures into the successful aging ethos of the Ambulatory Care Clinic. Similarly, to promote cultural integration, transcultural approaches are used for diet, mental challenges, self-efficacy, and social support. To further strengthen the importance of social support in successful aging, staff members are encouraged to participate in these groups. The hospital offers free yoga and smoking cessation programs to its staff.

The integration project emphasizes use of empirical measurement as a way to track progress and to provide reinforcing and corrective feedback to patients and staff.

The attending and resident physicians and the nurse practitioner manage medication. All patients receive education about diagnosis, treatment options (including alternative therapies), expected outcomes, and potential side effects. Again, measurement forms a core component to assure timely feedback to patients and staff.

Culturally competent staff provides the service in the patient's language to assure the complementing integration for patients who might otherwise not have had access to destigmatized mental and physical health care.

## CHALLENGES AND RESPONSES

Drs. Chen and Frankel had been practicing lifestyle medicine since 2001 and demonstrated clinical and financial gains, which generated organizational support for their projects. With the support of senior leadership, Drs. Chen and Frankel were able to resolve initial resistance by conveying a clear message that change would occur to those who saw only obstacles.

Drs. Chen and Frankel introduced the idea of floating workplace in response to being told that there was "no space." The continuum-of-practice became the front desk, waiting room area, vital signs room, various examination rooms, and the nursing discharge desk.

Changing the medical residents' training curriculum modified the attitude that behavioral health practice did not belong in primary care because Primary Care Providers are not comfortable with behavioral issues. The culture was changed with coursework on physical and mental health integration through East-West Life Style Medicine, on-site consultation with and supervision by the project psychiatrist and assigned psychosomatic fellow, and daily face-to-face feedback by the clinical coordinator, an adult nurse practitioner.

The problem of interrupted routine clinical work that increased time pressure on staff was managed by redefining job descriptions to include behavioral health factors, improving communication, streamlining documentation, and providing brief scripts to promote lifestyle conceptualizations to patients.

Challenges to interprofessional collaboration were managed with weekly interdisciplinary staff meetings and ongoing interactions with the behavioral health team.

There are short- and long-term financial challenges. The short-term ones are increasing billable visits by working with regulatory agencies to support sustainable billing practices and by lobbying Medicare, Medicaid, and insurance companies to reimburse Primary Care Providers for behavioral health care on parity with physical health care. The long-term challenge is to build a practice model that sustains geriatric integration services beyond the grant and across the entire life span.

## PRELIMINARY CLINICAL OUTCOMES

More than 300 English, Spanish, Chinese, and Korean-speaking patients over sixty-five were screened, assessed, and given brief lifestyle medicine counseling in more than 600 visits. After completing the PHQ-9 and GAD-7, patients were directly assessed, at which time false negatives were managed. The screening instruments stimulated communication among staff and patients. Additional screening instruments will be introduced—for example, the CAGE for alcohol and the MMSE for cognitive deficits. About 5 percent of assessed patients were prescribed medication.

### Initial Data

Age: The average age was seventy-four, with a range from sixty-five to ninety-three.

Gender: Sixty-nine percent were female, 31 percent male.

Language: Twenty percent spoke English, 54 percent Spanish, 9 percent Korean, 6 percent Hindi, 6 percent Chinese, and 5 percent spoke other languages.

Ethnicity: Six percent were white, 47 percent Hispanic, 24 percent Asian, 12 percent African American, 9 percent Native Hawaiian/Pacific Islander, and 2 percent were other ethnicities.

Identified issues: Sixty-four percent presented physical health issues, 33 percent mental health issues, 1 percent social issues, 1 percent financial issues, and 0.5 percent each identified cognitive and housing issues.

PHQ-9: The average score was 3 out of 27 with a range of 0 to 27.

GAD-7: The average score was 3 out of 21 with a range of 0 to 21.

### Collaboration about Behavioral Health Issues

Many PCPs expressed frustration about their patient's "noncompliance" with medical advice for overweight and obesity, hypertension, diabetes, high cholesterol, diet, exercise, taking medication, and showing up for appointments. Noncompliance was reframed and included in a group of mental disorders called Psychological Factors Affecting Physical Conditions.

For example, many patients had Maladaptive Health Behaviors Affecting Hypertension.

Frequent educational encounters and the reconceptualization of non-compliance as Maladaptive Health Behaviors Affecting a Physical Condition increased collaboration and enlisted the PCPs' cooperation in accepting behavioral health practices for their multicultural patients.

As a result, nearly 100 percent of screened and assessed patients were given brief individual, small-group, and couple-focused Eastern-Western lifestyle medicine counseling for maladaptive health behaviors. Cognitive techniques and meditation exercises such as tai chi and yoga were used.

### The Data-Gathering Plan

Gathering objective data is crucial to the project's success. The following data are being organized. First, relevant physiological indicators: weight, blood pressure, fasting blood glucose level and A1c, and lipid profile. Second, behavioral indicators: life style behaviors such as diet and exercise, meditative practices such as tai chi and yoga, smoking, substance and alcohol use, social activity, life quality measures, compliance with prescribed medication and treatment appointments, and other self-management skills. And third, medical utilization rates such as hospitalization for serious conditions.

### Long-Range Vision

Drs. Chen and Frankel are using the current project to plan their long-range vision: the Center for Integrated Eastern-Western Life Style Medicine. The Center will be an experimental space for people to acquire transcultural practices that best fit their self-management needs for longevity. Participants will be able to select from Eastern practices such as diet, acupuncture, acupressure, herbal medicine, tai chi, and yoga, and form Western practices such as diet, relaxation techniques, strength and aerobic training, Cognitive-Behavior Modification, and psycho- and self-analysis to assist their pursuit of longevity.

### IN SUMMARY

This voice from the community, the Flushing Hospital Medical Center's Physical Health–Mental Health Integration Project through Life Style Medicine, developed its roots in the dialogue between Drs. Chen and Frankel, who experienced themselves as part of the ongoing dialogue between Eastern and Western thinkers, recognizing, as did those before us, that there are more similarities than differences between these two great cultural traditions.

# REFERENCES

Confucius. 1953. *The sayings of Confucius.* New York: Mentor Books.

Engel, G. L. 1977. The need for a new medical model. *Science* 196:129–136.

Foucault, M. 1994. *The birth of the clinic: An archaeology of medical perception.* New York: Vintage Books.

———. 1998. *The care of the self: The history of sexuality, Volume 3.* New York: Vintage Books.

Harrison, G. G., Kagawa-Singer, M., Foerster, S. B., Lee, H., Kim, L. P., Nguyen, T.-U., Fernandez-Ami, A., Quinn, V., and Bal, D. G. 2005. Seizing the moment: California's opportunity to prevent nutrition-related health disparities in low-income Asian American populations. *Cancer* 104(12s): 2962–2968.

Hippocrates. 400 B. C. E. The Internet Classics Archives; Aphorisms by Hippocrates. http://classics.mit.edu/Hippocrates/aphorisms.1.i.html.

Ma, G. X. 1999. Between two worlds: The use of traditional and Western health services by Chinese Immigrants. *Journal of Community Health* 24(6): 421–437.

Mackenzie, E. R., Taylor, L., Bloom, B. S., Hufford, D. J., and Johnson, J. C. 2003. Ethnic minority use of complementary and alternative medicine (CAM): A national probability survey of CAM utilizers. *Alternative Therapies in Health and Medicine* 9(4): 50–56.

Murphy, Kate. 2007. Teaching doctors to teach patients about lifestyle. *New York Times,* April 17, Science section, New York edition.

*Oxford English Dictionary.* 2002. Oxford: Oxford University Press.

Rowe, J. W., and Kahn, R. L. 1989. *Successful aging.* New York: Pantheon Books.

Spinoza, B. D. 1996. *Ethics.* New York: Penguin Putnam.

U.S. Department of Health and Human Services. 2000. *Healthy People 2010.* 2nd ed. 2 vols. Washington, DC: U.S. Government Printing Office. http://search. msn.com/results.aspx?q=Healthy+People+2010&FORM=MNH.

# PART VIII

## Disparities and Opportunities

# Chapter 39

# Poor Health Outcomes in Asian American Communities: An Overview of Health Disparities

## Walter Tsou

According to the Centers for Disease Control's (CDC) Office of Minority Health and Health Disparities,

> Asian Americans represent both extremes of socioeconomic and health indices. While some enjoy high incomes, a significant minority of Asian Americans live in poverty. Asian Americans contend with numerous factors which may threaten their health. Some negative factors are infrequent medical visits due to the fear of deportation, language/cultural barriers, and the lack of health insurance. Asian Americans are most at risk for the following health conditions: cancer, heart disease, stroke, unintentional injuries (accidents), and diabetes. Asian Americans also have a high prevalence of the following conditions and risk factors: chronic obstructive pulmonary disease, hepatitis B, HIV/AIDS, smoking, tuberculosis, and liver disease (U.S. Dept of HHS 2006).

## A Closer Look at Income, Poverty, and Health Insurance

The U.S. Census Bureau publishes an annual report on U.S. income, poverty, and health insurance based on the annual Current Population Survey. In 2007, the median per capita income for Asians was $29,901, which was the second highest of all racial groups, except for non-Hispanic whites (DeNavas-Walt et al. 2007). However, in 2007 approximately

**Table 39.1** 2007 U.S. Income and Poverty Status by Race and Hispanic Origin

| Race | Median Income ($ dollars) | Per Capita Income | Number Below Poverty | Percent Below Poverty |
|---|---|---|---|---|
| White | $52,115 | $28,325 | 25,120,000 | 10.5% |
| White, not Hispanic | $54,920 | $31,051 | 16,032,000 | 8.2% |
| Black | $33,916 | $18,428 | 9,237,000 | 24.5% |
| **Asian** | **$66,103** | **$29,901** | **1,349,000** | **10.2%** |
| Hispanic (any race) | $38,679 | $15,603 | 9,890,000 | 21.5% |

*Source:* U.S. Census Bureau, Current Population Reports: *Income, Poverty, and Health Insurance Coverage in the United States: 2007.*

1,350,000 (10.2%) Asians lived below poverty (DeNavas-Walt et al. 2007). Furthermore, in 2007, 552,000 (4.2%) Asians lived below 50 percent of poverty, a condition of destitution.

In 2007, 2,234,000 (16.8%) Asians were uninsured during the year (DeNavas-Walt et al. 2007). This represented an increase from 2,045,000 (15.5%) in 2006. In 2007, 11.7 percent of Asian children under the age of 18 were uninsured. This was not statistically different from 2006.

## DEFINING HEALTH DISPARITIES

In its seminal book *Unequal Treatment: Confronting Racial and Ethnic Disparities in Healthcare* (Smedley et al. 2003), the Institute of Medicine defined disparities in health care as racial or ethnic differences in the quality of health care that are not due to access-related factors or clinical needs, preferences, and appropriateness of intervention. The committee focused on two levels of concern: (1) the operation of health care systems

**Table 39.2** 2006–2007 U.S. Health Insurance Status by Race and Hispanic Origin.

| Race | 2006 Uninsured | 2006 Percent Uninsured | 2007 Uninsured | 2007 Percent Uninsured |
|---|---|---|---|---|
| White | 35,486,000 | 14.9% | 34,300,000 | 14.3% |
| White, not Hispanic | 21,162,000 | 10.8% | 20,548,000 | 10.4% |
| Black | 7,652,000 | 20.5% | 7,372,000 | 19.5% |
| **Asian** | **2,045,000** | **15.5%** | **2,234,000** | **16.8%** |
| Hispanic (any race) | 15,296,000 | 34.1% | 14,770,000 | 32.1% |

*Source:* U.S. Census Bureau, Current Population Reports; Income, Poverty, and Health Insurance Coverage in the United States: 2007.

and the legal and regulatory climate in which health systems operate and (2) discrimination at the individual and provider levels.

Their analysis offers a framework for examining health disparities in the Asian American community and raises many important societal and political questions in seeking solutions to addressing these disparities.

Many factors therefore contribute to health disparities in Asian populations, including lack of financial resources, limited access to health insurance, difficulty in finding linguistically and culturally competent health professionals, hard-to-navigate immigration policies, unequal access to the opportunities of American life and education, and overt discrimination by individuals and organizations. This chapter acknowledges these factors, but it is beyond its scope to address all of them.

## Data Limitations

As noted earlier in this book, descriptions of disparities and poor health outcomes among Asian Americans are difficult to obtain because the data are usually not collected or analyzed, the sample size is too small to be statistically meaningful, or Asian Americans are almost invariably lumped together as a homogeneous population, obscuring significant differences between different subpopulations (Report 2007). Hence, published data on Asian Americans limit the ability to embark on detailed discussions on heath outcomes in Asian Americans. Dr. Marguerite Ro noted this difficulty in addressing issues related to the health of Asian American women (Ro 2002). The National Health Disparities Report found that only two-thirds of their core report measures of quality could be analyzed for Asians because of lack of data (National Healthcare Disparities Rep. 2007). The ability to find sufficient data to characterize poor health outcomes is limited with the use of currently available published data.

Most of the published data on health disparities show narrow measures for Asian Americans and do not reflect the difficulties encountered in obtaining needed health care services. In describing measurable health disparities, these facts merely reflect snapshots of the larger context in which Asian Americans live their lives in America.

## Snapshots from National Studies

Three national studies have collected data on health care disparities among Asian Americans: the National Healthcare Disparities Report, the National Center for Health Statistics, and the Commonwealth Fund. The National Healthcare Disparities Report is compiled by the Agency for Healthcare Research and Quality. The National Center for Health Statistics has compiled data on Asians as far as their status, behavior, and utilization of health, including Asian subpopulations. Finally, the Commonwealth

Fund's *Racial and Ethnic Disparities in U.S. Health Care: A Chartbook* has compiled data from these national studies as well as some of their own data into their chart book.

The National Healthcare Disparities report (2007) noted several areas where health outcomes for Asian Americans were worse. In particular, many of the disparities noted below were related to problems communicating with or understanding their health care providers. These disparities include:

## Immunizations

- Asian American adults age sixty-five and over were 50 percent more likely than non-Hispanic whites to lack immunization against pneumonia.

## Mental Health

- In 2005, the proportion of Asian Americans who received mental health treatment or counseling was less than a third compared to that of non-Hispanic whites (4% compared with 14%).

## Communication

- Asian American adults reported poor communication with health care providers.
- Asian American long-stay nursing home residents were more likely to be physically restrained.
- The percentage of hospice patients whose families reported that they did not receive the right amount of medicine for pain was significantly higher for Asian Americans (11.5%) than for non-Hispanic whites (5.6%) in 2006. The percentage whose families reported that they did not receive care consistent with their wishes was more than three times higher for Asian Americans (18.3%) compared with non-Hispanic whites (5.5%) (The National Healthcare Disparities Rep. 2007).
- From 2002 to 2004, the gap between Asian Americans and non-Hispanic whites in the proportion of adults who reported sometimes or never getting care for illness or injury as soon as they wanted remained the same. However in 2004, the proportion was about two times higher for Asian Americans than for non-Hispanic whites (26.7% compared with 13.1%).
- According to the 2003 National Assessment of Adult Literacy, Health Literacy Component, 13 percent of Asian Americans were "below basic" literacy, meaning they could understand no more than the most simple and concrete skills.

The 2007 National Health Disparities Report (NHDR) recognized the limitations of its national survey for understanding the Asian American community. Therefore, in 2001, 2003, and 2005 results from the California

Health Interview Survey (CHIS) were added to the NHDR national survey, to include more detailed data on Asian Americans. Some of the pertinent findings from the CHIS include:

## Mammography

- The proportion of women who reported having a mammogram in the past two years was significantly lower for Asian Americans than for non-Hispanic whites (74.6% compared with 80.7%). Among Asian subpopulations, the proportion was lowest for Koreans (58.1%).

## Diabetes

- In 2005, the proportion of Asian American adults in California with low English proficiency who received all three recommended services for diabetes (hemoglobin A1c, retinal exam, and foot exam) was less than half that of Asian American native English speakers (26.2% compared with 59.1%).

## Uninsured

- The proportion under age sixty-five who were uninsured all year was significantly higher for all Asian subgroups than non-Hispanic whites, except for South Asians. The proportion was over five times higher for Koreans than for non-Hispanic whites (29.7% compared with 5.8%).

The National Center for Health Statistics has published "Health Characteristics of the Asian Adult Population: United States, 2004–2006" (Barnes 2008). This comprehensive study based on data from the Family Core and the Sample Adult Core components of the 2004–2006 National Health Interview Survey examined a wide range of Asian American health data, including:

## Health Status

- Overall, over 60 percent of Asian adults and non-Hispanic whites adults were in excellent or very good health. However, Vietnamese adults (19%) were more than twice as likely as adults in other Asian subgroups to be in fair or poor health. Vietnamese women (28%) were more than twice as likely as Vietnamese men (11%) to be in fair or poor health.

## Health Behavior

- Most Asian adults had never smoked, with rates ranging from 65 percent, for Korean adults, to 84 percent, for Chinese adults. Korean adults (22%) were about two to three times as likely to be current smokers as were Japanese (12%), Asian Indian (7%), or Chinese adults (7%).

- Japanese adults (14%) were more likely to be current moderate or heavier drinkers compared with Filipino (9%), Chinese (7%), Asian Indian (6%), or Vietnamese adults (6%). Vietnamese adults (68%) had the highest percentage of lifetime abstinence from alcohol use; rates for adults in other Asian subgroups ranged from 32 percent, for Japanese, to 57 percent, for Asian Indians.
- Although the prevalence of obesity is low within the adult Asian population, Filipino adults (14%) were more than twice as likely to be obese as Asian Indian (6%), Vietnamese (5%), or Chinese adults (4%).
- Overall, about three in ten Asian adults engaged in regular leisure-time physical activity. Of the adults in Asian subgroups, Vietnamese adults (46%) were most likely to be inactive in their leisure time.

## Health Care Utilization

- Among Asian adults, Korean adults (25%) were most likely to be without a usual place for health care; rates for adults in other Asian subgroups ranged from 12 percent, for Japanese or Filipino adults, to 16 percent, for Chinese or Vietnamese adults.
- Among Asian adults with a usual place for health care, Vietnamese adults (23%) were more likely than Filipino (14%), Asian Indian (13%) or Japanese adults (13%) to consider a clinic or health care center as their usual place for health care.
- Asian adults (2%) and Hispanic adults (4%) were more likely to have never seen a dentist, compared with non-Hispanic whites (less than 1%) or black adults (1%).
- A larger percentage of Korean adults (12%) had not been to a dentist in the past five years compared with Japanese adults (4%).
- Filipino adults (8%) were more likely than Chinese adults (5%) to have lost all their natural teeth.

The Commonwealth Fund sponsored an extensive review of health disparities and published the *Racial and Ethnic Disparities in U.S. Health Care: A Chartbook (Mead et al. 2008)*. Data obtained from their Health Care Quality Survey found some poor outcomes for Asian Americans including the following:

- Hispanics and Asian Americans are less likely to get a same-day or next-day appointment to see a doctor than non-Hispanic whites (54% vs. 66%).
- Asian Americans and Hispanics are less likely to understand their doctor and less likely to feel their doctor listened to them than blacks and non-Hispanic whites (49% vs. 68%).

## Selected Poor Outcomes

Some well-known illnesses have higher prevalence in Asians.

**Table 39.3** Liver and Stomach Cancer Incidence and Death Rates by Race, 2000–2004.

| Racial/Ethnic Group | Liver and Bile Duct | | Stomach | |
|---|---|---|---|---|
| | Incidence | Death | Incidence | Death |
| All | 6.2 | 4.9 | 8.1 | 4.2 |
| African American/Black | 7.6 | 6.5 | 12.5 | 8.2 |
| Asian/Pacific Islander | 13.9 | 10.6 | 14.3 | 8.0 |
| Hispanic/Latino | **9.7** | **7.6** | **12.3** | **6.8** |
| American Indian/ Alaska Native | 9.7 | 8.4 | 11.5 | 7.2 |
| Non-Hispanic White | 5.2 | 4.5 | 7.1 | 3.7 |

Statistics are for 2000–2004, age adjusted to the 2000 U.S. standard million population, and represent the number of new cases of invasive cancer and deaths per year per 100,000 men and women.

## Cancer

According to the National Cancer Institute, two cancers in particular, stomach and liver, have higher incidence rates in Asian Americans than in any other racial or ethnic group. Asian Americans are twice as likely to die from these cancers as non-Hispanic whites.

Based on California survey data, large variations were found in cancer incidence and mortality in Asian subpopulations. McCracken et al. (2007) found in California higher age-adjusted liver cancer mortality for Asian Americans at 23.8% compared to 6.8% for non-Hispanic whites. Equally significant, within the Asian American male population, mortality rates for liver cancer varied by subgroup: 54.3% for Vietnamese, 33.9% for Koreans, 23.3% for Chinese, 16.8% for Filipinos, and 9.3% for Japanese.

Both stomach and liver cancers have links to infectious diseases, suggesting that they are preventable. Stomach cancer has been linked to possible *Helicobacter pylori* infection (NCI Fact Sheet 2006), and liver cancer is closely linked to chronic hepatitis B infection.

In 2005, a hepatitis B screening study in New York City among 1,836 mostly new Asian immigrants found that approximately 15 percent had chronic hepatitis B infection, a rate 35 times greater than that among the general U.S. population (Pollack et al. 2006).

The five-year relative survival rate for all cancers for Native Hawaiians is 47 percent, compared with 57 percent for non-Hispanic whites and 55 percent for all races (CDC 2002).

From 1988 to 1992, the highest age-adjusted incidence rate of cervical cancer occurred among Vietnamese American women (43 per 100,000), almost five times higher than the rate among non-Hispanic white women (7.5/100,000) (CDC 2004). Equally significant, in 2003, Asian American women (ages 18+) were the least likely to have had a Pap test (68.3%) compared with other racial/ethnic women (non-Hispanic white: 79.3%, black: 83.8%, Hispanic/Latino: 75.4%, American Indian/Alaska Native: 84.8%) (CDC 2007).

## Communicable Diseases

In the area of infectious diseases, the incidence of acute hepatitis B has decreased dramatically with the advent of vaccination. In 2006, acute hepatitis B incidence in Asian and Pacific Islanders (API) was similar to that in Hispanics and non-Hispanic whites (*MMWR*, Surveillance 2008). In 2007, Asians were 22.9 times more likely to have tuberculosis than non-Hispanic whites (*MMWR*, Trends 2008). Tuberculosis has a higher morbidity in Asian Americans and is directly related to the higher prevalence in foreign-born immigrants.

## SOCIOECONOMIC DETERMINANTS OF HEALTH

In general, the measurable health data for Asian Americans represent selected snapshots on the wide diversity of the population. Major differences can be found in subpopulations. Central to discussing health disparities is the need for a closer examination of the lives led by Asian Americans as well as of the environment in which many Asian Americans live. Poor health outcomes and health disparities are closely tied to social determinants such as housing, the availability of jobs, good schools and education, access to transportation, and a stable and safe neighborhood.

It is impossible to minimize the impact of two major societal forces, our health care system and immigration policies, which strongly impact health outcomes, particularly for Asians. First, our market-based health care system is overtly discriminatory against the poor and increasingly inadequate for even the insured population (Cunningham and Felland 2008). As noted, the rates of uninsured are higher among Asian Americans than among the U.S. population, and there are fewer linguistically and culturally competent health professionals available to provide them with adequate health care. One of the consequences of the difficulty in assimilating into American life is the inability to navigate the complexities of the health care system. Despite the great need, there are not enough health professionals who are linguistically and culturally competent. The 2004 National Sample Survey of Registered Nurses (HRSA 2006) reported that Asian Americans RNs were underrepresented relative to their proportion of the U.S. population (2.9% vs. 4.4%). Much more difficult is finding mental health professionals who are linguistically and culturally competent. Lack of linguistically competent health professionals contributes to dissatisfaction and perceptions of poor communication.

Second, we have no coherent immigration policy that encourages or recognizes the contribution to American life of immigrants. In particular, new Asian immigrants face multiple hurdles including changing attitudes about immigration, language and cultural barriers, lack of health insurance, and difficulty in navigating our health care system (Kagawa-Singer 2000). Much of U.S. immigration policy is directed at denying health benefits for undocumented immigrants (Carrasquillo et al. 2000) and restricting even legal immigrants from obtaining Medicaid benefits for five years (Personal Responsibility and Work Opportunity Reconciliation Act of 1996). Confused by such laws, immigrants live in fear of deportation and refrain from seeking medical attention. These barriers contribute to racial disparities.

There are too many Asian Americans who face discrimination in the opportunities of American life, a fact that deserves our full attention. Gee and colleagues (2007) noted in a national study that discrimination against Asian Americans was associated with chronic health conditions. However, to the extent that families are able to come together to create communities that consciously address these social determinants of health, we have a chance to give each generation a better life in the future.

## DANGER OF THE MODEL MINORITY MYTH

The ability to speak English and understand American culture is strongly correlated with taking advantage of opportunities in America. Many Asian Americans who have worked diligently and have been able to create businesses, start and raise families in supportive environments, and attend good schools, gaining a good education, have been able to live "the American dream."

However, the myth of Asian Americans as the model minority is mistaken (Asian Americans and Pacific Islanders Facts 2008). Assumptions of the success of Asian Americans epitomized by enrollment in the elite schools of America are not only incorrect but they also ignore that large segments of the Asian community struggle in American society. In 2008, New York University and the College Board analyzed U.S. college enrollment and found a wide distribution of Asian Americans across community colleges as well as prestigious universities. Many, particularly among the poor, do not have the resources to attend college (College Board 2008).

Relative to other groups in most communities, Asian Americans have far fewer linguistically or culturally appropriate resources. The danger of labeling Asian Americans as the "model minority" is reflected in false assumptions that Asians are inherently capable and that society can justifiably limit or redirect resources away from them. In particular for new immigrants or those who are linguistically isolated, America can be a fearful or frightening country.

In summary, we have evidence of two Americas for Asian Americans. Many have taken advantage of the educational opportunities in our country and prospered. But many have faced enormous difficulties in accessing health care, negotiating our immigration and work regulations, communicating with health professionals or officials, and have been unable to obtain needed medical care. The result is disparities in care, worsened by the lack of resources and language difficulties. It is to these Asian Americans that much of our efforts at improving access, care, and communication can have the greatest impact.

## REFERENCES

Barnes, P.M., Adams, P.F., and Powell-Griner, E. *"Health Characteristics of the Asian Adult Population: United States, 2004–2006."* NCHS, Advance Data, No. 394, January 22, 2008.

Carrsaquillo, O., Carrasquillo, A.I., and Shea, S. *"Health Insurance Coverage of Immigrants Living in the United States: Differences by Citizenship Status and Country of Origin."* AJPH 90, no. 6 (June 2000): 917–923.

Centers for Disease Control and Prevention (CDC), National Center for Chronic Disease Prevention and Health Promotion (NCCDPHP). *"Health Disparities among Native Hawaiians and Other Pacific Islanders Garner Little Attention."* Chronic Disease Notes and Reports 15 (2), Spring/Summer 2002, pg. 15, CDC.

CDC. Achieving Greater Health Impact. *"Health Disparities Affecting Minorities, Asian Americans."* Fact Sheet, Racial and Ethnic Health Disparities, CDC Media Relations, April 2, 2004.

CDC, NCHS, Health U.S. 2005, table 87. Highlights in Minority Health & Health Disparities, CDC Office of Minority Health & Health Disparities, May 2007. The College Board. *"Asian Americans and Pacific Islanders Facts, Not Fiction: Setting the Record Straight,"* June 2008. http://professionals.collegeboard.com/profdownload/08-0608-AAPI.pdf.

Cunningham, P.J., and Felland L. *"Falling Behind: American's Access to Medical Care Deteriorates, 2003–2007."* Center for Studying Health System Change, June 2008.

DeNavas-Walt, C., Protor, B.D., Smith, J.C., and U.S. Census Bureau. *"Current Population Reports, Income, Poverty and Health Insurance Coverage in the United States, 2007."* U.S. Government Printing Office, Washington, DC, 2008.

Gee, G.C., Spencer, M.S., Chen, J., and Takeuchi, D. *"A Nationwide Study of Discrimination and Chronic Health Conditions among Asian Americans."* AJPH 97, no. 7 (July 2007): 1275–1282.

HRSA. *"The Registered Nurse Population: Findings from the March 2004 National Sample Survey of Registered Nurses."* HRSA, June 2006.

Kagawa-Singer, M. *"A Socio-Cultural Perspective on Cancer Control Issues for Asian Americans."* Asian Am Pac Isl J Health 8, no. 1 (2000):12–17.

McCracken, M., Olsen, M., Chen, M.S., Jr., et al. *"Cancer Incidence, Mortality and Associated Risk Factors among Asian Americans."* CA Cancer J Clin 57, no. 4 (July–August 2007): 190–205.

Mead, H., Cartwright-Smith, L., Jones, K., et al. *Racial and Ethnic Disparities in U.S. Health Care: A Chartbook, The Commonwealth Fund,* March 13, 2008. http://www.commonwealthfund.org/usr_doc/mead_racialethnicdisparities_chartbook_1111.pdf.

*MMWR, "Surveillance for Acute Hepatitis B, United States 2006,"* March 21, 2008. Surveillance for Acute Viral Hepatitis-United States, 2006, *MMWR* Surveillance Summaries, Vol. 57, SS-2, March 21, 2008.

MMWR, "Trends in Tuberculosis–2007," 57(11), pp. 281–285, March 21, 2008.

National Cancer Institute Fact Sheet. *"H.pylori and Cancer,"* October 17, 2006. http://www.cancer.gov/cancertopics/factsheet/risk/h-pylori-cancer.

National Healthcare Disparities Report 2007. Agency for Healthcare Research and Quality, February 2008.

Personal Responsibility and Work Opportunity Reconciliation Act of 1996. http://thomas.loc.gov/cgi-bin/query/z?c104:H.R.3734.ENR.

Pollack, H., Wan, K., Ramos, R., et al. *"Screening for Chronic Hepatitis B among Asian Pacific Islanders in New York City, 2005."* MMWR 55, no. 16 (May 2006): 505–598.

Report by the President's Advisory Commission on Asian Americans and Pacific Islanders. *"Enhancing the Economic Potential of Asian Americans and Pacific Islanders (AAPI),"* May 7, 2007. US Dept. of Commerce. http://www.mbda.gov/?section_id=9&bucket_id=620&content_id=6207&well=entire_page.

Ro, M. *"Moving Forward: Addressing the Health of Asian American and Pacific Islander Women."* AJPH 92, no. 4 (April 2002): 516–519.

Smedley, Brian D., Stith, Adrienne Y., and Nelson, Alan R. (eds.). *Unequal Treatment: Confronting Racial and Ethnic Disparities in Health Care.* Committee on Understanding and Eliminating Racial and Ethnic Disparities in Health Care. Washington DC: National Academies Press, 2003.

U.S. Department of Health and Human Services (DHHS), Office of Minority Health. Asian American/Pacific Islander Profile. *"Highlights in Minority Health & Health Disparities,"* May 2006. http://www.cdc.gov/omhd/Highlights/2006/HMay06AAPI.htm.

# Chapter 40

# Health in Asian American Communities: Lessons to "Raise the Bar"

## William B. Bateman and Benjamin K. Chu

OVERVIEW

This chapter uses what is known about Asian American health to illustrate the changes needed in our health system to improve the health of all Americans. Three themes emerge.

1. Asian American health is predominantly threatened by the same chronic diseases that are the major sources of death and disability in all American ethnic groups.

2. Asian Americans cannot be viewed as a "model minority" uniformly thriving in America, but rather as group like whites, blacks, Hispanics, and Native Americans that comprises a highly diverse subpopulation in whom disease frequency, disease expression, disease susceptibility and access to health care services vary widely depending on genetics, lifestyle, and environment.

3. In addition to establishing universal access to basic health care services, our health care system must greatly improve our ability to address the specific, complex needs of our many subpopulations, and to better prevent, detect, and treat chronic diseases.

The goal to eliminate health disparities between minority and majority populations in America was set during the Clinton administration in Healthy People 2010 (U.S. Department of Health and Human Services,

2000). For the first time, America declared that it was no longer sufficient to accept improvement within racial and ethnic categories as evidence of an improving social and health care environment. Now, the gaps between majority and minority populations in both health outcomes and access to medical services were to be eliminated.

Lack of data, the stigma of the "model minority," and the aggregation of all Asians as a single population put Asian Americans at risk for being overlooked in this bold initiative. However, as thoroughly covered elsewhere in this book, these barriers have been identified, and the realities of poorer health outcomes and poorer access to health services occurring in Asian American populations is increasingly being revealed and addressed. But disparities are only part of the picture. In viewing the totality of Asian American health, a fuller picture of what is needed can be seen.

This chapter begins with an overview of the major sources of morbidity and mortality in Asian Americans and all Americans—namely, cardiovascular disease (CVD) and cancer. This will reveal both the dramatic differences in health that exist within the many different populations classified as Asians, and the similarities in health determinants among Asian Americans as well as the general population. CVD risk will be discussed by looking at type 2 diabetes mellitus, and cancer by exploring those cancers for which Asians are at greatest or increasing risk. (Type 2 diabetes is used to illustrate CVD, as it has not been discussed elsewhere in this book, and it provides an excellent method for seeing the interplay of genetics, lifestyle, and environment in the development of CVD in Asian Americans.)

The emerging picture is that improving the health of Asian Americans and all Americans requires a health care system that is more aware and responsive to the different needs in communities and individuals, as well as more capable of addressing the general needs that affect the health of all. The recommendations proposed by the Institute of Medicine to eliminate health disparities are used as a template for addressing the complex, individual-specific needs. The Chronic Care Model developed by Dr. Ed Wagner provides the framework for better managing chronic disease.

The purpose is to go beyond the issue of health disparities and explore how the health of all Americans, Asian and non-Asian, can be improved to "raise the bar" for health in America.

## HEALTH AMONG ASIAN AMERICANS—DIVERSITY AND COMPLEXITY

With the lowest reported age-adjusted mortality of any ethnic group (see Table 39.1), Asian Americans, when viewed as a total population, appear to have better health than any other ethnic or racial group in the United States. Non-Hispanic Asian adults are also least likely to be current smokers, be obese, have hypertension, delay or not receive medical care because of cost, be tested for HIV, or be in fair or poor health compared

**Table 40.1**

| Major Race Group | 2005 Age-Adjusted Death Rate Per 100,0000* |
|---|---|
| All | 798.8 |
| Non-Hispanic White population | 796.6 |
| Hispanic or Latino | 590.7 |
| Non-Hispanic Black population | 1,016.5 |
| Asian or Pacific Islander population (API) | 440.2 |
| American Indian or Alaska Native (AIAN) population | 663.4 |

*From Health: United States, 2007, Table 29, U.S. Department of Health and Human Services, Centers for Disease Control and Prevention, National Center for Health Statistics.

with non-Hispanic white, non-Hispanic black, non-Hispanic American Indian and Alaskan Natives (AIAN), or Hispanic adults. (Barnes et al. 2008).

However, these facts hide the very poor health and poor access to care of some Asian American subpopulations, and they divert attention from factors that could improve the health of Asian Americans.

Improving the health of Asian Americans requires that we learn much more about the health of specific subpopulations, and implement strategies that address the specific and often complex issues influencing health. Our health system must be reformed so that it is both accessible to the total population and more effective in the prevention and early detection of cancer and cardiovascular disease risk factors, and the management of chronic disease.

## Cardiovascular Disease

Cardiovascular disease (CVD) is the leading cause of death in the United States, accounting for 40 percent of all deaths, and it is the leading cause of death among Asian Americans and Pacific Islanders (AAPIs). However, AAPIs as a group are only 60 percent as likely to die from CVD as the general population, whereas South Asians and some Pacific Islander subgroups have many times the rates of CVD associated deaths. (National Heart, Lung and Blood Institute, National Institutes of Health, January 2000).

There is still much to be learned about the causes of these extreme differences, but the emerging picture is consistent for Asians and non-Asians alike. The differences are largely driven by the known risk factors for CVD: genetic predisposition, hypertension (high blood pressure), elevated LDL cholesterol ("bad" cholesterol), diabetes mellitus, cigarette smoking, obesity, lack of exercise, diet, and decreased access to medical services.

As the major killer, the risks for cardiovascular diseases cannot be ignored in any American population, and for some Asian American groups, the prevalence of risk factors can be surprisingly high. For example, 155 Southeast Asian refugees were assessed in a primary care clinic in Seattle, Washington. About 1 in 4 smoked or had hypertension, and roughly 1 in 7 warranted treatment for hypercholesterolemia; 44 percent had low levels of HDL, the good cholesterol (Dodson et al. 1995).

Diabetes mellitus, commonly known as "sugar diabetes," is characterized by having higher than normal amounts of glucose in the blood, the sugar the body uses for fuel. If the glucose level is high enough, the sugar spills into urine. Hence, many Asian cultures understand the disease by its tendency to cause sweet urine.

Diabetes provides an excellent model for explaining the interplay of genetics, environment, and lifestyle for CVD risk factors. Diabetes is caused or made worse by the same environmental and lifestyle issues that influence other major CVD risk factors—namely, hypertension and cholesterol. It is itself a major, independent risk factor for CVD. Alone, it is a serious disease capable of causing crippling or lethal problems including blindness, kidney failure, and amputations. Diabetes is a very serious problem: besides being itself a risk factor for CVD, it is caused or worsened by the factors that similarly influence CVD—obesity, hypertension, hyperlipidemia (high bad cholesterol or increased fat in the blood), smoking, and a sedentary lifestyle.

There are three types of diabetes mellitus: type 1, type 2 and gestational (diabetes during pregnancy). Type 1 was formerly known as "childhood-onset diabetes" because of its predilection to start early in life. It is caused by the failure of the pancreas to produce insulin, the hormone that controls blood sugar. Type 1 is not genetically determined, and its prevalence in Asian Americans is not changing. Type 2 used to be called "adult-onset diabetes" because of its tendency to start in later life, but that has changed. It is now rapidly increasing in children, paralleling the rise in obesity in children. Type 1 and type 2 diabetes cause the same severe problems. The outcomes are determined by the duration of the disease and how well it is treated, not the type of diabetes.

Type 2 diabetes is strongly influenced by genetics, meaning that the tendency to develop it is largely inherited. However, it is increasing in Asian Americans because of changes in lifestyles, not because of a shift in the gene pool. The underlying cause of type 2 diabetes is resistance to the effects of insulin. Insulin resistance is largely moderated by body fat, especially fat around the organs in the abdomen (visceral abdominal fat).

More specific information is emerging about genetic influences on the impact of obesity as a risk for type 2 diabetes. A study compared 679 non-immigrant South Asians in India with 1083 migrant South Asians in Dallas, Texas, and 858 nonmigrant Caucasians in Dallas. Subjects carrying a particular gene, the polymorphic ENPP1 121Q allele, were more likely to have type 2 diabetes in all of the groups (Abate et al. 2005).

Metabolic syndrome describes a group of cardiovascular risk factors, cardiovascular disease, and type 2 diabetes that tend to develop in combination and predict a higher risk for disease. These risk factors include dyslipidemia, central obesity, hypertension, and hyperinsulinemia. A study of 432 individuals from 68 Japanese American families was conducted to estimate the heritability of these factors and found them to be strongly influenced by genetics (Austin et al. 2004).

Type 2 diabetes is the most common form of diabetes, and its prevalence and incidence are increasing. A review of Medicare fee-for-service beneficiaries, sixty-seven years of age or older, from 1993 to 2001, showed the general prevalence was 145 per 1000 in 1993. By 2001, it was 197 per 1000, an increase of 36 percent. For Asian Americans, the increase was by 68 percent, the highest increase in prevalence among any ethnic group. The actual rate was 243 per 1000 in 2001 as compared to 184/1000, 296/1000, and 334/1000 for whites, blacks, and Hispanics, respectively. (McBean et al. 2003). The increasing prevalence of type 2 diabetes in the United States and the rest of the industrialized world is associated with the increase in obesity caused by changes in diet and activity levels.

Certain Asian populations, especially those coming from the Indian Subcontinent, are particularly susceptible to this (Abate and Chandalia 2007). An Atlanta, Georgia–based study surveyed 1046 Asian Indian immigrants and found that 22.5 percent of men and 13.6 percent of women reported having diabetes. These are significantly higher rates than found on national surveys of whites, blacks, and Hispanics (Venkataraman et al. 2004).

The reasons why certain populations, including many Asians, are genetically prone to developing type 2 diabetes mellitus are still being debated. A commonly expressed theory is that of a "thrifty genotype." This theory proposes that populations subjected to starvation over multiple generations pass along a genetic tendency to store calories more effectively, making them prone to obesity and type 2 diabetes when food is not scarce. Another theory is that because people of European descent have been exposed to high animal fat diets over many generations, they have developed an inherited resistance to these foods, which our species was not originally equipped to eat and maintain good health (Baschetti 1998). Whatever the cause, it is clear that genetics plays a significant role, but the interplay of environment, eating habits, and physical activity is the defining factor.

## Diabetes and Obesity

Because it is easy to measure, the relationship between weight and height is used to define obesity, but the health problems caused by obesity relate to an excess in body fat, and more specifically, excessive body fat around the waist and the internal organs. Araneta compared the association between body fat around the internal organs, visceral adipose tissue (VAT), and type 2 diabetes risk in three ethnic populations of women age fifty-five to eighty years: Filipina, African American, and white. Of the three, Filipinas had the lowest average weights in relation to their heights (Body Mass Index [BMI], weight in kilograms divided by the height in meters squared [kg/m$^2$]), but their VAT was significantly higher than that of either African Americans or whites, and they were over twice as likely to have diabetes than the African American women, and seven times more likely than the white women (Araneta and Barrett-Connor 2005).

Very strong evidence for the sensitivity of Asian American health to weight gain and a diet high in fat, saturated fat, and sugar comes from the Nurses' Health Study. This prospective study carefully monitored the health of 78,419 nurses from 1980 to 2000. The nurses were in apparent good health in 1980. There were 801 Asian Americans in this population. During the study period, the Asians were 1.43 times as likely as whites to develop diabetes. The risk among other minorities was greater, 1.76 for Hispanics and 2.18 for blacks. However, when the data were adjusted so that Body Mass Index (BMI) did not influence the outcome, Asians became the most at risk for developing diabetes, with a risk 2.26 times that of whites, and 1.86 and 1.34 that of Hispanics and blacks, respectively, indicating that small weight gains in Asians are more likely to cause diabetes. Specifically, for each five kilograms (eleven pounds) of weight gained after the age of eighteen and the onset of the study in 1980, the risk of diabetes increased by 84 percent in Asians, 44 percent for Hispanics, 38 percent in blacks, and 37 percent in whites. Healthy diets and weight control are extremely important for Asians (Shai et al. 2006).

The Behavioral Risk Factor Surveillance System (BRFSS) is a population-based telephone survey of the health status and health behaviors of Americans in all fifty states, Guam, Puerto Rico, and the U.S. Virgin Islands. In 2001, assessing subjects thirty years of age or older, Asian Americans as a group were found to have the same rate of diabetes mellitus as whites, and roughly one-half the rates as blacks or Hispanics. However, when adjusted for body mass index, age, and sex, the rates for blacks and Hispanics were less than 20 percent higher, and the rate in Asian Americans were 60 percent higher than that for whites, again indicating that a higher BMI, an indicator of obesity and body fat, is much stronger in increasing the risk for diabetes in those of Asian descent (McNeely and Boyko 2004).

It appears that the propensity for Asian Americans to develop diabetes at lower BMIs than other ethnic groups relates to a greater tendency to accumulate fat around the waist and abdominal organs, the so-called central adiposity. As BMI is the measure generally used to assess risk, this raises a question about its use in Asian Americans. Should there be a different guideline in defining overweight and obesity for people of Asian descent? (McNeely et al. 2001)

A Canadian study strongly suggests there should be. Thirty kilograms of weight per meter of height squared (BMI = kg/m$^2$) has been validated as a point where cardiovascular and diabetes risk increases in those of European descent. Canadian researchers randomly sampled four ethnic groups (289 South Asians, 281 Chinese, 207 Native people, and 301 Europeans) from four regions of Canada. From the data, ethnic specific "cut points" were derived based on their association with markers of cardiovascular risk. This "cut point" was a BMI of twenty-four for the Chinese, South Asian, and Native people, six points lower than that for those of European descent (Razak et al. 2007).

Researchers in India have also assessed the upper limit of normal for BMI, waist circumference and waist-hip ratios, using a statistically significant association with developing diabetes to determine where normal ends and abnormal begins. As in the Canadian study, they found dramatically different values than those validated on people of European descent, which are widely applied in the United States. A BMI of twenty-three was the higher limit of normal for this population (Snehalatha et al. 2003), a result very similar to that of the Canadian study.

A study of Japanese Americans in the state of Washington, a group also known to have a high prevalence of type 2 diabetes, further illustrates the importance of abdominal fat as a cause of diabetes. In it, 146 second-generation Japanese American men were followed for up to thirty months. Fifteen of them developed type 2 diabetes, and they had significantly higher levels of abdominal fat on entry to the study when compared with those who did not develop diabetes. This study gave further insight into how abdominal fat led to diabetes by showing a correlation between higher levels of abdominal fat and markers of increased insulin resistance, the hallmark of type 2 diabetes (Bergstrom et al. 1990).

Looking at the incidence and predictors of diabetes among 7,210 Japanese American men between the ages of forty-five and sixty-eight in the Honolulu Heart Program, body mass index and physical inactivity were found to be independent predictors of developing diabetes. This association was stronger for those over fifty-five, suggesting that obesity and inactivity become more dangerous with age (Burchfiel et al. 1995).

The implication is that many Asian Americans are genetically prone to type 2 diabetes at much lower BMIs than European and African Americans. Thus, lifestyle-related factors, diet, weight control, and exercise are especially relevant to their health.

## Lifestyle, Diabetes, and Interventions

Evidence shows that lifestyle changes can prevent the onset of type 2 diabetes among Asians who are at high risk. For example, a group of

Asian Indians with a prediabetic condition called impaired glucose tolerance were divided into four groups: Group 1 (the control group) received
no new attention to lifestyle modification; Group 2 was given lifestyle
modification advice about diet and exercise (LSM); Group 3 was given a
medication (Metformin); and Group 4 was given both LSM and the medication. Whereas 55 percent of the control group developed diabetes during the study period of about three years, the rate was only 39.3 percent
for Group 2 (LSM) and roughly the same for Groups 3 and 4 (Ramachandran
et al. 2006).

Second-generation Japanese American men have four times the rate of
type 2 diabetes compared to same-age Japanese men. Both groups consume a similar amount of calories on a daily basis, but Japanese American
men eat diets higher in fat and protein, and those with diabetes eat more
fat and protein than those who do not (Tsunehara et al. 1990).

The importance of maintaining the sound dietary practices of the traditional cultures is especially apparent when looking at the nutritional
status of American children. In an extensive literature review looking at
the nutritional status of ethnically diverse children including Asians, the
underserved, ethnically diverse populations were found to have an
increased risk over the general population for obesity, increased bad cholesterol levels, and dietary habits not meeting the Dietary Guidelines for
Americans. This is even more alarming considering that U.S. children in
general do not eat well. More than 80 percent consume more than the recommended amounts of total fat and saturated fats, the major dietary
sources of obesity and cardiovascular risk (Bronner 1996). It appears that
the children in underserved, ethnic minority groups have the unhealthi-
est eating habits among all American children, a population that eats
poorly in general.

On the hopeful side, data from the 2001 California Health Interview
Survey was used to compare the health habits of Asian, Latino, and white
adolescents, age 12 to 17, and assessed across first-, second-, third- and
later-generation immigrants. First-generation Asian Americans showed
less healthy habits than whites, lower participation in preventive behaviors, less physical activity, and more game playing and television watching. However, the Asian adolescents' health habits improved with each
generation. The eating habits of Asian American adolescents were better
than that of whites across all generations, showing a higher consumption
of fruits and vegetables and lower consumption of sodas. Unfortunately,
this favorable trend does not hold for all new immigrants, as first generation Latino adolescents also showed better eating habits than whites, but
over successive generations, their habits deteriorated to below the level of
white adolescents (Allen et al. 2007).

Physical activity is also very important to the prevention of diabetes.
This is shown in many studies, including one from the Honolulu Heart Program, which also looked at Japanese American men. Here the age-adjusted

six-year cumulative incidence of diabetes decreased with increasing exercise from nearly 74 per 1000 in the 25 percent exercising the least, to just over 34 per 1000 in the 25 percent exercising the most. The effect of exercise was independent of other risk factors for diabetes and heart disease, including weight, and it was as significant for those over fifty-five as it was for the younger men (Burchfiel et al. 1995).

Taken together, these studies indicate that Asian Americans are extremely sensitive to changes in diet and activity, which may lead to diabetes mellitus and CVD risk in general.

### Effects of Environment: Moving from East to West

A key issue for Asian Americans, as well as other immigrant groups, is the tendency for health to deteriorate in the social and cultural environment of the United States. The reasons for both the "new immigrant vigor" and the deterioration of health over subsequent generations provide important insights into the role of lifestyle and social environment on health.

The Hawaii-Los Angeles-Hiroshima Study is a longitudinal analysis that began in 1970. It is designed "mainly to determine the effects of environmental changes on various diseases by comparing Japanese-Americans with native Japanese subjects" (Nakanishi et al. 2004). As Japanese Americans who live in Hawaii and Los Angeles originate mainly from Hiroshima, Japan, these groups are genetically identical to native Japanese. The findings have been invaluable to the general understanding of the interplay of genetics and environment in determining health for all Americans, and they are of special significance to Asian Americans. These findings show that Japanese Americans adopt a relatively high fat and simple carbohydrate diet with low physical activity as compared to native Japanese, and that the prevalence of type 2 diabetes among Japanese Americans and their death rates from ischemic heart disease are higher.

It also reveals that the insulin levels in the blood are higher among Japanese Americans, even when the serum glucose levels were not statistically different as compared to native Japanese. Based on this, Japanese Americans are thought to have high insulin resistance, a precursor of type 2 diabetes. However, similar to Japanese subjects, but unlike American whites, Japanese Americans have a low initial insulin response after a glucose load. The total cholesterol and triglyceride levels are also higher among Japanese Americans. These results support the conclusion that the insulin resistance brought on by the dietary and activity changes found in the Japanese Americans combine with the apparently genetically regulated weakness of pancreatic beta cell function needed to provide increased insulin to produce the observed increased risk for diabetes. These data indicate that, for genetically similar people, environmental factors strongly influence the development of diabetes mellitus and cardiovascular disease (Nakanishi et al. 2004).

However, this negative health effect of "Westernization" can be mitigated. For example, the higher rates of type 2 diabetes and coronary heart disease found in Japanese American men as compared to same-aged men in Japan is reduced in those with a higher education (Leonetti et al. 1992).

Achievement in school is generally associated with better health. Evidence of this starting early in life can be seen from a study of Vietnamese adolescents in California: 783 Vietnamese adolescents living in four counties were interviewed over the phone. Thirty-nine percent of the interviews were conducted in Vietnamese. The health risk behaviors assessed included ever smoking a cigarette, sedentary versus an active lifestyle, consumption of fruits and vegetables, consumption of foods high in fat, ever drinking alcohol, and ever engaging in sexual behavior. The girls tended to be more sedentary than the boys, but the boys were more likely to have experimented with smoking and drinking. However, indicators of school performance were associated with less health-compromising behaviors for both boys and girls. For boys, better grades were associated with the healthier behaviors; for girls, it was extracurricular activities that predicted the healthier behaviors (Kaplan et al. 2003).

Utilization of health care services also varies among different ethnic groups. A Philadelphia study looking at low-income patients with diabetes who had access to primary health care services showed that Asian Americans and Hispanics were least likely to be admitted to a hospital, and non-Hispanic whites the most likely. The chief conclusion drawn in this study was that low-income people with diabetes who had access to regular medical care had hospital care patterns similar to higher income diabetics (Robbins and Webb 2006). In other words, access to routine health care successfully countered the generally negative influence that low-income has on health.

There are also successful examples of health care providers overcoming socioeconomic, language, and cultural barriers to improve the management of type 2 diabetes. Wang describes an approach tailored to the needs of Chinese Americans. Forty Chinese Americans with type 2 diabetes were recruited to participate in a ten-session program that integrated Chinese cultural values into a Western diabetes management program. Thirty-three, or 83 percent of them attended all ten sessions; 75 percent understood the course content; 70 percent were able to identify diabetes management skills; 83 percent could demonstrate them. Most impressive is that 44 percent were able to lose five or more pounds, most lowered their blood pressure, and the average glucose control improved from a little worse than the treatment goal to meeting it. Significant improvements in their expressed quality of life were also achieved (Wang and Chan 2005). The authors concluded that their method of culturally sensitive health education needs to be tried on a larger scale and tested against a control group, but their ability to produce a better outcome on all important levels—including self-management skills, biological outcome, and improving quality of life—is already demonstrated.

Although Asian Americans as a whole are less likely to die from CVD than all other major ethnic groups, CVD and diabetes mellitus (DM) are major sources of morbidity and mortality for Asian Americans. People of Asian descent—including South Asians, Southeast Asians, and Far East Asians—are genetically prone to CVD and DM risk factors at much lower weights (BMIs) than European Americans. Both diet and exercise are strong mediators of these health hazards. Living in the United States is associated with increased risks that can be mitigated by education, maintenance of original dietary and exercise habits, as well as by having access to linguistically and culturally responsive health care.

## Cancers

Cancers are the second leading cause of death in the United States, and the same is true for Asian Americans. Here again, collectively AAPIs are roughly 60 percent as likely as the general population to die from cancer, with age-adjusted death rates from all cancers 115.5 per 100,000 for AAPIs and 192.7 for the total population. However, a closer look at cancer rates reveals important disparities. AAPIs have twice the death rate for liver cancer, at 10.6 per 100,000, as opposed to 4.9 for the total population. They are also more likely to develop stomach cancer than any other racial or ethnic group, a rate more than 80 percent higher than whites, and they are twice as likely as whites to die from it (Ries et al. 2006).

It is also alarming that, although AAPIs have lower incidence and mortality rates than whites for the most common cancers in the United States—lung and bronchus, colon and rectum, breast and prostate—their rate of decline in incidence from 1996 to 2005 is consistently lower than those for both whites and all races (see Table 39.2). This implies that whatever factors

**Table 40.2** Age-Adjusted Average Percentage Change 1996–2005 in Top Cancer Sites by Race/Ethnicity

| Type of Cancer | AAPI | White | Black | Hispanic | All Races |
|---|---|---|---|---|---|
| Breast | −0.4 | −1.6* | −0.8* | −0.8* | −1.5* |
| Prostate | −0.3 | −0.5 | −1.9* | −0.7 | −0.6 |
| Colorectal | −1.6* | −2.2* | −0.9 | −1.2* | −2.0* |
| Lung-Bronchus | −0.7* | −1.3* | −1.7* | −2.0* | −1.4 |

*The Average Percentage Change is significantly different from zero ($p < .05$).
*Source:* Trends are from thirteen SEER areas (San Francisco, Connecticut, Detroit, Hawaii, Iowa, New Mexico, Seattle, Utah, Atlanta, San Jose–Monterey, Los Angeles, Alaska Native Registry, and Rural Georgia).

are driving the decline are not as effective with AAPIs as with the general population.

Although much more research is needed, it is clear that the cause for increased incidence of liver and stomach cancer relates to factors from life in Asia, and the lower rate of decline in the cancers more prevalent in the United States relates to factors encountered in America. To improve the health of Asian Americans, both issues must be addressed. As with CVD, preventing cancer and deaths related to cancer requires attention to the same factors for both Asians and non-Asians. Genetic predisposition needs to be understood, exposure to cancer-causing factors needs to be decreased, and early detection and entry into the most effective treatment needs to be promoted.

Liver cancer in Asian Americans is largely secondary to chronic liver infection with the hepatitis B virus, a problem mostly affecting first-generation Asian Americans. This subject is well reviewed elsewhere in this textbook. Hepatitis B can be prevented by a vaccine, and the risk of developing liver cancer in those with chronic hepatitis can be reduced with treatment. However, this requires knowledge in the community about access to these services and a responsive health care system. Much more work is needed in both areas.

Gastric cancer also is more common in new immigrant Asian Americans, but its causes and prevention are not as well known. It too is well reviewed elsewhere in this textbook. Again, the best available approaches require a knowledgeable community and a responsive health care system, the same factors resulting in the decline of the most common cancers in other ethnic groups.

This starts with increasing the awareness among Asian Americans of health issues and services. Data from the Health Information National Trends Survey reveal that much needs to be done. It shows that Asian Americans have a lower awareness of the National Institutes of Health and the American Cancer Society, are less likely to think that not smoking or quitting smoking would reduce cancer risk, are less knowledgeable about colon cancer screening, and consider their personal cancer risk to be low. This is despite their using the media similarly to whites and having an overall high level of trust of cancer information from doctors. This survey, though limited by small numbers of many at-risk Asian groups, provides our most authoritative insights into this issue (Nguyen and Bellamy 2006).

Clinical trials play a critical role in advancing the treatment of cancer by testing new drugs and approaches that may benefit patients. For those whose cancers have not responded to conventional treatment, participating in a research study may provide access to a beneficial intervention. Clinical trials are also an essential component of the way in which cancer treatment is improved.

However, the evidence is that Asian Americans are less likely to have heard the term *clinical trial* and are more likely than non-Asians to define a clinical trial as "an experiment" or as "a test procedure in a clinic." They are also less likely to have been involved in or to know someone in a trial, and they report less willingness than white respondents to consider trial participation (Paterniti et al. 2005).

Interest in establishing culturally responsive approaches to health promotion is growing, as is the knowledge of how to accomplish this. Whereas health education generally focuses on convincing someone of the importance of establishing, replacing, or stopping a particular behavior, that is not always what is needed. In one report, eight focus groups were conducted of low-income Hmong families with children aged five to fourteen to inform the development of a community-wide campaign aimed at increasing physical activity and the consumption of fruits and vegetables. They found that, like most Asians, these families valued physically active lifestyles and diets high in fruits and vegetables, but what they needed to maintain these habits was access to safe spaces and adequate time for physical activity, access to land to grow fresh produce, and time at home to prepare food. They also expressed concern over the marketing their children are exposed to that promotes unhealthy foods (Pham et al. 2007).

Much more work is needed to determine the most effective means for educating Asian Americans about the risks, prevention, early detection, and treatment of cancers. Despite the fact that Asian Americans as a whole are less likely to die from cancer than all other ethnic groups—including white non-Hispanics—new-immigrant Asian Americans suffer disproportionately from liver and gastric cancers, and later-generation Asian Americans are not experiencing the same decline in incidence of the cancers most common in the United States experienced by the other ethnic and racial populations. Both issues need specific attention to improve the health of Asian Americans.

## Conclusions: Lessons from the Health Status of Asian Americans

Health, good and bad, is the result of complex interactions of human biology, environment, lifestyle, and health care services (LaLonde 1981). All of these factors vary with ethnicity and race, socioeconomic status, level of education, and community, among other factors.

Asian Americans, like Americans in general, are a highly diverse group, genetically, culturally, and in their personal histories. Those who are new immigrants face challenges to their health that originated in their countries of origin, as well as those brought on by the stresses of immigration. Beyond first-generation immigrants, the threats to health rapidly change to the same lifestyle-driven, chronic diseases that create the major morbidity and mortality for the general population. Improving the health of Asian Americans requires a health and medical care system that addresses the specific and complex needs of each individual, while also effectively diagnosing and treating the common chronic diseases, and providing early detection and entry into treatment for the most common cancers.

## BARRIERS TO HEALTH AND HEALTH CARE FOR ASIAN AMERICANS

For Asians, life in America tends to reduce the health risks from infectious diseases that are more dominant in Asian countries, and replace them with the lifestyle-related chronic diseases that are dominant in the United States. Improving the health of Asian Americans requires specific attention to both the conditions that are connected with country of origin, and those developing in the United States. Those that relate to country of origin tend to show up as health disparities. Those related to life in America do not. Health activists, the health care system, and health care providers serving Asian Americans must directly address both these issues and remove the specific barriers to such care that Asian Americans experience.

To address these barriers, we can turn to the recommendations contained in the Institute of Medicine publication that provided the first comprehensive picture of health disparities in America, *Unequal Treatment: Confronting Racial and Ethnic Disparities in Healthcare*. For the emerging problems that relate more to life in America, we will review the status of chronic disease management in the U.S. health system, and the approaches that are being either proposed or used to improve it.

### Institute of Medicine (IOM) Recommendations for Eliminating Health Disparities: A Template for Addressing Complex and Diverse Health Problems in America

The IOM's report contains general recommendations, as well as recommendations for legal, regulatory, and policy interventions; health system interventions; patient education and empowerment recommendations; and recommendations for cross-cultural education in the health professions; data collection and monitoring; and research needs. The recommendations are aimed at eliminating health disparities for ethnic minorities, but here they are presented as a means for addressing the complex and diverse problems that adversely affect American health. They are listed in Table 39.3. Commentary relating to their role in addressing the barriers to care and improving Asian American health follows.

#### Recommendation 2-1: Increasing Awareness of Racial and Ethnic Disparities

Nearly every chapter in this textbook identifies the significant limitations in our understanding of Asian American health. As a population, Asian Americans are only recently included in the large, national epidemiological studies that monitor our nation's health, and the oversampling needed to

**Table 40.3** Summary of Recommendations from the IOM*

*General Recommendations*

| | |
|---|---|
| **Recommendation 2-1:** | Increase awareness of racial and ethnic disparities in healthcare among the general public and key stakeholders. |
| **Recommendation 2-2:** | Increase healthcare providers' awareness of disparities. |

*Legal, Regulatory and Policy Interventions*

| | |
|---|---|
| **Recommendation 5-1:** | Avoid fragmentation of health plans along socioeconomic lines. |
| **Recommendation 5-2:** | Strengthen the stability of patient-provider relationships in publicly funded health plans. |
| **Recommendation 5-3:** | Increase the proportion of underrepresented U.S. racial and ethnic minorities among health professionals |
| **Recommendation 5-4:** | Apply the same managed care protections to publicly funded HMO enrollees that apply to private HMO enrollees. |
| **Recommendation 5-5:** | Provide greater resources to the U.S. DHHS Office for Civil Rights to enforce civil rights laws. |

*Health Systems Interventions*

| | |
|---|---|
| **Recommendation 5-6:** | Promote the consistency and equity of care through the use of evidence-based guidelines. |
| **Recommendation 5-7:** | Structure payment systems to ensure an adequate supply of services to minority patients, and limit provider incentives that may promote disparities. |
| **Recommendation 5-8:** | Enhance patient-provided communication and trust by providing financial incentives for practices that reduce barriers and encourage evidence-based practice. |
| **Recommendation 5-9:** | Support the use of interpretation services where community need exists. |
| **Recommendation 5-10:** | Support the use of community health workers. |
| **Recommendation 5-11:** | Implement multidisciplinary treatment and preventive care teams. |

*Patient Education and Empowerment*

| | |
|---|---|
| **Recommendation 5-12:** | Implement patient education programs to increase patients' knowledge of how to best access care and participate in treatment decisions. |

*Cross-Cultural Education in the Health Professions*

| | |
|---|---|
| **Recommendation 6-1:** | Integrate cross-cultural education into the training of all current and future health professionals. |

*Data Collection and Monitoring*

| | |
|---|---|
| **Recommendation 7-1:** | Collect and report data on health care access and utilization by patients' race, ethnicity, socioeconomic status, and where possible, primary language. |

**Table 40.3** (Continued)

| | |
|---|---|
| IOM Recommendation: | Include measures of racial and ethnic disparities in performance measurement. |
| **Recommendation 7-2:** | Include measures of racial and ethnic disparities in performance measurement. |
| **Recommendation 7-3:** | Monitor progress toward the elimination of health-care disparities. |
| **Recommendation 7-4:** | Report racial and ethnic data by OMB categories, but use subpopulation groups where possible. |
| *Research Needs* | |
| **Recommendation 8-1:** | Conduct further research to identify sources of racial and ethnic disparities and assess promising intervention strategies. |
| **Recommendation 8-2:** | Conduct research on ethical issues and other barriers to eliminating disparities. |

*Unequal Treatment: Confronting Racial and Ethnic Disparities in Healthcare.* Institute of Medicine of the National Academies, The National Academies Press 2003, pp. 20–21.

get statistically reliable results is just starting. The vast diversity of the people classified as Asian American, and the need to assess the subgroups is highly challenging, but also extremely important. Awareness is made still more difficult because many Asian Americans, like other ethnic and racial groups, are of mixed race and ethnicity and not only of Asian descent. The interactions of this diversity and the influence of the many other powerful determinants of health add further to the complexity.

Increasing awareness of Asian American health among the general population and stakeholders requires strong and creative action. National and regional population health assessments need to be formed and funded to routinely oversample the Asian populations. Creative concepts such as enclaves as a unit of analysis, as described in the chapter by Dr. Tom Chung in this textbook, need to be used and further validated.

Also, disparities should not be the only focus of intense ethnic and racial study. As seen in this chapter, health strengths within ethnic minorities can also yield highly important findings.

## Recommendation 2-2: Increasing Healthcare Providers' Awareness of Disparities

The many barriers to health care faced by Asian Americans are well described in nearly every chapter of this book. Language, immigration status, income, lack of health insurance, lack of access to services, and a low understanding of how to use the health care system, especially for preventive health care, present significant problems for many. Health care providers, especially those serving large Asian American communities, not only need to be aware of these disparities, they also must develop programs that specifically address them.

### Recommendations 5-1 and 5-2: Improving Health Plans and Publicly Subsidized Care, and Strengthening Relationships Between Patients and Healthcare Providers.

Even when insured, low-income Asian Americans and other racial and ethnic minorities tend to have access only to health plans that pay less for services and set more limits on the types of services available (Phillips 2000). Among other problems, these health plans also often fail to provide minority patients with a "medical home," a health care provider with whom a consistent relationship is developed. The federal Agency for Healthcare Research and Quality has found that continuity of care with a primary care provider is associated with an increased use of preventive services. This relationship with a medical provider allows for an understanding and trust between patient and provider, an essential element in providing culturally competent care. Although these "lower-end" health plans are often required to provide access to a specific primary care provider, the fact that they are low-paying plans tends to produce a fragmentation of care.

The ability to communicate in the language the patient prefers for medical care is obviously essential. Providing interpreting services adds to the expense of care, and there are not enough bilingual providers to meet the total demand. It is also not reasonable to expect all bilingual providers to work in low-income settings. Although delivering primary care to multilingual, low-income populations is likely to cost more than delivering care to an English-speaking, higher-income population, it generally is less well supported, leading to further fragmentation of care.

Regulation and parity between private and public plans alone will not adequately address the language barriers. We need more bilingual health care professionals, better payment for primary care, and direct support for linguistic and cultural competence in the health care settings serving populations speaking languages other than English. The optimal care of linguistically and culturally diverse populations costs more than services to a monolingual population.

### Recommendations 5-3 and 5-9: Importance of Bilingual Providers and Interpreting Service

For Asian American communities, the major issue is the need for more bilingual Asian American health care professionals, and the ability to access high-quality medical interpreting programs when a bilingual provider is not available. Here too, the fact that the Civil Rights Act and regulatory agencies require that patients receive care in their preferred language is not sufficient to make it happen. Although Asian Americans comprise a significant portion of today's health care workforce, many are not medically competent in an Asian language, and with over 100 languages to cover, it is not feasible that a bilingual workforce alone will adequately support a stable patient-provider relationship for all Asian Americans. Readily accessible, affordable, and highly competent medical interpreting programs are essential. Most of the available services that meet regulatory standards do not meet these standards.

Interpreting in health care settings can be achieved in four ways:

1. Proximal, consecutive—in-room interpreters speaking in sequence. The interpreter tells the other person what is being said after one person says something.

2. Proximal, simultaneous—in-room interpreters interpreting at the same time each person is talking. The interpreter tells the other person what is being said as it is being spoken, like at the United Nations, except the interpreter is in the room.

3. Remote, consecutive—interpreters not in the room, available via phone or video-conferencing devices, speaking in sequence. The interpreter tells the other person what is being said after one person says something.

4. Remote, simultaneous—interpreters not in the room, available via phone or video-conferencing devices, interpreting at the same time each person is talking, like at the United Nations.

In all cases, the approach fails if the interpreter is not fluent in both an Asian language and English, and knowledgeable of medical vocabulary and the ethics and responsibilities of interpreters. Although regulation insists on using assessed and trained interpreters, there are no consistent standards, and most interpreting still involves undertested and undertrained people, doing proximal, consecutive interpreting.

The well-established services that do exist generally rely on a proximal, consecutive, or less frequently, a simultaneous approach. Although proximal interpreting has been shown to produce superior results when compared to using no interpreting, the communication is far from what happens when provider and patient speak the same language. With the interpreter in the room, the interpreter becomes the main person that each relate to, rather than each other.

Strengthening the stability of patient-provider relationships for Asian Americans will require the development of an interpreting process that mimics what happens when provider and patient speak the same language, as well as producing a health care workforce that ethnically and racially mirrors the community served. Remote, simultaneous interpreting, using carefully assessed, trained, and quality-controlled interpreters is the method most like a concordant language visit. With it, there is no interpreter to look at, the interpreting simulates a direct conversation, and the provider and patient relate as if they were talking directly. Such a system exists in the TEMIS program (Team/Technology Enhanced Medical Interpreting System) in the South Manhattan Healthcare Network of New York City's public hospital system. However, New York City is still the only place that has invested in this approach, and its funding is still insufficient to make it widely available. Expanding the availability of truly bilingual and culturally responsive providers and the use of remote, simultaneous interpreting is fundamental to improving the health of Asian Americans.

## Recommendation 5-5: Greater Resources to the U.S. DHHS Office for Civil Rights to Enforce Civil Rights Laws.

Enforcement of civil rights laws is a major, if not the main, factor that has produced both awareness of and the significant improvements in ethnic and racial minority health. Asian American health concerns and the recognition of bilingual Asians as an underrepresented minority in health professions need to be on the agenda.

## Recommendation 5-6: Use of Evidence-Based Guidelines

The disparities seen in Asian Americans concerning the use of evidence-based, guideline-driven services such as Pap smears and mammograms should not just be the subject of research publications. Every health care setting must begin to assess adherence to guidelines for every ethnic and racial group they serve, seek parity among populations, and promote improvement in general compliance.

## Recommendation 5-10: The Use of Community Health Workers

This recommendation has special relevance to Asian Americans, especially new immigrant communities. The complex linguistic, social, political, economic, and cultural barriers between health care providers and some Asian American communities require liaisons between community and health care service. Community health workers, people hired from the community and trained to connect health care services with the community, are essential. This approach will support better understanding of community in the health care setting and vice versa, as well as provide needed jobs.

## Recommendation 5-11: Multidisciplinary Treatment and Preventive Care Teams

Health care is a team effort requiring different disciplines—such as doctors, nurse practitioners, physician assistants, nurses, social workers, case managers, and clerical and nursing assistants—for it to function well. Such interdisciplinary teams are needed in all levels of care, including primary care where most health-promotive and disease-preventive services are delivered. Asian Americans are needed in all of these disciplines.

### Recommendation 5-12: Patient Education Programs

When the major sources of morbidity and mortality were infectious diseases, patients played a small role in their care, and simply following the doctor's advice was sufficient. As chronic diseases strongly related to lifestyle are now the major sources of disability and death, the competence of the patient in preventing or managing the problem is essential. When someone has diabetes, hypertension, or elevated cholesterol, it is their diet and activity levels in addition to using prescribed medication that determines the outcome. Simply being respectful to the doctor is not sufficient. The patient needs to know what to do, why to do it, and how to do it. This requires both education and participation in treatment decisions, something that some Asian American populations are not accustomed to, but all can benefit from.

### Recommendation 6-1: Cross-Cultural Education Training of All Current and Future Health Professionals

The impact of this training will be entirely dependent on how it is done. It will improve care for Asian Americans to the extent that it gives health professionals an understanding that their approach to health care is itself culturally driven, and with that, an appreciation that there is a wide range of beliefs that governs lifestyles and the use of health care services. Through this understanding, they will hopefully be in a better position to understand their Asian American patients, and with that understanding, be more effective in diagnosing and treating their problems.

However, if the cross-cultural education results only in an understanding of various traditional Asian cultures, stereotyping and miscommunication will be the outcomes. Although it is important for health care providers to know something about traditional Asian cultures, this knowledge by itself would not serve Asian Americans well.

### Recommendation 7-1: Collecting and Reporting Data, and Monitoring Progress

There is a very important principle for operating any complex system, such as a health care system. If you measure it, you can manage it better. In our recent past, demographic data such as race and ethnicity were too often used for prejudicial reasons, resulting in a reluctance to carefully monitor patient race, ethnicity, socioeconomic status, and primary language. Now, it must be tracked so that variation within subpopulations can be seen, understood, addressed, and resolved.

*Recommendation 8-1: Research on Disparities and
Promising Intervention Strategies*

Promoting health in Asian Americans requires attention to both areas of disparities and better health. We believe that this is true for all ethnic and racial minorities, for the same reason we believe it for Asian Americans. The strengths of a population that create superior health outcomes are likely to be useful in overcoming disparities, and not just for the group being studied. It will be exciting to see in much greater detail the sources of both worse and better health, and the approaches that "raise the bar."

*Recommendation 8-2: Ethical Issues and Other
Barriers to Eliminating Disparities*

The fact that ethical issues sometimes prevent the collection of data required to assess the impact of race, ethnicity, and socioeconomic status is a testimony to how far offtrack our past has taken us. It is a shame that variables used to help define a population have been sources of discrimination and bias. Hopefully, we will overcome this problem.

For Asian Americans, the significant barriers include finding a way to better define the subpopulations of Asian Americans; overcoming the view that research is always an experiment and best avoided; and changing the notion that Asians are such a distinct group that they should not be included in studies meant to inform us about health in the general population. It will be interesting to see research on these as well as other barriers in order to improve health in Asian American communities.

However, addressing the health disparities and barriers to better manage the unique health problems faced by Asian Americans will be a necessary, but not sufficient, component of the reform needed to improve their general health status. It will not be sufficient to improve the general health of the American population either. To raise the bar, we need a health system that addresses these complexities and delivers effective chronic disease prevention and management.

## Chronic Disease Management in our Health System

In 2000, 45 percent of the U.S. population had a chronic condition, and almost half of those had multiple chronic conditions. It is expected that these numbers will continue to increase. In fact, it is expected that nearly half of all Americans will have a chronic condition by 2020; yet our health system is poorly organized for preventing, detecting, and managing these problems (Anderson 2004).

Even with 43 million Americans lacking health insurance, the United States spends more for health care per person than any other country—fully 16 percent of our gross domestic product, also the highest in the world. Seventy-five percent of these expenditures are to pay for the medical care of people with chronic diseases (Halvorson 2007). The American health care system is widely recognized for being in the forefront in treating acute diseases, but it lags behind other developed nations in disease prevention and the management of chronic diseases. One reason is the absence of universal health care.

From 2001 to 2007, the number of adults under the age of sixty-five who lacked health insurance for some part of the year grew from 38 million to 50 million, or from 24 percent of the population to 28 percent. In 2007, 72 million, or 41 percent of working-age adults, reported a problem with paying their medical bills, up from 58 million (34%) in 2005. These financial barriers to care impede both the detection and the treatment of chronic diseases, but even when they are removed, we do not perform well.

In 2006, a RAND publication reported that "all adults in the United States are at risk for receiving poor health care, no matter where they live; why, where, and from whom they seek care; or what their race, gender, or financial status is" (RAND Health 2006). Reporting on people with private health care insurance, the National Committee on Quality Assurance found weak performances in chronic disease management including diabetes management and cancer screening. Only 13 percent of diabetics had their LDL-C (bad cholesterol) at acceptable levels, 21 percent had poor glucose control and only 36 percent had the expected eye examinations. These all-inclusive statistics obscure the fact that there was a wide range in performance, such that if all plans could perform as well as the top ten, they estimated that between 7,100 and 15,900 deaths could be avoided by better glucose control; between 4,400 and 9,400 by better cholesterol management, and between 9,200 and 22,800 by better blood pressure control. If cancer screening was performed by all, as well as in the top-ten plans, the estimated avoidable yearly deaths would be between 200 and 700 for breast cancer, 600 and 800 for cervical cancer, and 6,000 and 12,600 for colorectal cancer (National Committee for Quality Assurance 2007).

For these and other reasons, it is no surprise that in his 2004 testimony to the U.S. Senate Committee on Health, Education, Labor, and Pensions, Robert H. Brook of RAND Health stated, "In essence, the U.S. health care system is out of control. It wastes money because it provides care that is not needed, and it causes a great deal of harm because care that is needed is not provided" (Brook 1999). Brook is far from the first and certainly not the last high-level health system expert to share this low opinion of our health system, and the general public feels the same way. A 2008 survey conducted by Harris Interactive, Inc. for the Commonwealth Fund concluded that 80 percent of adults believe that our health system "needs to be fundamentally changed, or completely rebuilt" (How et al. 2008).

Our health system's approach to chronic disease management is one of the areas that is already undergoing fundamental change, but there is a long way to go. The Chronic Care Model, developed by Dr. Ed Wagner under funding from the Robert Wood Johnson Foundation, was developed with the recognition that the conventional approach for detecting and managing chronic diseases, relying heavily on doctor visits, is in a large way failing to detect and adequately treat chronic disease. Cardiovascular risk factors such as diabetes mellitus, hypertension, and hyperlipidemia are going unrecognized and are often undertreated even when recognized. Doctor office attempts to promote smoking cessation are only modestly effective. A more multidimensional model is needed. The Chronic Care Model refers to six different levels of attention.

1. Self-Management
2. Decision Support
3. Delivery System Design
4. Clinical Information System
5. Organization of Health Care
6. Community

Table 39.4 contains a description of each of these components and Figure 39.1 shows how they interact to produce better outcomes. All Americans, including Asian Americans, need this multifaceted approach focused on them.

## CONCLUSION

The state of health in the United States for the majority of the population is well below that in much of the world, despite the fact that we have and spend more resources on health than any other nation. We have proposed that the health of all Americans can be improved by better understanding and addressing the differences, both positive and negative, of the health between and among ethnic and racial minorities. The available information on Asian American health provides insights into why this is so and how this can be achieved. We need a transformed approach, and we cannot expect different results by continuing to do the same thing. We need a health system that informs and empowers individuals and communities, eliminates prohibitive financial barriers to routine and preventive services, addresses the diverse language and health practices in the communities served, and uses the "medical home" concept as well as computer technology to decrease the fragmentation of care.

An intense focus on the health of Asian Americans, as well as on that of all ethnic and racial groups, allows us to better understand the many subtle factors that are needed to accomplish this system reform. The role of socioeconomic status, education, and lifestyle in health can only be well understood by knowing more about our various subpopulations. We need to understand and proactively apply awareness of these factors to

**Table 40.4**

**Self-Management**
Effective self-management is very different from telling patients what to do. Patients have a central role in determining their care, one that fosters a sense of responsibility for their own health.

**Decision Support**
Treatment decisions need to be based on explicit, proven guidelines supported by at least one defining study. Health care organizations creatively integrate explicit, proven guidelines into the day-to-day practice of the primary care providers in an accessible and easy-to-use manner.

**Delivery System Design**
The delivery of patient care requires not only determining what care is needed but also clarifying roles and tasks to ensure the patient gets the care; making sure that all the clinicians who take care of a patient have centralized, up-to-date information about the patient's status; and making follow-up a part of standard procedure.

**Clinical Information System**
A registry—an information system that can track individual patients as well as populations of patients—is a necessity when managing chronic illness or preventive care.

**Organization of Health Care**
Health care systems can create an environment in which organized efforts to improve the care of people with chronic illness take hold and flourish.

**Community**
To improve the health of the population, health care organizations reach out to form powerful alliances and partnerships with state programs, local agencies, schools, faith organizations, businesses, and clubs.

strategies designed to intervene, prevent, and treat chronic diseases for all, not just for the elimination of health disparities among minorities.

The recommendations from the IOM and the Chronic Care Model provide frameworks for the two types of reforms needed in service delivery. Following the IOM recommendations will enable us to better address the wide variety of disease risk and barriers to health care and health practices that exist in all American ethnic and racial groups. The Chronic Care Model better addresses the major sources of morbidity and mortality affecting all Americans.

It is well established that higher socioeconomic status, education, a well-functioning community, access to health care—including having a "medical home" (continuity of care)—the right diet, exercise, limited or no use of harmful substances such as tobacco and alcohol, and behavioral health result in better health outcomes. The health care system must address those factors which it can influence: access, continuity of care, and healthy behaviors. Making it happen requires a reformed health

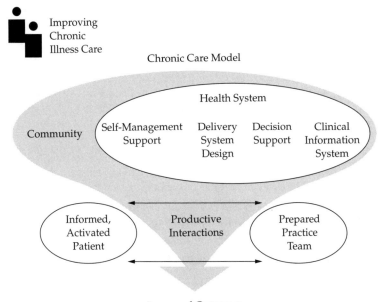

**Figure 40.1** Wagner, E.H. Chronic disease management: What will it take to improve care for chronic illness? *Effective Clinical Practice.* 1998;1(1):2–4.

system that supports access to all for basic services, including preventive and chronic disease management; more knowledge of the genetic determinants of disease, as well as ethnic and cultural influences; and better implementation of what is known. It is through a focus on health and behavioral factors within and among minority populations, in our case Asian Americans, that we will be able to raise the bar on health for both the fastest-growing minority population and all Americans.

## REFERENCES

Abate, N., and M. Chandalia. 2007. Ethnicity, type 2 diabetes and migrant Asian Indians. *Indian Journal of Medical Research* 125, (3) (Mar): 251–8.

Abate, N., M. Chandalia, P. Satija, B. Adams-Huet, S. M. Grundy, S. Sandeep, V. Radha, R. Deepa, and V. Mohan. 2005. ENPP1/PC-1 K121Q polymorphism and genetic susceptibility to type 2 diabetes. *Diabetes* 54, (4) (Apr): 1207–13.

Allen, M. L., M. N. Elliott, L. S. Morales, A. L. Diamant, K. Hambarsoomian, and M. A. Schuster. 2007. Adolescent participation in preventive health behaviors, physical activity, and nutrition: Differences across immigrant generations for Asians and Latinos compared with whites. *American Journal of Public Health* 97, (2) (Feb): 337–343.

Anderson, G. Horvath. 2004. The growing burden of chronic disease in America. *Public Health Reports* 119, (3): 263–270 (May–June).

Araneta, M. R., and E. Barrett-Connor. 2005. Ethnic differences in visceral adipose tissue and type 2 diabetes: Filipino, African-American, and white women. *Obesity Research* 13, (8) (Aug): 1458–1465.

Austin, M. A., K. L. Edwards, M. J. McNeely, W. L. Chandler, D. L. Leonetti, P. J. Talmud, S. E. Humphries, and W. Y. Fujimoto. 2004. Heritability of multivariate factors of the metabolic syndrome in non-diabetic Japanese Americans. *Diabetes* 53, (4) (Apr): 1166–1169.

Barnes, P. N., Adams, P. F., Powell-Griner, E., Division of Health Interview Statistics. 2008. *Health characteristics of the Asian adult population: United states, 2004–2006.* Washington, DC: National Center for Health Statistics, 394.

Baschetti, R. 1998. Diabetes epidemic in newly Westernized populations: Is it due to thrifty genes or to genetically unknown foods? *Journal of the Royal Society of Medicine* 91, (12) (Dec): 622–625.

Bergstrom, R. W., L. L. Newell-Morris, D. L. Leonetti, W. P. Shuman, P. W. Wahl, and W. Y. Fujimoto. 1990. Association of elevated fasting C-peptide level and increased intra-abdominal fat distribution with development of NIDDM in Japanese-American men. *Diabetes* 39, (1) (Jan): 104–11.

Bronner, Y. L. 1996. Nutritional status outcomes for children: Ethnic, cultural, and environmental contexts[erratum appears in *Journal of the American Dietetic Association* 97, (6): 584]. *Journal of the American Dietetic Association* 96, (9) (Sep): 891–903.

Brook, R. H. 1999. *Ensuring delivery of necessary care in the United States: Testimony presented to the Senate Committee on Health, Education, Labor, and Pensions.* RAND Health, CT-152.

Burchfiel, C. M., J. D. Curb, B. L. Rodriguez, K. Yano, L. J. Hwang, K. O. Fong, and E. B. Marcus. 1995. Incidence and predictors of diabetes in Japanese-American men. The Honolulu Heart Program. *Annals of Epidemiology* 5, (1) (Jan): 33–43.

Burchfiel, C. M., D. S. Sharp, J. D. Curb, B. L. Rodriguez, L. J. Hwang, E. B. Marcus, and K. Yano. 1995. Physical activity and incidence of diabetes: The Honolulu Heart Program. *American Journal of Epidemiology* 141, (4) (Feb 15): 360–368.

Chesla, C. A., and K. M. Chun. 2005. Accommodating type 2 diabetes in the Chinese American family. *Qualitative Health Research* 15, (2) (Feb): 240–255.

Copenhagen, WHO. 1984. *Health promotion: A discussion document.*

Culhane-Pera, K., K. A. Peterson, A. L. Crain, B. A. Center, M. Lee, B. Her, and T. Xiong. 2005. Group visits for Hmong adults with type 2 diabetes mellitus: A pre-post analysis. *Journal of Health Care for the Poor & Underserved* 16, (2) (May): 315–327.

Dodson, D. J., T. M. Hooton, and D. Buchwald. 1995. Prevalence of hypercholesterolaemia and coronary heart disease risk factors among Southeast Asian refugees in a primary care clinic. *Journal of Clinical Pharmacy & Therapeutics* 20, (2) (Apr): 83–89.

Halvorson, G. C. 2007. *Health care reform now! A prescription for change.* San Francisco, CA, www.josseybass.com, Jossey-Bass.

How, S. K. H., A. Shih,, J. Lau,, and C. Schoen. 2008. *Public views on U.S. health system organization: A call for new directions.* Commonwealth Fund, 1158.

Kaplan, C. P., D. Zabkiewicz, S. J. McPhee, T. Nguyen, S. E. Gregorich, C. Disogra, J. F. Hilton, and C. Jenkins. 2003. Health-compromising behaviors among Vietnamese adolescents: The role of education and extracurricular activities. *Journal of Adolescent Health* 32, (5) (May): 374–383.

Lalonde, Marc. 1981. *A new perspective on the health of Canadians—A working document.* Canada: Minister of Supply and Services, Cat. No. H31-1374.

Leonetti, D. L., C. H. Tsunehara, P. W. Wahl, and W. Y. Fujimoto. 1992. Educational attainment and the risk of non-insulin-dependent diabetes or coronary heart disease in Japanese-American men. *Ethnicity & Disease* 2, (4): 326–336.

McBean, A. M., Z. Huang, B. A. Virnig, N. Lurie, and D. Musgrave. 2003. Racial variation in the control of diabetes among elderly Medicare managed care beneficiaries. *Diabetes Care* 26, (12) (Dec): 3250–3256.

McNeely, M. J., and E. J. Boyko. 2004. Type 2 diabetes prevalence in Asian Americans: Results of a national health survey. *Diabetes Care* 27, (1) (Jan): 66–69.

McNeely, M. J., E. J. Boyko, J. B. Shofer, L. Newell-Morris, D. L. Leonetti, and W. Y. Fujimoto. 2001. Standard definitions of overweight and central adiposity for determining diabetes risk in Japanese Americans. *American Journal of Clinical Nutrition* 74, (1) (Jul): 101–107.

Nakanishi, S., M. Okubo, M. Yoneda, K. Jitsuiki, K. Yamane, and N. Kohno. 2004. A comparison between Japanese-Americans living in Hawaii and Los Angeles and native Japanese: The impact of lifestyle Westernization on diabetes mellitus. *Biomedicine & Pharmacotherapy* 58, (10) (Dec): 571–577.

National Committee for Quality Assurance. 2007. *The state of health care quality 2007.*

National Heart, Lung and Blood Instititute, National Institutes of Health. January 2000. *Addressing cardiovascular health in Asian Americans and Pacific Islanders— A background report.* NIH Publication No. 00-3647.

Nguyen, G. T., and S. L. Bellamy. 2006. Cancer information seeking preferences and experiences: Disparities between Asian Americans and whites in the health information national trends survey (HINTS). *Journal of Health Communication* 11, (Suppl 1): 173–180.

Paterniti, D. A., M. S. Chen Jr, C. Chiechi, L. A. Beckett, N. Horan, C. Turrell, L. Smith, et al. 2005. Asian Americans and cancer clinical trials: A mixed-methods approach to understanding awareness and experience. *Cancer* 104, (12 Suppl) (Dec 15): 3015–3024.

Pham, K. L., G. G. Harrison, and M. Kagawa-Singer. 2007. Perceptions of diet and physical activity among California Hmong adults and youths. *Preventing Chronic Disease* 4, (4) (Oct): A93.

Phillips KA, Mayer ML, Aday LA. 2000. Barriers to care among racial/ethnic groups under managed care. *Health Affairs* 19: 65–75.

Ramachandran A., C. Snehalatha, S. Mary, B. Mukesh, A. D. Bhaskar, V. Vijay. Indian Diabetes Prevention Programme (IDPP). 2006. The Indian diabetes prevention programme shows that lifestyle modification and metformin prevent type 2 diabetes in Asian Indian subjects with impaired glucose tolerance (IDPP-1). *Diabetologia* 49, (2) (Feb): 289–297.

RAND. *The first national report card on quality of health care in America. Research highlights.* RAND, 2006.

Razak, F., S. S. Anand, H. Shannon, V. Vuksan, B. Davis, R. Jacobs, K. K. Teo, M. McQueen, and S. Yusuf. 2007. Defining obesity cut points in a multiethnic population. *Circulation* 115, (16) (Apr 24): 2111–2118.

Ries L. A. G, D. Melbert, M. Krapcho, A. Mariotto, B. A. Miller, E. J. Feuer, L. Clegg, M. J. Horner, N. Howlader, M. P. Eisner, M. Reichman, B. K. Edwards (eds.). SEER Cancer Statistics Review, 1975–2004, National Cancer Institute. Bethesda, MD, http://seer.cancer.gov/csr/1975_2004/, based on November 2006 SEER data submission, posted to the SEER Web site, 2007.

Robbins, J. M., and D. A. Webb. 2006. Hospital admission rates for a racially diverse low-income cohort of patients with diabetes: The urban diabetes study. *American Journal of Public Health* 96, (7) (Jul): 1260–1264.

Shai, I., R. Jiang, J. E. Manson, M. J. Stampfer, W. C. Willett, G. A. Colditz, and F. B. Hu. 2006. Ethnicity, obesity, and risk of type 2 diabetes in women: A 20-year follow-up study. *Diabetes Care* 29, (7) (Jul): 1585–1590.

Snehalatha, C., V. Viswanathan, and A. Ramachandran. 2003. Cutoff values for normal anthropometric variables in Asian Indian adults. *Diabetes Care* 26, (5) (May): 1380–1384.

Tsunehara, C. H., D. L. Leonetti, and W. Y. Fujimoto. 1990. Diet of second-generation Japanese-American men with and without non-insulin-dependent diabetes. *American Journal of Clinical Nutrition* 52, (4) (Oct): 731–738.

Venkataraman, R., N. C. Nanda, G. Baweja, N. Parikh, and V. Bhatia. 2004. Prevalence of diabetes mellitus and related conditions in Asian Indians living in the United States. *American Journal of Cardiology* 94, (7) (Oct 1): 977–980.

U.S. Department of Heath and Human Services. November 2000. *Healthy people 2010.* 2nd ed. Washington, DC: U.S. Government Printing Office.

Wang, C. Y., and S. M. Chan. 2005. Culturally tailored diabetes education program for Chinese Americans: A pilot study. *Nursing Research* 54, (5) (Sep–Oct): 347–353.

WHO, Geneva. 1946. *Constitution of the World Health Organization.*

Wu, A. H., M. C. Yu, C. C. Tseng, F. Z. Stanczyk, and M. C. Pike. 2007. Diabetes and risk of breast cancer in Asian-American women. *Carcinogenesis* 28, (7) (Jul): 1561–1566.

# About the Editors

**William B. Bateman Jr., MD,** is the Director of Medical and Professional Affairs at Gouverneur Healthcare Services, the largest non-hospital-based ambulatory center in New York City with a 210-bed Skilled Nursing Facility. He is a Clinical Associate Professor of Medicine at the New York University School of Medicine and an Associate Director for NYU's Institute for Community Health and Research, where he also directed the Sino-American Health Care Exchange Program until 2007. He is a graduate of the University of Michigan College of Medicine.

He served as Chief of Medicine and Medical Director of the Gouverneur Diagnostic and Treatment Center from 1990 to 1999. From 1999 to 2007, he was the Director of Business Development for the South Manhattan Healthcare Network, which includes Bellevue Hospital Center, Coler-Goldwater Memorial Hospital, and Gouverneur Healthcare Services. During that time he also served as the Chief Learning Officer for the Urban Learning Academy, a "corporate university" located in Bellevue dedicated to providing a workplace-based learning environment that improves the quality of services, as well as staff and patient satisfaction. Before moving to NYU in 1990, he was an Assistant Professor of Medicine and of Epidemiology and Social Medicine at the Albert Einstein College of Medicine, and Director of the Social Internal Medicine Residency Program at Montefiore Medical Center in the Bronx. This program received a national award from the Pew Family Foundation for its outstanding contributions to the advancement of primary care.

Throughout his career, Dr. Bateman has focused on improving access to care and the health status of the vulnerable populations of New York City. Among many other projects, this led him to organize and lead the development of a remote, simultaneous medical interpreting system called TEMIS (Team/Technology Enhanced Medical Interpreting System), which provides an interpreting method that most closely simulates direct communication between patients and their healthcare providers when they do not speak the same language. He was the author and Project Director for Bellevue Hospital Center's Speaking Together Program, a national collaborative funded by the Robert Wood Johnson Foundation of ten hospitals applying quality improvement methods to interpreting services.

**Noilyn Abesamis-Mendoza, MPH,** is the Manager of Health Policy for the Coalition for Asian American Children & Families (CACF), the nation's only policy advocacy organization dedicated to improving the health and well-being of Asian Pacific American children. Noilyn leads CACF's health advocacy efforts on language access, culturally responsive health services, and health care affordability. Among the major programs she coordinates is Project CHARGE (Coalition for Health Access Reaching Greater Equity), a pan-Asian network of fourteen partners.

Prior to joining CACF, Noilyn served as the Deputy Director of Outreach & Programs for the NYU Center for the Study of Asian American Health (CSAAH). She developed and oversaw key outreach, educational, and community-based initiatives for CSAAH, which included managing the development of seven ethnic-specific community health needs and resource assessments; coordinating over forty workshops, conferences, and training opportunities; and fostering and strengthening relationships with key stakeholders, healthcare institutions, businesses, media and government agencies.

In 2004, Noilyn co-founded the Kalusugan Coalition, a Filipino health collaborative, where she currently serves as the Board Chair. Noilyn has also served as a board member or advisor for the API Caucus of APHA; CACF's Action Council; Peace of Heart Choir; NIH/NHLBI Filipino Healthy Heart; Healthy Family Initiative; and St. Peter's College Center for Personal Development. She was a recipient of the New American Leaders Fellowship Program and the United Way of NYC Nonprofit Leadership Development Institute's Senior Fellow Program. She received a BA in Environmental Analysis & Design from the University of California, Irvine, and an MPH, Sociomedical Sciences from the Columbia University Mailman School of Public Health.

**Henrietta Ho-Asjoe, MPS,** has been the Administrator and the Director of Community Development for the Center for the Study of Asian American Health (CSAAH) at the NYU Langone Medical Center since 2004. In her current position Ms. Ho-Asjoe directs CSAAH's programmatic, educational, training, and outreach cores. Externally, she represents the Center to key local and national stakeholders, at site visits, as a panelist, on Advisory Boards, and to the media. At the Medical Center, her expertise is called upon to advise deans, physicians, and medical students.

Prior to NYU, Ms. Ho-Asjoe directed the Chinese Community Partnership for Health at New York Downtown Hospital, where she led a multicultural team committed to assisting Chinese Americans overcome barriers to healthcare access. In addition to awards and appointments to boards locally and nationally, she received a Proclamation for her dedication to healthcare from the Manhattan Borough President's Office.

# Index

Note: All page numbers followed by a *t* refer to tables and/or figures on the indicated page. For example, 17*t* refers to a table on page 17.

AAHC, 73–82
AAPCHO, 227, 231, 547–548
Abdominal fat, 55, 92, 782, 783
Academic achievement. *See*
    Educational attainment
Academic institutions, 355
Access to health care. *See* Health
    care access
Acculturation
  alcohol, 377, 491
  cancer, 39, 49
  cardiovascular diseases, 90
  converging trends, 586
  cultural identity, 283,
    317–318
  family, 294, 511
  gambling, 376
  illicit substances, 373
  immigrant advantage, 552
  mental health, 280, 292, 301,
    335, 481–482, 630
  physician-patient relationship,
    312–313
  sexual behavior, 494
  smoking, 369, 734
  suicide, 413–414
  traditional Asian medical
    practices, 713–714
  treatment adherence, 231

  verbal communication, 290
  violence and, 390, 392, 633
ACE inhibitors, 106, 109, 112, 118
Acid reflux, 62
ACIP, 192
Acquired immunodeficiency
    syndrome. *See* HIV/AIDS
ACT-UP, 247
Acupressure, 714
Acupuncture
  bloodletting, 708
  clinical studies, 709
  hepatitis B virus,188
  prevention, 664
  roots, 710
  use of, 711, 712, 714, 715
Add Health, 464
Addictive disorders
  alcohol, 305, 578, 639
  children, 354, 482, 491–492
  converging trends, 586
  diagnosis, 320
  disparities, 281, 633
  prevalence and presentation, 305,
    412
  socioeconomic status, 580
  substance use and affect, 365–378
  suicide and, 408
  treatment outcomes, 352

ii